DIAGNOSTIC IMAGING

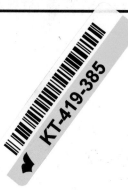

PETER ARMSTRONG
MB, BS, FRCR
Professor of Radiology,
St Bartholomew's Hospital, London;
Formerly Professor and Vice-Chairman,
Department of Radiology, University of Virginia,
Charlottesville, Virginia, USA

MARTIN L. WASTIE
MB, BChir, FRCP, FRCR
Consultant Radiologist,
University Hospital, Nottingham

THIRD EDITION

FOUR DRAGONS

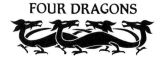

OXFORD

BLACKWELL SCIENTIFIC PUBLICATIONS

LONDON   EDINBURGH   BOSTON

MELBOURNE   PARIS   BERLIN   VIENNA

© 1981, 1987, 1989, 1992
Blackwell Scientific Publications
Editorial Offices:
Osney Mead, Oxford OX2 0EL
25 John Street, London WC1N 2BL
23 Ainslie Place, Edinburgh EH3 6AJ
238 Main Street, Cambridge
    Massachusetts 02142, USA
54 University Street, Carlton
    Victoria 3053, Australia

Other Editorial Offices:
Librairie Arnette SA
2, rue Casimir-Delavigne
75006 Paris
France

Blackwell Wissenschafts-Verlag GmbH
Meinekestrasse 4
D-1000 Berlin 15
Germany

Blackwell MZV
Feldgasse 13
A-1238 Wien
Austria

First published as *X-ray Diagnosis* 1981
Reprinted 1982, 1983 (twice), 1985
Second edition published as *Diagnostic Imaging* 1987
Reprinted 1989
International Student Edition 1989
Indonesian translation 1990
Third edition 1992
Four Dragons edition 1992
Reprinted 1993

Set by Setrite Typesetters, Hong Kong
Printed and bound in Great Britain
by The Alden Press, Oxford

DISTRIBUTORS

Marston Book Services Ltd
PO Box 87
Oxford OX2 0DT
(*Orders*: Tel: 0865 791155
            Fax: 0865 791927
            Telex: 837515)

USA
Blackwell Scientific Publications, Inc.
238 Main Street
Cambridge, MA 02142
(*Orders*: Tel: 800 759-6102
            617 876-7000)

Canada
Times Mirror Professional Publishing, Ltd
130 Flaska Drive
Markham, Ontario L6G 1B8
(*Orders*: Tel: 800 268-4178
            416 470-6739)

Australia
Blackwell Scientific Publications Pty Ltd
54 University Street
Carlton, Victoria 3053
(*Orders*: Tel: 03 347-5552)

A catalogue record for this book is available from
the British Library

ISBN 0−632−03093−3 BSP
ISBN 0−632−03095−X (Four Dragons)

Contents

Preface

Medical students can be forgiven their bewilderment when faced with the daunting array of information which goes under the heading 'Diagnostic Imaging'. Conventional radiology remains the mainstay of most imaging departments and we have once again given it due emphasis in this edition of *Diagnostic Imaging*. Since the previous edition was published 5 years ago there has been a great increase in the use of ultrasound, computed tomography (CT) and particularly magnetic resonance imaging (MRI). When the previous edition was written, MRI was in its infancy but now it is an important imaging method and has even become the imaging modality of choice in certain conditions. We believe that every doctor must now be familiar with all these techniques as well as with conventional radiology.

It has been our intention to indicate the potential of each imaging modality but we have not attempted to describe any of the techniques in detail, otherwise the book would be too unwieldy. We realise that some of our recommendations will not be applicable in every hospital since so much depends on the personal preference of clinicians and radiologists as well as on the available equipment and expertise.

We have once again tried to meet the needs of the medical student and young doctor in training, by explaining the techniques used in diagnostic imaging and the indications for their use. As before much of the book is devoted to helping the reader understand the principles of interpretation, both of plain films and the images obtained with other imaging modalities.

It is unfortunately beyond the scope of a small book, such as this one, to describe fully the pathology responsible for the various appearances. Similarly, to have dealt adequately with the role of imaging in clinical management would have necessitated large sections on surgery, medicine and pathology. Consequently, this book cannot be read in isolation; it must be accompanied by the study of these other subjects.

Acknowledgements

It would not have been possible to prepare this edition without the help of the many radiologists who have given ideas, valuable comments and inspiration. We would like to thank the staff of the Radiology Departments at the University Hospital, Nottingham, the University of Virginia Medical Center and St Bartholomew's Hospital, London. We would particularly like to thank Drs R. H. A. Gregson, A. R. M. Wilson, P. J. McMillan, B. J. Preston, S. C. Whitaker, J. E. Dacie, R. W. Kerslake and T. E. Keats. Drs T. Jaspan, I. M. Holland and Wayne Cail unstintingly provided many neuroradiological pictures.

Dr Keith Dewberry of Southampton; Drs Paul Dee, Spencer Gay and Denny Watson of the University of Virginia; Drs Brent Harrison, Scott McPhierson and their colleagues of the University of Mississippi; Drs G. Kumar, M. Paramsothy and Professor Joginder Singh of Kuala Lumpur, Malaysia; Professor Donald Longmore of the National Heart Hospital; Dr Andreas Adam of the Royal Postgraduate Medical School and IGE, UK, were all most generous in providing illustrations for the book. Drs Norman A. G. Brenbridge and Tony Buschi, formerly at the University of Virginia, assisted greatly in the previous editions with the sections on ultrasound and computed tomography.

Our particular thanks go to Dr Andrew A. McLeod and Mark J. Monaghan MSc, both of King's College Hospital, London, who provided several of the illustrations for the cardiac chapters, and to Dr Janet Husband of the Royal Marsden Hospital, Surrey, who so willingly provided many CT images.

We owe a big debt of gratitude to Drs O. Nylén and B. Lindén of Falun, Sweden, who have gone to great efforts to provide many of the MRI pictures.

We must also thank most sincerely the photographers in the Departments of Medical Illustration at the University of Virginia, University Hospital, Nottingham, and at St Bartholomew's Hospital, London, who prepared the photographic prints.

This book would have been totally impossible without the endless typing and retyping undertaken by Linda McGurk of Nottingham, Mrs Sherry Deane and Mrs Pat West of the University of Virginia, and Mrs Julie Jessop of St Bartholomew's Hospital, London, and we thank them most heartily for all their help.

Finally, we would like to express our gratitude to Mr Peter Saugman and Ms Vicky Murray of Blackwell Scientific Publications.

Peter Armstrong
Martin L. Wastie

1

Introduction

The use of the imaging department

X-ray and imaging departments need to be well run and efficiently utilised in order to minimise radiation hazard and be cost-effective. Organising the department is in the hands of radiologists and radiographers, but the use to which it is put is largely decided by the referring clinicians. Good communication between clinician and radiologist is vital. The radiology staff need to know and understand the clinical problem in order to carry out appropriate tests and to interpret the results in a meaningful way. The clinicians need to understand the strengths and limitations of the answers provided.

Another important aspect is sensible selection of investigations. There are two basic philosophies which take opposite paths to achieve a diagnosis. One approach is to request a battery of investigations, aimed vaguely in the direction of the patient's symptoms, hoping something will turn up. The other approach is 'trial and error': decide one or two likely diagnoses and carry out the appropriate test to support or refute these possibilities. Each course has its proponents; we favour the selective approach since there is little doubt that the answers are usually obtained less expensively and with less distress to the patient. This approach depends on critical clinical evaluation; the more experienced the doctor, the more accurate he or she becomes in choosing appropriate tests.

Laying down precise guidelines for requesting the various imaging examinations is difficult because patients are managed differently in different centres and the information required varies significantly.

• An examination should only be requested when there is a reasonable chance that it will affect the management of the patient. There should be a question attached to every request, e.g. for a chest radiograph — what is the cause of this patient's haemoptysis?

• The time interval between follow-up examinations should be sensible, e.g. once pneumonia has been diagnosed, chest films to assess progress can safely be left 7–10 days, unless clinical features suggest a complication.

• One should be specific about the localisation of problems. X-raying the clavicle, shoulder, humerus, elbow and forearm is clearly inappropriate for a patient whose symptoms are clinically those of an abnormality in or immediately adjacent to the shoulder. It may be reasonable to construct a programme of investigations but the radiologist should always be asked to cancel any remaining tests once the desired positive result is obtained.

• Consider carefully which diagnostic imaging procedure will give the relevant information most easily, e.g. radionuclide bone scans should be the initial screening method in a search for asymptomatic bone metastases rather than skeletal survey.

• Whenever possible, the choice of examination should minimise the amount of radiation given.

X-rays

Production of x-rays (Fig. 1.1)

X-rays are part of the electromagnetic spectrum. They are used for all conventional radiography and for computed tomography (CT). They are produced when high-speed electrons decelerate rapidly. This is

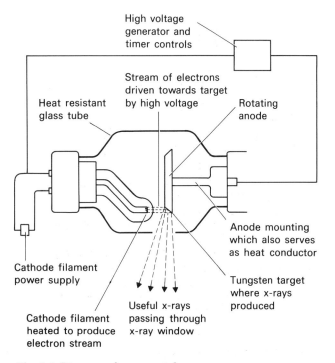

High voltage
generator and
timer controls

Stream of electrons
driven towards target
by high voltage

Heat resistant
glass tube

Rotating
anode

Anode mounting
which also serves
as heat conductor

Cathode filament
power supply

Tungsten target
where x-rays
produced

Useful x-rays
passing through
x-ray window

Cathode filament
heated to produce
electron stream

Fig. 1.1 Diagram of an x-ray tube.

achieved by passing a very high voltage across two terminals placed in an evacuated tube. One of the terminals, the cathode, is a tungsten alloy filament. The other terminal, the anode, is a tungsten alloy target set in a disc of copper. The cathode is heated to incandescence and it liberates free electrons. When a high voltage, usually in the range of 50–150 kV, is applied across the two terminals, the electrons are attracted towards the anode at high speed. They hit the tungsten target and x-rays are produced.

Only a small portion of the x-ray beam escapes through an opening in the metal casing surrounding the tube; the remainder are absorbed by the casing.

Absorption of x-rays

Radiographic images depend on the fact that x-rays are absorbed to a variable extent as they pass through the body. The visibility of structures and disease de-

pends on this differential absorption. With conventional radiography, where an image of the resulting shadows is recorded on film or viewed on a fluorescent screen (fluoroscopy), there are four basic densities— gas, fat, other soft tissues and calcified structures. X-rays that pass through air are least absorbed and therefore cause the most blackening of the radiograph, whereas calcium absorbs the most and so the bones and other calcified structures appear virtually white. The soft tissues, with the exception of fat, e.g. the solid viscera, muscle, blood, bowel wall, etc., all have the same absorptive capacity and appear the same shade of grey on the conventional radiograph. Fat absorbs slightly fewer x-rays and, therefore, appears a little blacker than the other soft tissues.

Computed tomography expands the number of visible densities to more than 2000 shades of grey by using computer manipulation of information received from multiple projections.

Conventional radiography

Photographic effect

X-rays cause blackening of the emulsion of a developed photographic film. In practice, the effects of the x-ray beam are usually intensified by the use of fluorescent screens which emit light when exposed to x-rays. The photographic film is sandwiched between two fluorescent screens in a special light tight cassette. When exposed to x-rays it is mainly the light emitted from the fluorescent screens that causes the blackening of the developed film.

Projections in conventional radiography

Projections are usually described by the path of the x-ray beam. Thus a posteroanterior (PA) view is where the beam passes from the back to the front; the standard projection for a routine chest film. An AP view is one taken from the front. The term 'frontal' refers to either PA or AP projection.

The image on an x-ray film is two-dimensional. All

the structures along the path of the beam are projected on to the same portion of the film. Therefore it is often necessary to take at least two views to gain information about the third dimension.

Precise localisation of a shadow requires more than one view, usually at right-angles to one another, e.g. the PA and lateral chest film. Sometimes two views at right-angles are not appropriate and oblique views are substituted.

Horizontal ray films

Air-fluid levels are an important radiological sign. Their detection requires a projection using a horizontal x-ray beam, e.g. an erect or a lateral-decubitus film. The reason that air-fluid levels can only be seen on a film taken with a horizontal beam can best be understood by analogy with the fluid level in a glass of water. The only way to see the air-fluid level is to look at it from the side, i.e. in a horizontal direction.

Grids

When x-rays strike an object, some of the beam is scattered thus reducing the quality of the x-ray image. To overcome this problem a grid is used, consisting of a large number of parallel, thin strips of lead held apart by material which allows the primary beam of radiation to pass unimpeded, the obliquely scattered radiation being absorbed by the lead strips in the grid (Fig. 1.2).

Portable films

Films can be taken of patients in bed or in the operating theatres using portable x-ray machines. Such machines have substantial limitations on the exposures they can achieve. This usually means longer exposure times and poorer quality films. The positioning and radiation protection of patients in bed is often inferior to that which can be achieved within the x-ray department. Consequently, portable films should only be requested when the patient cannot be moved to the x-ray department.

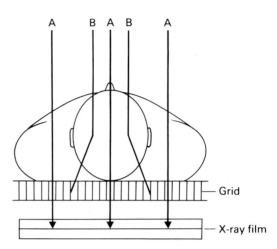

Fig. 1.2 Principle of the grid. The beams labelled A pass through both the patient and the grid to strike the film. The two beams labelled B are scattered (deflected) within the body; they are absorbed by the slats of the grid and, therefore, do not reach the film.

Magnification in radiography

All conventional x-ray images show some magnification, because the x-ray tube sends out a diverging beam of x-rays. The closer the object is to the film, the less the magnification.

Conventional tomography

The aim of a tomogram (laminogram) is to blur out overlying structures, but to keep a selected plane of the body in sharp focus. This is achieved by moving the x-ray tube and film about an axis which can be located at the level of interest.

Computed tomography (see p. 8) has now replaced most conventional tomographic examinations.

Contrast agents in conventional radiography and CT

Radiographic contrast agents are used to visualise structures or disease processes that would otherwise be invisible. Barium is widely used to outline the gastrointestinal tract; all the other radio-opaque media rely on iodine in solution to absorb x-rays and so act as a contrast agent. The same substances are used for urography, angiography and contrast enhancement at computed tomography. Usually they are given in large doses, often with rapid rates of injection. Since their only purpose is to produce opacification, ideally they should be pharmacologically inert. This has not yet been totally achieved, though the introduction of low-osmolality agents, such as the non-ionic media, is a big step in the right direction. The advantage of the newer agents is that they have a lower osmolality than the ionic contrast media previously in general use. The disadvantage of the newer agents is that they are considerably more expensive than their prede-cessors and the high cost has led many institutions to introduce limitations on their use. Many of the adverse effects are intimately related to the osmolality of the agent and with the new low-osmolality media these are much less frequent and often much less severe. The following discussion applies particularly to the older ionic agents.

Most patients experience a feeling of warmth spreading over the body as the contrast medium is injected; a few find this feeling objectionable. Some-times, particularly with slow injections of the more concentrated solutions, pain occurs in the upper arm and shoulder due to stasis in the veins. When this occurs it is helpful to raise the patient's arm at the end of the injection. Contrast inadvertently injected outside the vein is very painful indeed and therefore should be carefully guarded against.

Nausea, vomiting or light-headedness are experi-enced by a few patients and some will develop an urticarial rash. All these phenomena usually subside spontaneously.

Bronchospasm, laryngeal oedema or hypotension occasionally develop and may be so severe as to be life threatening. It is, therefore, essential to be prepared for these dangerous reactions and to have available the equipment and drugs to cope with them. Approxi-mately one in 160 000 patients dies as a consequence of ionic contrast agents, a risk which, though small, should not be ignored.

Patients with known allergic manifestations, par-ticularly asthma, are more likely to have an adverse reaction. Even normal people develop clinically occult bronchospasm, so it is not surprising that asthmatic patients may show an exacerbation of their asthma and, on occasion, experience a life-threatening attack. Similarly, patients who have had a previous reaction to contrast agents have a higher than average risk of problems during the examination. Such patients are usually premedicated with steroids, preferably for at least 18 hours prior to the examination. Antihistamine drugs may also be given shortly before the contrast injection.

Patients with a higher than average risk of compli-cations from intravenous contrast injections include:
- Infants, who are at risk from a rapid rise in plasma osmolality because of the high osmolality of the in-jected contrast agent. Even with low-osmolality agents the injection rate in infants should, when possible, be slow.
- Elderly patients, who often tolerate the injected contrast medium poorly.
- Those with known heart disease. Arrhythmias are a risk in patients with heart disease.
- Those with renal failure, myeloma or severe dia-betes. Such patients are more likely to show a deterio-ration of renal function due to the contrast medium if they are deprived of fluids prior to the examination.

In many centres, these high-risk groups are given low-osmolality agents to help minimise complications from contrast injections.

Ultrasound

In diagnostic ultrasound examinations, very high fre-quency sound is directed into the body from a trans-ducer placed in contact with the skin. In order to make good acoustic contact, the skin is smeared with a jelly-like substance. As the sound travels through the body, it is reflected by the tissue interfaces to produce echoes which are picked up by the same transducer and converted into an electrical signal.

Since air, bone and other heavily calcified materials

→ cystic structures :- Acoustic Enhancement.
→ Solid structures :- Acoustic Shadow.

absorb nearly all the ultrasound beam, ultrasound plays little part in the diagnosis of lung or bone disease. The information from abdominal examinations may be significantly impaired by gas in the bowel which interferes with the transmission of sound.

Fluid is a good conductor of sound and ultrasound is, therefore, a particularly good imaging modality for diagnosing cysts, examining fluid-filled structures such as the bladder and biliary system, and demonstrating the fetus in its amniotic sac. Ultrasound can also be used to demonstrate solid structures which have a different acoustic impendence from adjacent normal tissues, e.g. metastases.

Ultrasound is often used to determine whether a structure is solid or cystic (Fig. 1.3). Cysts or other fluid-filled structures produce large echoes from their walls but no echoes from the fluid contained within them. Also, more echoes than usual are received from the tissues behind the cyst; an effect known as 'acoustic enhancement'. Conversely, with a calcified structure,

e.g. a gall stone, there is a great reduction in the sound that will pass through, so a band of reduced echoes, referred to as an 'acoustic shadow', is seen behind the stone.

Ultrasound is produced by causing a special crystal to oscillate at a predetermined frequency. Very short pulses of sound lasting about a millionth of a second are transmitted about 500 times each second. The crystal not only transmits the pulses of sound but also 'listens' to the returning echoes, which are electronically amplified to be recorded as signals on a television monitor. Photographic reproductions of the image on the monitor can provide a permanent record.

Acoustic signals ↓ Electrical impulses.

The time taken for each echo to return to the transducer is proportional to the distance travelled. Knowledge of the depth of the interface responsible for the echoes allows an image to be produced. Also by knowing the velocity of sound in tissues it is possible to measure the distance between interfaces. This is of great practical importance as, for example, in obstetrics where the measurement of the fetal head has become the standard method of estimating fetal age.

$T \propto d$

During the scan, the ultrasound beam is electronically swept through the patient's body and a section of the internal anatomy is instantaneously displayed. The resulting image is a slice (Fig. 1.3), so in order to obtain a three-dimensional assessment a number of slices must be created by moving or angling the transducer.

Unlike other imaging modalities there are no fixed projections and the production of the images and their subsequent interpretation depend very much on the observations of the operator during the examination.

At the energies and doses currently used in diagnostic ultrasound no harmful effects on any tissues have been demonstrated.

Doppler effect

Sound reflected from a mobile structure shows a variation in frequency which corresponds to the speed of movement of the structure. This shift in frequency, which can be converted to an audible signal, is the

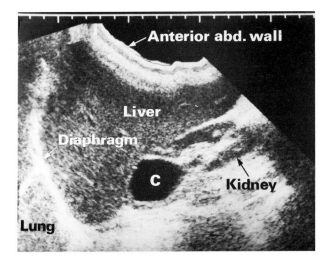

Fig. 1.3 Ultrasound scan. The distance marker at the top is in centimetres. The image represents a longitudinal section through the lower lung, liver and right kidney. A cyst (C) is present in the upper pole of the kidney.

principle underlying the Doppler probe used in obstetrics to listen to the fetal heart.

The Doppler effect can also be exploited to image blood flowing through the heart or blood vessels. Here the sound is reflected from the blood cells flowing in the vessels (Plate 1, opposite page). If blood is flowing towards the transducer the received signal is of higher frequency than the transmitted frequency, whilst the opposite pertains if blood is flowing away from the transducer. The difference in frequency between the sound transmitted and received is known as the Doppler frequency shift.*

During the examination the flow velocity waveform can be displayed and recorded. As the waveforms from specific arteries and veins have characteristic shapes, flow abnormalities can be detected. If the Doppler angle (Plate 1) is known then the velocity of the flowing blood can be calculated and blood flow can be calculated provided the diameter of the vessel is also known.

A further development is colour Doppler, namely the superimposition of Doppler information in colour on a standard ultrasound image (Plate 2, opposite page 7). The direction of blood flow can readily be determined and flow towards the transducer is by convention coloured red, whereas blue indicates flow away from the transducer.

Doppler studies are used to detect venous thrombosis, arterial stenosis and occlusion, particularly in the carotid arteries. In the abdomen, Doppler techniques can determine whether a structure is a blood vessel and can help in assessing tumour blood flow. In obstetrics, Doppler ultrasound is used particularly to determine fetal blood flow through the umbilical artery. With Doppler echocardiography it is possible to demonstrate regurgitation through incompetent

---

* The formula is: $\text{frequency shift} = \dfrac{2\,\text{IF} \times \text{FV} \times \cos \Theta}{c}$

(As c, the speed of sound in tissues, and IF, the incident frequency of sound, are constant and if Θ, the Doppler angle is kept constant, the frequency shift depends directly on the blood flow velocity FV.)

valves and pressure gradients across valves can be calculated.

Radionuclide imaging

The radioactive isotopes used in diagnostic imaging emit gamma rays as they decay. Gamma rays are electromagnetic radiation, similar to x-rays, produced by radioactive decay of the nucleus. Many naturally occurring radioactive isotopes, e.g. potassium-40, uranium-235, have half lives of hundreds of years and are, therefore, unsuitable for diagnostic imaging. The radioisotopes used in medical diagnosis are artificially produced and most have short half lives, usually a few hours or days. To keep the radiation dose to the patient to a minimum, the smallest possible dose of an isotope with a short half life should be used. Clearly, the radiopharmaceuticals should have no undesirable biological effects and should be rapidly excreted from the body following completion of the investigation.

Radionuclide imaging depends on the fact that certain substances concentrate selectively in different parts of the body. Radionuclides can be chemically tagged to these substances. Occasionally, the radionuclide in its ionic form will selectively concentrate in an organ, so there is no need to attach it to another compound. The radionuclide most commonly used is technetium-99m (^{99m}Tc). It is readily prepared, has a convenient half life of 6 hours and emits gamma radiation of a suitable energy for easy detection. Other radionuclides that are used include indium-111, gallium-67, iodine-123 and thallium-201.

Technetium-99m can be used in ionic form (as the pertechnetate) for thyroid and vascular imaging, or ^{99m}Tc can be tagged to other substances, e.g. a complex organic phosphate labelled with ^{99m}Tc will be taken up by the bones and can be used to visualise the skeleton (Fig. 1.4). Particles are used in lung perfusion images; macroaggregates of albumin with a particle size of 10–75 μm when injected intravenously are trapped in the pulmonary capillaries. If the macroaggregates are labelled with ^{99m}Tc then the blood flow to the lungs can be visualised. It is also possible to label the

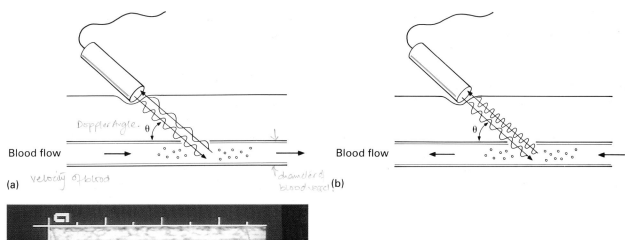

(a) Doppler Angle. θ

Blood flow

velocity of blood

diameter of blood vessel

(b) θ

Blood flow

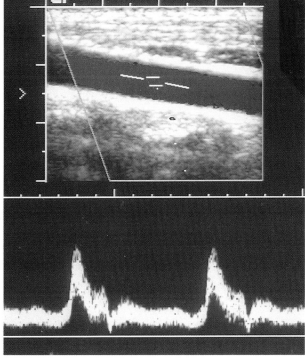

(c)

Plate 1 Principle of Doppler ultrasound. (a) With blood flowing away from the transducer, the frequency of the received sound is reduced. (b) With blood flowing towards the transducer, the frequency of the received sound is increased. (θ is the angle between the vessel and the transmitted sound wave: an angle known as the Doppler angle.) (c) Flow velocity waveform of normal internal carotid artery. The peaks represent systolic blood flow. The waveform has been taken from the gate within the artery shown in the colour Doppler image. The angle of the beam is indicated by the fine zig-zag line.

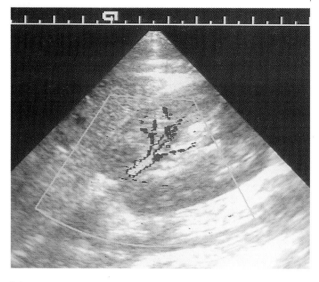

(a)

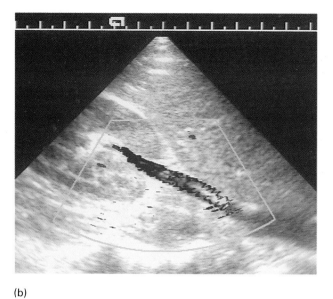

(b)

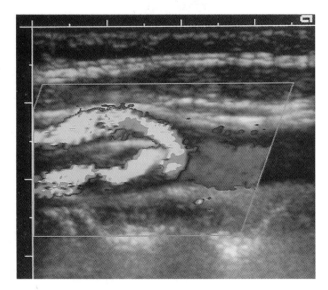

(c)

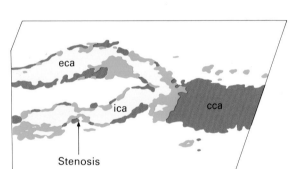

Plate 2 Colour Doppler. (a) Normal renal artery. (b) Normal renal vein. (c) Bifurcation of common carotid artery showing stenosis of internal carotid artery. The flowing blood is revealed by colour. The precise colour depends on the speed and direction of the blood flow. cca, common carotid artery; eca, external carotid artery; ica, internal carotid artery.

patient's own red blood cells with ^{99m}Tc to assess cardiac function, or the white cells with indium-111 for abscess detection. Small quantities of radioactive gases, such as xenon-133, xenon-127 or krypton-81m can be inhaled to assess ventilation of the lungs. All these radiopharmaceuticals are free of side effects.

The gamma rays emitted by the isotope are detected by a gamma camera enabling an image to be produced. A gamma camera consists of a circular sodium iodide crystal, usually 40 cm in diameter coupled to a number of photomultiplier tubes. Light is produced when the gamma rays strike and activate the sodium iodide crystal, and the light is then electronically amplified and converted to an electrical pulse. The electrical pulse is further amplified and analysed by a processing unit so that a recording can be made. Invariably, some form of computer is linked to the gamma camera to enable rapid serial images to be taken and to perform computer enhancement of the images when relevant.

In selected cases emission tomography is performed. In this technique the gamma camera moves around the patient. A computer can analyse the information and produce sectional images similar to CT. Emission tomography can detect lesions not visible on the standard views. Because only one usable photon for each disintegration is emitted this technique is also known as single photon emission computed tomography (SPECT).

Nuclear medicine techniques are used to measure function and to produce anatomical images. Even the anatomical images are dependent on function, e.g. a bone scan depends on bone turnover. The anatomical information they provide, however, is limited by the relatively poor spatial resolution compared to conventional radiography, ultrasound or CT.

Positron emission tomography

Positron emission tomography (PET) uses short-lived positron emitting isotopes. Two gamma rays are produced from the annihilation of each positron which can be detected by a specialised gamma camera. The resulting images reflect the distribution of the isotope.

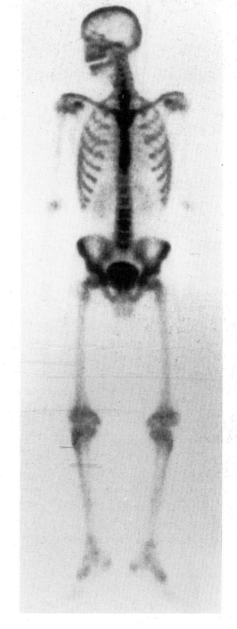

Fig. 1.4 Normal radionuclide bone scan. The patient has received an intravenous injection of a ^{99m}Tc-labelled bone scanning agent (a complex organic phosphate). This agent is taken up by the bone in proportion to bone turnover and blood flow.

By using isotopes of biologically important elements such as carbon or oxygen, PET can be used to study physiological processes such as blood perfusion of tissues, metabolism of substances such as glucose, as well as complex biochemical pathways such as neurotransmitter storage and binding. Changes in metabolism of diseased tissue can also be studied.

A cyclotron is needed to produce the necessary isotopes, and, therefore, PET is currently restricted to large research centres.

Computed tomography

Computed tomography differs from conventional radiography in that it uses a more sensitive x-ray detection system than photographic film, namely gas or crystal detectors, and then manipulates the data from the detectors using a computer. Both systems use x-rays generated in much the same way. The x-ray tube rotates around the patient. In some systems the detectors also move, but in others they are arranged as a stationary ring around the patient (Fig. 1.5). The outstanding feature of CT is that very small differences in x-ray absorption values can be visualised. Compared to conventional radiography, the range of densities recorded is increased from approximately 20 with standard film to 2000 or more with CT. The density resolution is such that not only can fat be distinguished from other soft tissues, but gradations of density within soft tissues can also be recognised, e.g. brain substance from cerebrospinal fluid (CSF), and tumour from surrounding normal tissues. This revolutionary technique, which was first introduced in the 1970s, substantially altered the diagnostic approach to many diseases, particularly intracranial disorders.

The patient lies with the part to be examined within the gantry housing the x-ray tube and detectors. Although other planes are sometimes practicable, horizontal (axial) sections are by far the most commonly employed. The section level and thickness to be imaged are selected by the radiographer; the usual thickness is between 1.0 and 10 mm. By moving the patient through the gantry, multiple adjacent sections can be imaged allowing a picture of the body to be built up. Thinner sections provide more accurate information, but more sections are then required for a given volume of tissue.

The data obtained from each set of exposures are reconstructed into an image by computer manipulation. The computer calculates the attenuation (absorption) value of each picture element (known in computer jargon as a pixel). Each pixel is 0.25−0.6 mm in diameter, depending on the resolution of the machinery, with a height corresponding to the section thickness chosen. Since each pixel has a definite volume, the attenuation value recorded represents the mean value of that volume of tissue (voxel). The resulting images are displayed on a television monitor and photographs of the images are used for the permanent record. Additionally, the basic data can be stored on an optical disc or on magnetic tape.

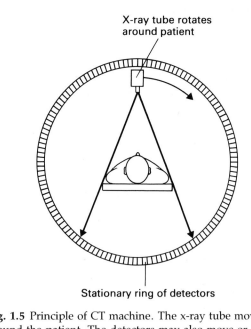

X-ray tube rotates around patient

Stationary ring of detectors

Fig. 1.5 Principle of CT machine. The x-ray tube moves around the patient. The detectors may also move or, as in this example, remain stationary. The time taken for the tube to travel the full 360° is usually 1−2 seconds.

The attenuation values are expressed on an arbitrary scale (Hounsfield units) with water density being 0, air density being minus 1000 units and bone density being plus 1000 units. The range and level of densities to be displayed can be selected by controls on the computer. The range of densities visualised on a particular image is known as the *'window width'* and the mean level as the *'window level'* or *'window centre'*.

The human eye can only appreciate a limited number of shades of grey. With a wide window all the structures are visible, but fine details of density difference cannot be appreciated. With a narrow window width, variations of just a few Hounsfield units can be recognised, but much of the image is either totally black or totally white and in these areas no useful information is provided. The effects of varying window width and level are illustrated in Figures 1.6 and 2.6 (p. 20).

Reconstruction to other planes

Computed tomography is usually performed in the axial plane. It is possible, however, to reconstruct images in planes other than those used to obtain the original sections. The computer has in its memory attenuation values for every voxel imaged and can present the data in any desired plane, e.g. coronal or sagittal. The problem is that though the voxel is very narrow, it usually has a considerable height and so the image is composed of long narrow blocks and consequently has poor spatial resolution. If the section thickness is very small, e.g. 1.5 mm, then reconstructions of reasonable spatial resolution can be obtained.

Partial volume effect

Since each voxel has a definite height, often 10 mm, a structure or lesion may be partly in and partly out of the section. The image displayed uses the mean attenuation for the entire voxel, so the density of a structure 'partially in the volume' may not be truly representative of that structure, nor may its size be correctly represented (Fig. 1.7).

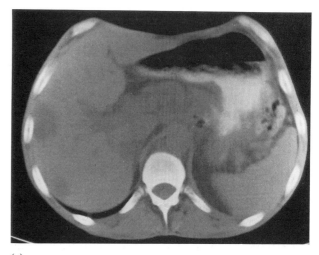

(a)

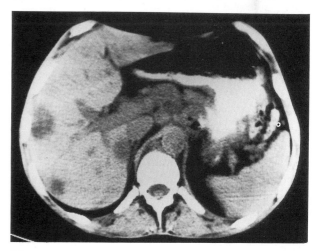

(b)

Fig. 1.6 Effect of varying window widths. In (a) and (b) the level has been kept constant at 30 HU. The window width in (a) is 600 HU, whereas in (b) it is only 100 HU. Note that with the narrow window in image (b) it is possible to appreciate minor density differences in the liver and so diagnose the metastases relatively easily, but much of the image is either white or black and in these areas little information is available. The effect of varying window level is shown in Figure 2.6, page 20.

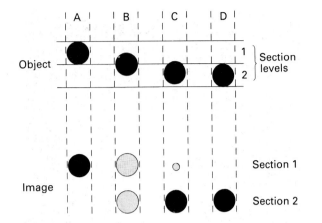

Fig. 1.7 Partial volume effect. Objects A and D occupy the full height of the section and, therefore, their diameter and density are accurately represented on the images of Sections 1 and 2. Object B lies half in Section 1 and half in Section 2. Its image will indicate the correct diameter, but the density will be half the true density of the object on *both* images. Object C lies largely in Section 2 but projects into Section 1. The upper image will underestimate the diameter *and* the density, whereas the lower image will be accurate apart from a minor underestimate of density. By using narrower sections, 'partial volume' inaccuracies are reduced, but more sections are then necessary to cover the same volume of tissue.

Artefacts

As might be anticipated, there are numerous artefacts that can occur with CT. Two frequently seen artefacts are those produced by movement (each exposure usually takes 1 or 2 seconds) and those from objects of very high density such as barium in the bowel, metal implants or surgical clips. Both types give rise to radiating linear streaks. The major problem is the resulting degradation of the image of the surrounding structures.

Magnetic resonance imaging

Magnetic resonance imaging (MRI) is a new system of imaging which depends on the magnetic properties of the nuclei of certain elements.

The basic principles of MRI depend on the fact that the nuclei of certain elements behave like small, spinning bar magnets and align with the magnetic force when placed in a strong magnetic field. At the field strengths currently used in medical imaging, hydrogen nuclei (protons) in water molecules and lipids are responsible for producing anatomical images. If a radiofrequency pulse at an appropriate frequency (resonant frequency) is applied, a proportion of the protons change their alignment, flipping through a preset angle, and rotate in phase with one another. Following this radiofrequency pulse, the protons return to their original positions. As the protons realign (relax) they induce a radio signal which, though very weak, can be detected by coils placed around the patient. The site of origin of this radio signal can be determined and an image representing the distribution of the hydrogen protons can be built up (Fig. 1.8). The strength of the signal depends not only on proton density but also on two relaxation times, T_1 and T_2; T_1 depends on the time the protons take to return to the axis of the magnetic field, and T_2 depends on the time the protons take to dephase. A T_1-weighted image is one in which the contrast between tissues is due mainly to their T_1 relaxation properties, while in a T_2-weighted image the contrast is due to the T_2 relaxation properties. Some sequences produce mixed (often called 'balanced') images which approximate to proton density. Most pathological processes show increased T_1 and T_2 relaxation times and these processes, therefore, appear lower in signal (blacker) on a T_1-weighted scan and higher in signal (whiter) on a T_2-weighted scan than the normal surrounding tissues. The T_1 and T_2 weighting of an image can be selected by appropriately altering the timing and sequence of radiofrequency pulses.

An MRI scanner (Fig. 1.9) consists of a large circular magnet. Inside the magnet are the radiofrequency transmitter and receiver coils, as well as gradient coils to allow spatial localisation of the MRI signal. Ancillary equipment converts the radio signal into a digital form which is then processed by a computer to form a final image. One advantage of MRI over CT is that the

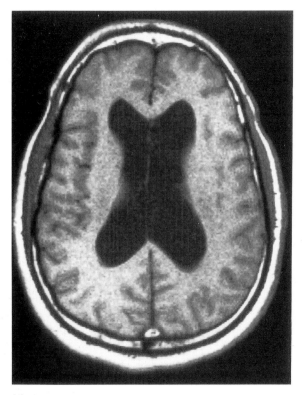

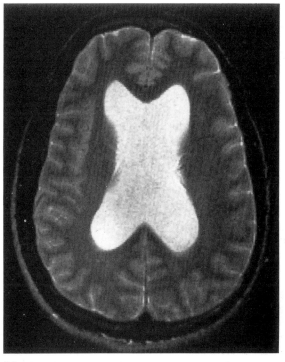

(b)

(a)

Fig. 1.8 MRI images of the brain. Axial sections through the level of the lateral ventricles in a patient with substantial ventricular dilatation. (a) T_1-weighted image. (b) T_2-weighted image. The CSF is dark on the T_1-weighted image and white on the T_2-weighted image. Note also that the intensity of the white and grey matter of the brain differs on the two images.

Fig. 1.9 Diagram of an MRI machine. The patient lies within a strong magnet (usually a cylindrical magnet). The radiofrequency transmitter coils send radiowaves into the patient and the same coils receive signals from within the patient. The intensity and source of these signals can be calculated and displayed as an image.

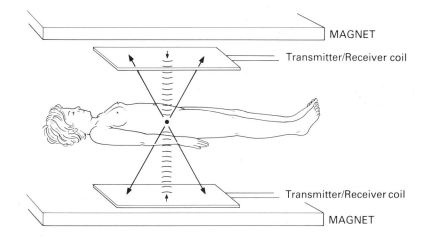

information can be directly reconstructed in any plane. Currently MRI is, in most instances, a slow process (often several minutes) requiring a long scan time compared to CT, with the disadvantage that it is necessary to keep the patient still during the scanning procedure. Unavoidable movements due to breathing, cardiac pulsation and peristalsis often degrade the image. Techniques for limiting the effect of such motion with significantly shorter scan times and various electronic gating devices are being actively developed. Cardiac gating is already widely available.

In the same way that contrast media have been of great value in CT, magnetic contrast media are providing useful diagnostic information with MRI. These agents depend on magnetic and paramagnetic properties to produce contrast. The most widely used agent is gadolinium DTPA which dramatically decreases the T_1 relaxation time.

Magnetic resonance imaging gives very different information to CT. Its place in medical practice is changing rapidly. The earliest successful application of MRI was in scanning of the brain and spinal cord, where it has significant advantages over CT and few disadvantages. It is now also an established technique for imaging the heart, spine, bones and joints. At first sight it may seem rather surprising that MRI is providing valuable information in skeletal disease since calcified tissues do not generate any signal at MRI. This seeming paradox is explained by the fact that MRI provides images of the bone marrow directly (Fig. 1.10) and demonstrating the bone marrow is important in many skeletal disorders.

The physical basis of vascular MRI is complicated and beyond the scope of this book. Suffice it to say that, with some sequences, fast flowing blood produces no signal, whereas with others it produces a bright signal. This 'motion effect' can be exploited to image the vascular system, e.g. large arteriovenous malformations can be readily demonstrated without contrast media (Fig. 1.11), hilar vessels can be distinguished from masses, and even stenoses of blood vessels can be demonstrated. Recently, special flow sequences have been developed which give images of vessels, resembling a conventional angiogram without the need for contrast media. This technique is known as magnetic resonance angiography (Fig. 1.12) and it may eventually replace conventional angiography. MRI of the heart uses electronic gating to obtain images during a specific proportion of the cardiac cycle. With this technique it is possible to limit the degradation of the image by cardiac motion and, therefore, demonstrate the cardiac chambers, valves and myocardium. Recently developed rapid scanning techniques allow the beating heart to be directly visualised as a cine image.

One of the advantages of MRI is that it involves no ionising radiation, and no adverse biological effects from diagnostic MRI have been demonstrated. It is, however, contraindicated at present in patients with

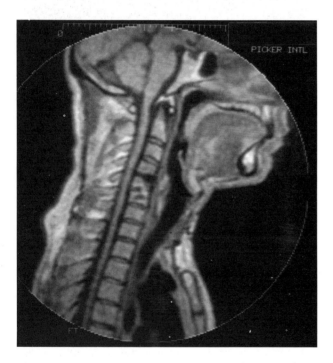

Fig. 1.10 Magnetic resonance image—sagittal section of upper thorax, neck and base of brain. The spinal cord and brain are very well seen. Note that with this signal sequence central nervous tissue is grey, CSF is black, fat is white and bone produces no signal (it is the fat in the bone marrow that produces the signal).

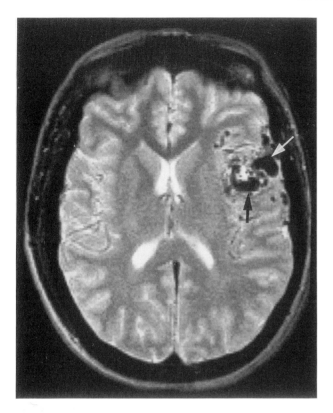

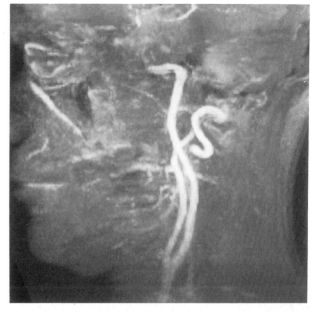

Fig. 1.12 MR angiogram of the left carotid arterial tree. Note that no contrast medium is used to obtain this image.

Fig. 1.11 MRI of head showing an arteriovenous malformation (arrows) in the left cerebral hemisphere. The fast-flowing blood in the malformation is responsible for absence of signal (signal void). The image is a T_2-weighted image, and is normal apart from the arteriovenous malformation.

certain types of aneurysm clips and cardiac pace-makers, because of the strong magnetic fields involved.

Radiation hazards

X-rays and other ionising radiation are harmful. Natural radiation from the sun, radioactivity in the environment, and atmospheric radioactivity from nuclear bombs and other man-made sources contribute a genetic risk over which the individual doctor has no control. However, radiation for medical purposes is several times greater than all other sources of man-made radiation and is under the control of doctors. It is their responsibility to limit the use of x-rays for medical purposes to those situations where the benefit clearly outbalances the risks. Unnecessary radiation is to be deplored. This is prevented by using appropriate equipment and good technique—limiting the size of the x-ray beam to the required areas, limiting the number of films to those that are necessary and keeping repeat examinations to a minimum. Just as important as these factors, all of which are really the province of those who work in the x-ray department, is avoiding unnecessary requests for x-ray examinations, particularly those that involve high radiation exposure such as barium enema and lumbar spine examination.

Radiation is particularly harmful to dividing cells. Genetically adverse mutations may occur following radiation of the gonads, resulting in congenital malformations and a genetic risk to the population. There is no threshold for the mutation rate, hence there is no such thing as a safe radiation dose.

Radiation to the developing fetus can have catastrophic effects. As well as the increased incidence of malformations induced in the developing fetus, it has been shown that the frequency with which leukaemia and other malignant neoplasms develop within the first 10 years of life is increased in children exposed to diagnostic x-rays while *in utero*, probably by about 40% compared to the normal population. X-raying a fetus should, therefore, be kept to the absolute minimum and preferably avoided.

Radiation-induced cancer is of general concern. If all radiation reducing methods were followed, including the elimination of unnecessary examinations, then in the UK it might be possible to reduce the number of cancer fatalities by over 100 cases per year.

2

Chest

The plain chest radiograph

The routine chest radiograph comprises a postero-anterior (PA) and a lateral view (Fig. 2.1). Ideally, both should be exposed on full inspiration with the patient in the upright position. Films taken on expiration are difficult to interpret because in expiration the lung bases appear hazy and the heart shadow increases in size (Fig. 2.2).

Even though chest films are the commonest x-ray examinations performed, they are also one of the most difficult plain films to interpret. The trained radiologist often scans the film in an apparently random fashion and if he finds an abnormality his subsequent thoughts are dictated by the possibilities that come to mind for that particular shadow. For example, if he sees a nodule representing a possible lung carcinoma, he analyses the shape of the nodule itself, and looks for other lung lesions and for evidence of spread of disease to the hilum, pleura or rib cage and so on. This problem-orientated approach—the observer constantly asking himself questions, not only about the shadows he sees but also about the patient's clinical findings—is the quickest and most accurate way of achieving a diagnosis. However, this approach takes time to learn and in the early stages a routine is necessary in order to avoid missing valuable radiological signs. The order in which one looks at the structures is unimportant; what matters is to follow a routine, otherwise important abnormalities will be overlooked. One way of examining the frontal and lateral chest films is presented below.

Trace the diaphragm

The upper surfaces of the diaphragm should be clearly visible from one costophrenic angle to the other, except where the heart is in contact with the diaphragm. On a good inspiratory film, the dome of the right hemidiaphragm is at the level of the anterior end of the sixth rib, the right hemidiaphragm being up to 2.5 cm higher than the left.

Check the size and shape of the heart

See p. 109 for the details.

Check the position of the heart and mediastinum

Normally, the trachea lies midway, or slightly to the right of the midpoint, between the medial ends of the clavicles. The position of the heart is very variable; on average one-third lies to the right of the midline, but anything from one-half to one-fifth of the heart lying to the right of the midline is within the normal range.

Look at the mediastinum

The right superior mediastinal border is usually straight or slightly curved as it passes downward to merge with the right heart border. The left superior mediastinal border is ill defined above the aortic arch.

The outline of the mediastinum and heart should be clearly seen except where the heart lies in contact with the diaphragm.

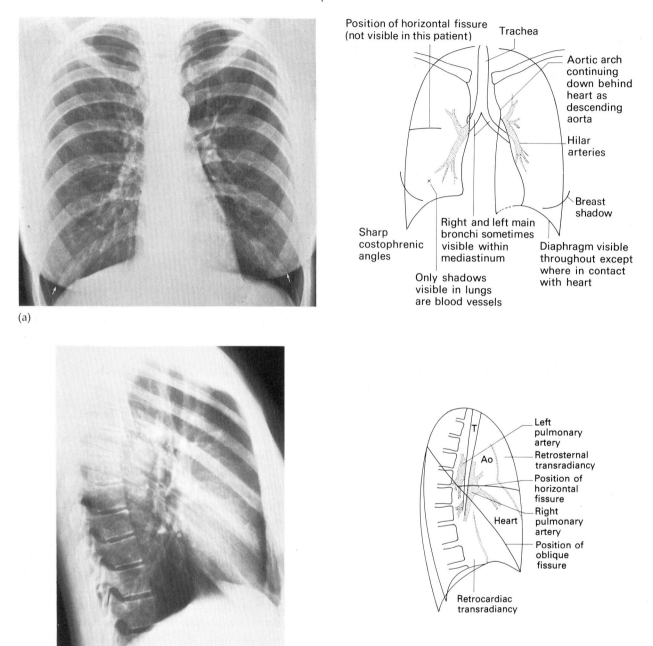

(a)

(b)

Fig. 2.1 Normal chest. (a) PA view. The arrows are on the breast shadows of this female patient. (b) Lateral view. Note that the upper retrosternal area is of the same density as the retrocardiac areas, and the same as over the upper thoracic vertebrae. The vertebrae are more transradiant (i.e. blacker) as the eye travels down the spine, until the diaphragm is reached. Ao, aorta; T, trachea.

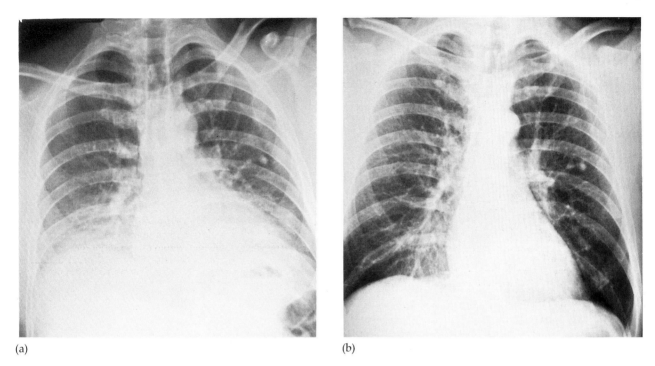

(a)

(b)

Fig. 2.2 Effect of expiration on chest film. Two films of the same patient taken one after the other. (a) Expiration. (b) Inspiration. On expiration the heart appears larger and the lung bases are hazy.

In young children, the normal thymus is clearly visualised. It may be very large and should not be mistaken for disease (Fig. 2.3).

Examine the hilar shadows

The hilar shadows represent the pulmonary arteries and veins. Air within the major bronchi can be recognised but their walls are not usually visible. The hilar lymph nodes in the normal patient are too small to recognise as discrete shadows.

The left hilum is usually slightly higher in position than the right.

Examine the lungs

The only structures that can be identified within normal lungs are the blood vessels, the interlobar fissures, and the walls of certain larger bronchi seen end-on. The fissures can only be seen if they lie tangential to the x-ray beam; they are after all composed of just two layers of pleura. Usually, only the horizontal fissure (minor fissure) is visible in the frontal projection, running from the right hilum to the sixth rib in the axilla. There is no equivalent to the horizontal fissure on the left. The oblique fissures (major fissures) are only visible on the lateral view. The fissures form the boundaries of the lobes of the lungs so a knowledge of their position is essential for an appreciation of lobar anatomy (see Fig. 2.16, p. 28). In about 1% of people there is an extra fissure visible in the frontal view—the so-called azygos lobe fissure (Fig. 2.4).

Look for abnormal pulmonary opacities or translucencies. Do not mistake the pectoral muscles, breasts (Fig. 2.5) or plaits of hair for pulmonary shadows. Skin lumps or the nipples may mimic pulmonary nodules. The nipples are usually in the fifth anterior rib space,

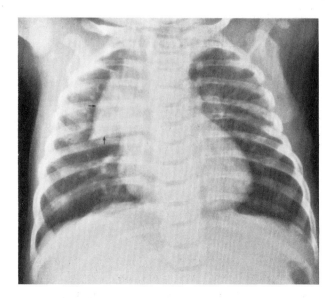

Fig. 2.3 Normal but prominent thymus in a child aged 3 months. The thymus shows the characteristic 'sail shape' projecting to the right of the mediastinum (arrows). This appearance should not be confused with right upper lobe consolidation or collapse.

but they are, in practice, rarely misdiagnosed provided one remembers that, in general, if one nipple is visible the other will also be seen.

A good method of finding subtle shadows on the frontal film is to compare one lung with the other, zone by zone. Detecting ill-defined shadows on the lateral view can be difficult. A helpful and reliable feature is that as the eye travels down the thoracic vertebral bodies, each body should appear more lucent than the one above until the diaphragm is reached.

Check the integrity of the ribs, clavicles and spine and examine the soft tissues

In females, check that both breasts are present. Following mastectomy the breast shadow cannot be defined. The reduction in the soft tissue bulk leads to an increased transradiancy of that side of the chest, which should not be confused with pulmonary disease.

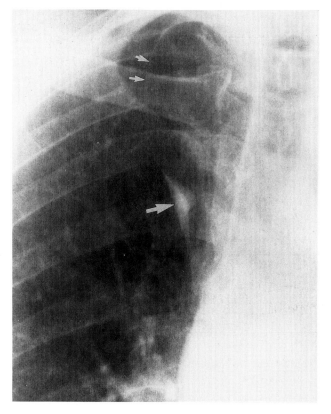

Fig. 2.4 The azygos lobe fissure. During normal intrauterine development the azygos vein migrates through the lung from the chest wall to lie within the mediastinum. In patients with an azygos 'lobe', the vein (large arrow) fails to reach the tracheo-bronchial angle and, therefore, lies in the lower end of the azygos fissure (small arrows). This variant is of no clinical significance.

Assess the technical quality of the film

Technical factors are important since incorrect exposure or faulty centring or projection may hide or mimic disease. The correctly exposed routine PA chest film is one in which the ribs and spine behind the heart can be identified but the lungs are not overexposed. Unless one can see through the heart, lower lobe lesions may be completely missed. A straight film is one where the medial ends of the clavicles are equidistant from the pedicles of the thoracic vertebrae.

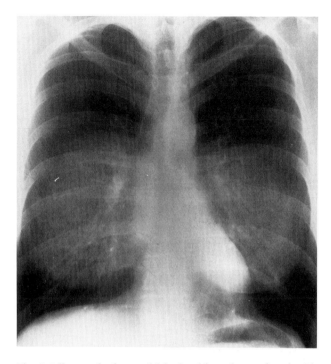

Fig. 2.5 Breast shadows which should not be confused with pulmonary consolidation. In this instance the patient has had mammary implants.

Extra views

Oblique views. Films taken with the patient turned to one or other side are useful for demonstrating the chest wall and, occasionally, for showing intrathoracic shadows to better advantage.

Lateral decubitus views are not, as the name would suggest, lateral views; they are frontal projections taken with the patient lying on one or other side using a horizontal x-ray beam. Their purpose is to demonstrate free pleural fluid which will collect along the dependent chest wall (see Fig. 2.46, p. 48).

Expiration films. A frontal film may be deliberately exposed on expiration in order to demonstrate diaphragmatic movement or the ability of the lung to deflate. A pneumothorax may be more obvious on an expiration than an inspiration film.

Fluoroscopy

The image at *fluoroscopy* is poor compared to that which can be achieved with x-ray film. It is rarely used and is limited to observing the movement of the diaphragm and demonstrating air trapping in cases of suspected inhalation of a foreign body.

Computed tomography

The greatest value of CT in chest disease is:
• To show the presence and extent of mediastinal masses and other mediastinal abnormalities. It is widely used to demonstrate enlarged lymph nodes when staging patients with neoplastic disease, particularly lung cancer and lymphoma. Sometimes CT can even determine the nature of the mediastinal abnormality. Knowing the shape and the precise location of an abnormality may make a particular diagnosis highly likely. One of the advantages of CT is that it can distinguish vascular from non-vascular structures, e.g. an aneurysm from a solid mass. Also CT allows one to recognise fat, which is useful in diagnosing fatty tumours and in excluding significant abnormalities when mediastinal widening is due merely to excess fat deposition.
• To show the shape of an intrapulmonary or pleural mass and to detect any calcification that may be present in the mass, when this is not evident or doubtful on plain chest radiographs.
• To localise a mass prior to biopsy.
• To demonstrate the presence of disease when the plain chest radiograph is normal in those cases where the possibility of intrathoracic abnormality is suspected on other grounds, e.g. in the detection of pulmonary metastases; finding a primary carcinoma in patients whose sputum cytology shows neoplastic cells; and demonstrating thymic tumours in patients with myasthenia gravis.
• To document the presence, extent and severity of

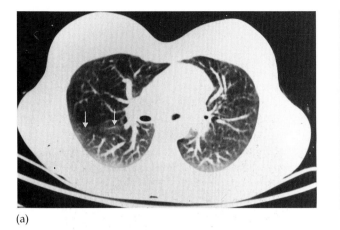

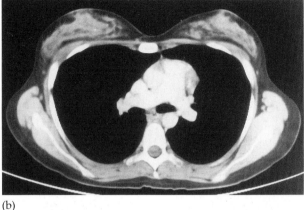

(a)   (b)

Fig. 2.6 Chest CT illustrating the different window centres (levels) used for the lungs and mediastinum. (a) Lung settings. A negative centre (−700 HU) shows the lungs to advantage, but detail of mediastinal structures is minimal, the mediastinum being virtually white. In this example, the lung vessels are the only identifiable shadows originating from within the lung. The position of the right oblique (major) fissure is arrowed. (b) Mediastinal settings. A centre close to average soft-tissue density (30 HU) and a narrow window width (300 HU) shows the structures within the mediastinum clearly, but the lungs are blacked out. Mediastinal adenopathy is present.

bronchiectasis and certain pulmonary parenchymal processes, such as fibrosing alveolitis.

Technique

A routine examination consists of adjacent sections 1 cm thick taken through the area of interest. To examine the entire chest from the posterior costo-phrenic recesses to the lung apices involves approximately 30 sections. Intravenous contrast medium is given in many cases when the purpose of the examination is to visualise the mediastinum or hilum; it is of no value for examining the lungs. The images are usually viewed at two distinct window settings (Fig. 2.6) (see p. 9 for explanation of CT windows and levels). If the CT scan has been performed to see bone lesions then bone settings are used.

Thinner sections can be used to produce images with higher spatial resolution in so-called 'thin-section CT', also known as high resolution CT (HRCT). High resolution CT is a specialised application being used with increasing frequency to show details of pulmonary parenchymal disease and bronchiectasis.

Normal images (Fig. 2.6a)

Just as with the plain chest radiograph and conventional tomograms, the only structures seen within the normal lungs are the blood vessels, the pleural fissures and the walls of the larger bronchi. Vessels within the lung are recognised by their shape rather than by contrast opacification. When seen in cross section they appear round and may be indistinguishable from small lung nodules. Fortunately most metastases and granulomas are located peripherally where the vessels are smallest.

The fissures are seen either as a line or their position may be recognisable only as a relatively avascular zone within the lung. The CT appearances of the normal mediastinum and hila are discussed on p. 57.

Conventional tomography

Conventional tomography has now been almost entirely replaced by CT. It can be used to investigate masses in the lungs and hilum in much the same way as CT, but has few other indications.

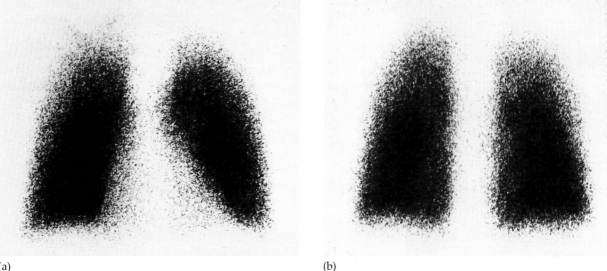

(a)   (b)

Fig. 2.7 Normal radionuclide perfusion scan using ^{99m}Tc-labelled macroaggregates of albumin. (a) Anterior view. (b) Posterior view.

Radionuclide lung scanning

There are two major types of lung scan, namely perfusion and ventilation scans.

For perfusion scans, macroaggregates of albumin with an average particle size of 30 µm, labelled with an isotope such as technetium-99 m, are injected intravenously. These particles become trapped in the pulmonary capillaries; the distribution of radioactivity, when imaged by a gamma camera, accurately reflects blood flow (Fig. 2.7).

For ventilation scans, the patient inhales a radioactive gas such as xenon-133, xenon-127 or krypton-81 m and the distribution of radioactive gas is imaged using a gamma camera (Fig. 2.8) Aerosols labelled with technetium-99 m may be used instead of gases.

The major indication for lung scanning is to diagnose or exclude pulmonary embolism (see p. 85).

Bronchography

Bronchography involves introducing an iodinated contrast material into the bronchial tree. The only

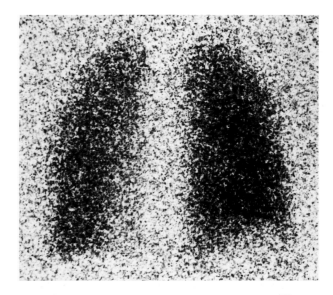

Fig. 2.8 Normal radionuclide ventilation scan using ^{133}Xe; posterior scan.

remaining indication is for the assessment of selected cases of bronchiectasis (see p. 81).

Pulmonary angiography

The pulmonary arteries and veins can be demonstrated by taking serial films following the rapid injection of angiographic contrast medium into the pulmonary arterial circulation through a catheter. The catheterisation is carried out under fluoroscopic control with continuous electrocardiographic and pressure monitoring, by an operator skilled in cardiac catheterisation. It carries a small but definite risk to the patient.

Its major use is to diagnose pulmonary emboli. Occasionally, it is needed to demonstrate congenital vascular anomalies.

Diseases of the chest with a normal chest radiograph

Serious respiratory disease may exist in patients with a normal chest radiograph. Sometimes it is only possible to detect abnormality by comparison with previous or later examinations, e.g. minor elevation of one hemidiaphragm due to pulmonary embolism, or subtle pulmonary shadows due to pulmonary fibrosis. Respiratory disease with a normal chest radiograph can be conveniently divided into:

1 *Obstructive airways disease*. Asthma and acute bronchiolitis may produce overinflation of the lungs, but in many cases the chest film is normal. Emphysema, when severe, gives rise to the signs described on p. 80 but when moderate, the chest radiograph may be normal or very nearly so. Uncomplicated acute or chronic bronchitis does not produce any radiological signs, so if a patient with chronic bronchitis has an abnormal film, he either has some other disease or he has developed a complication, e.g. pneumonia or cor pulmonale. A proportion of patients with productive cough due to bronchiectasis show no plain film abnormality.

2 *Small lesions*. It is usually impossible to see solitary lung masses or consolidations of less than 1 cm in diameter. Even 2–3 cm lung cancers may be very dif-

ficult to identify on routine films if they are hidden behind overlapping rib and clavicle shadows or behind the heart or diaphragm.

Endobronchial lesions, such as carcinoma, cannot be diagnosed on routine films unless they cause collapse/consolidation or considerable obstructive emphysema.

3 *Pulmonary emboli without infarction*. The chest radiograph is often normal in such patients, even with life-threatening emboli.

4 *Infections*. Most patients with acute bacterial pneumonia present with recognisable consolidation, but in other infections, notably *Pneumocystis carinii* pneumonia, the consolidation may only develop after the onset of symptoms. Patients with miliary tuberculosis may initially have a normal chest film.

5 *Diffuse pulmonary* disease, particularly pulmonary fibrosis of many different aetiologies, may be responsible for breathlessness with substantial alteration in lung function tests before any clear-cut radiological abnormalities are evident.

6 *Pleural abnormality*. Dry pleurisy will not produce any radiological findings; even 300 ml of pleural fluid may be impossible to recognise on standard PA and lateral chest films.

The abnormal chest

When faced with an abnormal examination of the chest, be it a plain chest film or even a CT or MRI scan, the first questions to ask oneself are 'where is the abnormality?' and 'how extensive is it?' Only then does one move on to the question 'what is it?' Clearly, the differential diagnosis for pulmonary lesions is quite different from that for mediastinal, pleural or chest wall disease. The first step is to examine all available films. Usually, the location of any lesion will then be obvious. If the shadow is surrounded on all sides by aerated lung it must arise within the lung. Similarly, many masses will clearly be within the mediastinum. However, when a lesion is in contact with the pleura or mediastinum it may be difficult to decide where it originated.

If the shadow has a broad base with smooth convex

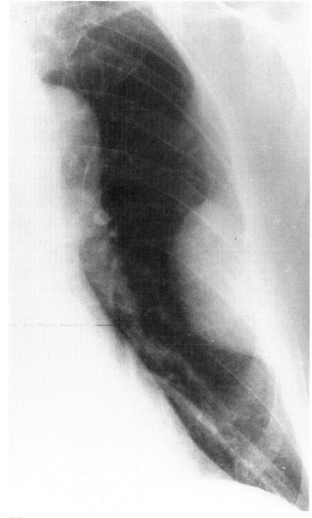

(a)

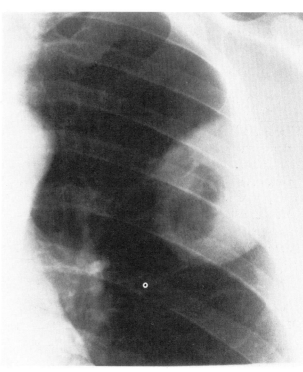

(b)

Fig. 2.9 (a) Extrapleural mass. The mass has a smooth convex border with a wide base on the chest wall (a myeloma lesion arising in a rib). This shape is quite different from a peripherally located pulmonary mass such as (b) a primary carcinoma of the lung.

borders projecting into the lung and a well-defined outline it is likely to be pleural, extrapleural or mediastinal in origin (Fig. 2.9).

Particular care is needed when evaluating shadows in the hilar region on a frontal chest radiograph. It is always essential to check on the lateral film whether the shadow is *at* the hilum or just projected over it (Fig. 2.10), since the causes and subsequent investigation of hilar enlargement are different to those of pulmonary shadows.

The silhouette sign (Fig. 2.11)

The silhouette sign is an invaluable sign for localising disease from the plain chest radiograph. The information on a chest film is largely dependent on the contrast between the radiolucent air in the lungs compared with the opacity of the heart, blood vessels, mediastinum and diaphragm. An intrathoracic lesion touching a border of the heart, aorta or diaphragm will obliterate that border on the chest radiograph. This sign was named 'the silhouette sign' by Felson and has two important applications:

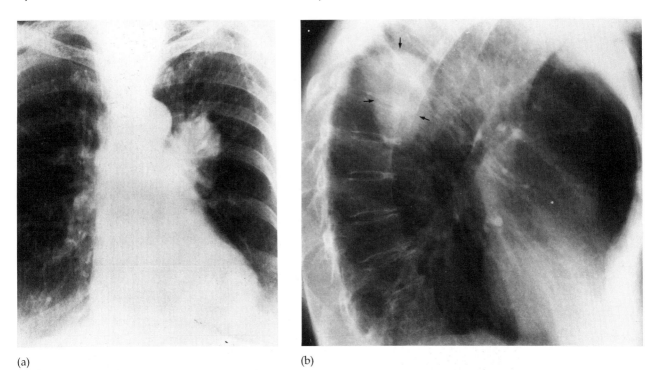

(a)   (b)

Fig. 2.10 Mass in apical (superior) segment of the left lower lobe. (a) PA film. The mass is projected over the left hilum. (b) Lateral film. Unless one studies the lateral film, it would be easy to misdiagnose this lesion as a hilar mass rather than as a peripherally located intrapulmonary mass (arrows). (The diagnosis in this instance was primary carcinoma of the bronchus.)

1 It is often possible to localise a shadow by observing which borders are lost, e.g. loss of the heart border must mean that the shadow lies in the anterior half of the chest. Alternatively, loss of part of the diaphragm outline indicates disease of the pleura or of the lung in direct contact with the diaphragm, usually the lower lobes.

2 It makes it possible, on occasion, to diagnose disorders such as pulmonary consolidation or collapse even when one is uncertain as to the presence of an opacity. It is a surprising fact that a wedge or lens-shaped opacity may be very difficult to see because of the way the shadow fades out at its margins, but if such a lesion is in contact with the mediastinum or diaphragm it causes loss of their normally sharp outline.

The lungs

When looking at a chest radiograph or a CT scan it is of practical help to try and place any abnormal intrapulmonary shadows into one or more of the following broad categories:
- Air-space filling
  (a) pulmonary oedema
  (b) pulmonary consolidation
- Pulmonary collapse (atelectasis)
- Spherical shadows
- Line shadows
- Widespread small shadows.

  The presence of cavitation or calcification should be noted.

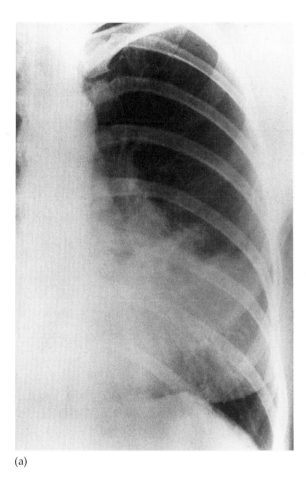

(a)

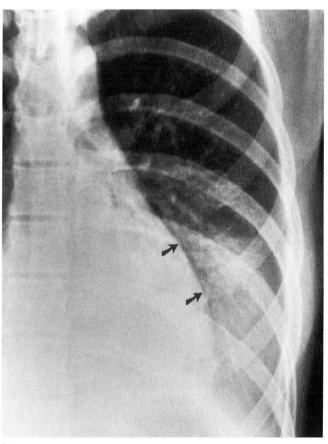

(b)

Fig. 2.11 'The silhouette sign'.
(a) The left heart border is invisible
because it is in contact with
consolidation in the adjacent lingula.
(b) The left heart border can be seen
because the consolidation is in the
left lower lobe and air in the lingula
preserves the visibility of the cardiac
silhouette (arrows). Note that now it
is the diaphragm outline that is
invisible. (c) The relationships of the
lingula and lower lobes to the heart
and diaphragm are best appreciated
in the lateral projection.

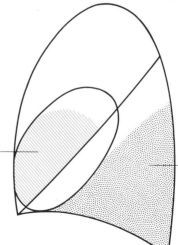

Consolidation in the
lingula obliterates
the left heart border
but leaves the
diaphragm visible

Consolidation in
the left lower lobe
obliterates the
diaphragm but leaves
the heart border
visible

(c)

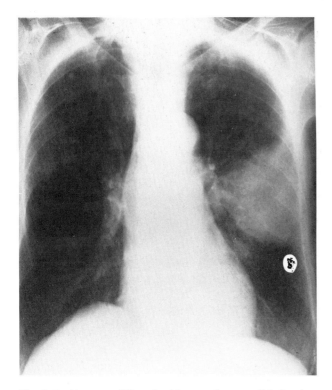

Fig. 2.12 Air-space filling. In this case the consolidation in the left lung is due to a pulmonary infarct.

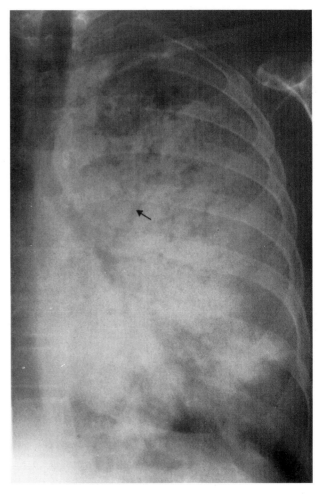

Fig. 2.13 The air bronchogram sign. An extensive air bronchogram is seen in this patient with pneumonia. The arrow points to some bronchi that are particularly well seen.

Air-space filling

'Air-space filling' means the replacement of air in the alveoli by fluid or, rarely, by other materials. 'Infiltrate' is a commonly used but less satisfactory term. The fluid can be either a *transudate* (pulmonary oedema) or an *exudate*. The causes of an alveolar exudate include infection, infarction, pulmonary contusion, haemorrhage, collagen disease and allergy.

The signs of 'air-space filling' are:
- A shadow with ill-defined borders (Fig. 2.12) except where the disease process is in contact with a fissure, in which case the shadow has a well-defined edge.
- An air bronchogram (Fig. 2.13). Normally, it is not possible to identify air in the bronchi within the lung substance because the walls of the bronchi are too thin and they are surrounded by air in the alveoli, but if the alveoli are filled with fluid, the air in the bronchi contrasts with the fluid in the lung. This sign is seen to great advantage in CT scans (Fig. 2.14).
- The silhouette sign, namely loss of visualisation of the adjacent mediastinal or diaphragm outline (see above for explanation of this sign).

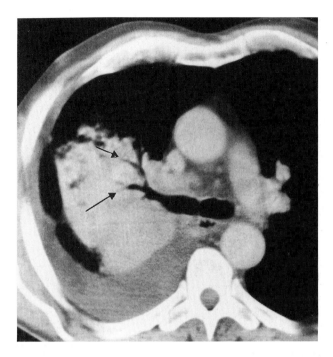

Fig. 2.14 CT scan showing an air bronchogram (arrows). This patient had pneumonia and also had a pleural effusion.

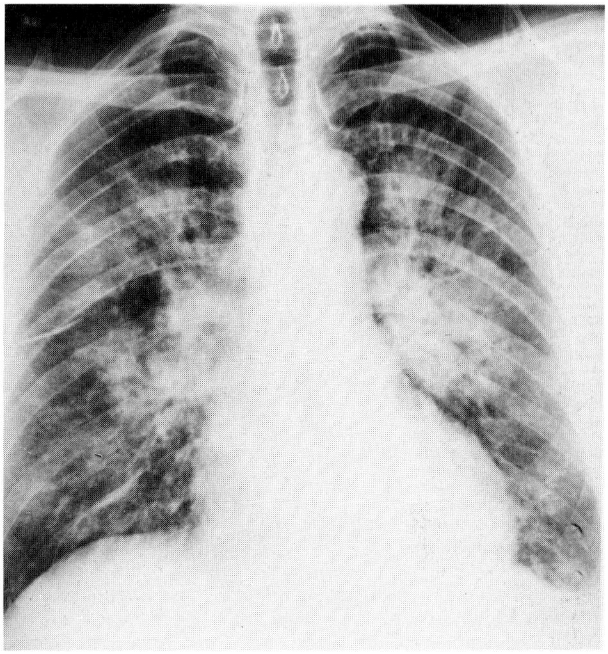

Fig. 2.15 Alveolar pulmonary oedema. Typical 'bat's wing' pattern. The shadows are bilateral and maximal in the perihilar region, fading towards the periphery of the lobes.

Pulmonary oedema

There are two radiographic patterns of pulmonary oedema: alveolar and interstitial. Since the oedema fluid initially collects in the interstitial tissues of the lungs, all patients with alveolar oedema also have interstitial oedema. Alveolar oedema is always acute. It is almost always bilateral (Fig. 2.15), and involves all the lobes. In the early stages, the shadowing is maximal close to the hila and fades out peripherally, leaving a relatively clear zone around the edges of the lobes. This pattern of oedema is sometimes called the 'butterfly' or the 'bat's wing' pattern. (Interstitial oedema is discussed on p. 118.)

The causes of pulmonary oedema are broadly divided into those due to circulatory disorders, e.g. acute left ventricular failure, mitral stenosis, renal failure and overtransfusion, and so-called 'non-cardiogenic pulmonary oedema' in which increased capillary permeability is the important mechanism. This mechanism of oedema is seen in adult respiratory distress syndrome (ARDS), aspiration of gastric contents, and inhalation of noxious gases. The appearance may initially be identical to that seen with cardiogenic pulmonary oedema, but in ARDS (see p. 85) the pulmonary shadowing becomes uniform over a period of days, until eventually all parts of the lungs are fairly equally affected.

One helpful feature in distinguishing cardiogenic pulmonary oedema from the non cardiogenic varieties and from widespread exudates, such as pneumonia, is the speed with which the oedema appears and disappears. Substantial improvement in a 24 hour period is virtually diagnostic of cardiogenic pulmonary oedema.

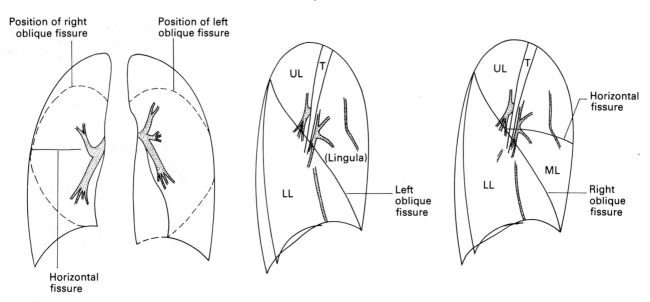

Fig. 2.16 Diagram showing the position of the lobes and fissures. The oblique (major) fissure is similar on the two sides. The oblique fissures are not visible on the frontal view; their position is indicated by the dotted line. In the left lung (centre diagram), the oblique fissure separates the upper lobe (UL) and lower lobe (LL). In the right lung, there is an extra fissure — the horizontal (minor) fissure, which separates the upper lobe (UL) and middle lobe (ML). (The lingular segments of the upper lobe are analogous to the segments of the middle lobe.) T, trachea.

Pulmonary consolidation (alveolar infiltrates)

Pure consolidation shows no loss of volume but consolidation is often accompanied by collapse.

Consolidation of a whole lobe or the majority of a lobe is virtually diagnostic of bacterial pneumonia. The recognition of lobar consolidation requires an appreciation of the radiological anatomy of the lobes (Fig. 2.16). Lobar consolidation produces an opaque lobe, except for air in the bronchi (air bronchograms). Since the consolidated lobe is airless, the fissure between it and the normal lung does not appear as a line, but is seen as a clear-cut border to the opacity. Because of the silhouette sign, the boundary between the affected lung and the adjacent heart, mediastinum and diaphragm will be invisible. The appearance of lobar consolidation is seen in Figure 2.17.

Patchy consolidation, i.e. one or more patches of ill-defined shadowing (Fig. 2.18), is usually due to:
- infection
- infarction
- contusion
- immunological disorders.

There is no reliable way of telling from the films which of these possibilities is the cause. In most instances the clinical and laboratory findings point to one of these alternatives.

When consolidation is spherical in shape it may be difficult to distinguish from a lung tumour, but usually serial films show a change over a short interval if the shadow is due to consolidation, whereas no change will be apparent if it is due to a tumour. An air bronchogram is a very helpful sign here, since it is common in pneumonia and very rare in tumours.

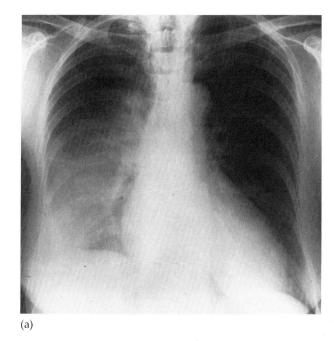

(a)

Fig. 2.17 Consolidation of the right lower lobe. Note the application of the silhouette sign here. (a) PA view. The heart border and the medial half of the right hemidiaphragm are visible, whereas the lateral half is invisible. On the lateral view (b), the oblique fissure forms a well-defined anterior boundary and the right hemidiaphragm is ill defined. Only the left hemidiaphragm is seen clearly.

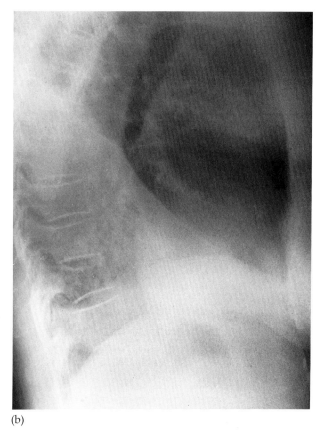

(b)

Cavitation (abscess formation) within the consolidated areas in the lung may occur with many bacterial infections (Fig. 2.19), but the organisms that are particularly liable to produce cavitation are staphylococci, klebsiella, *Mycobacterium tuberculosis*, anaerobic bacteria and various fungi. Abscess formation is only recognisable once there is communication with the bronchial tree, allowing the liquid centre of the abscess to be coughed up and replaced by air. The air is then seen as a transradiancy within the consolidation and an air–fluid level may be present (Fig. 2.20). CT is much more sensitive than plain films for demonstrating cavitation.

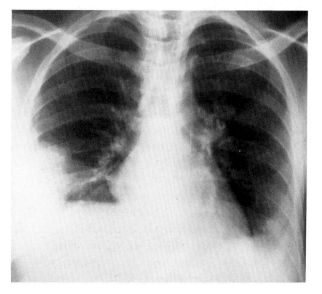

Fig. 2.18 Patchy consolidation in both lower lobes in a patient with bronchopneumonia.

Chapter 2

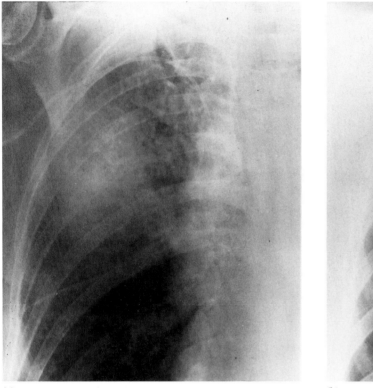

(a)

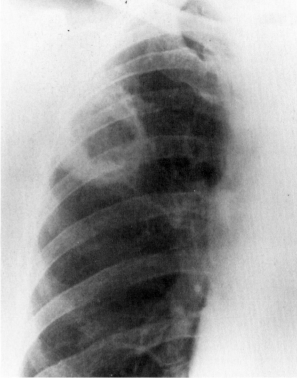

(b)

Fig. 2.19 Cavitation in staphylococcal pneumonia. (a) A round area of consolidation which, 7 days later (b), shows central translucency due to the development of cavitation.

Cavitation is occasionally seen in other forms of pulmonary consolidation, e.g. infarction and Wegener's granulomatosis.

Pneumatoceles (Fig. 2.21) are thin-walled air cysts which are associated with a number of consolidative processes; staphylococcal pneumonia and pulmonary contusion are the commonest. Pneumatoceles may increase or decrease in size very rapidly or, alternatively, they may persist for many years after the original consolidation has resolved, but eventually almost all of them will disappear.

Pulmonary collapse (atelectasis)

Collapse (loss of volume of a lung or lobe) may be due to any of the following:
- bronchial obstruction
- pneumothorax or pleural effusion
- fibrosis of a lobe, usually following tuberculosis
- bronchiectasis
- pulmonary embolus.

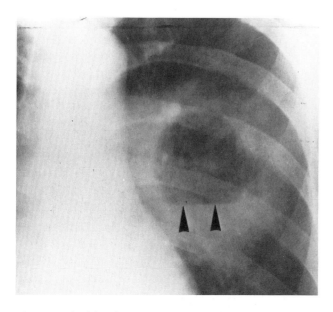

Fig. 2.20 Fluid level (arrows) in a lung abscess. Fluid levels are only visible if the chest radiograph is taken with a horizontal x-ray beam.

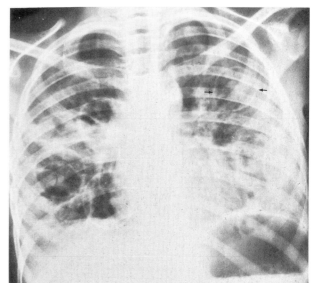

Fig. 2.21 Pneumatocele formation in staphylococcal pneumonia. The pneumatoceles are seen as large air-containing ring shadows. One in the left upper zone is arrowed.

Collapse due to bronchial obstruction

Collapse due to bronchial obstruction occurs because no air can get into the lung to replace the air absorbed from the alveoli. The commoner causes are:

1 Bronchial wall lesions
  - usually primary carcinoma
  - rarely, other bronchial tumours such as carcinoid
  - rarely, endobronchial tuberculosis
2 Intraluminal occlusion
  - mucus plugging, particularly in postoperative, asthmatic or unconscious patients, or in patients on artificial ventilation
  - inhaled foreign body
3 Invasion or compression by an adjacent mass
  - malignant tumour
  - enlarged lymph nodes.

The signs of collapse are:
- the shadow of the collapsed lobe
- the silhouette sign

- displacement of structures to take up the space normally occupied by the collapsed lobe.

Consolidation almost invariably accompanies lobar collapse, so the resulting shadow is usually obvious. Occasionally, the loss of volume is very severe and the lobe becomes so shrunken that unless it is precisely tangential to the x-ray beam it may be difficult to see on plain chest radiograph. The silhouette sign can be very useful in this situation, since the mediastinal and diaphragmatic borders will be ill defined adjacent to the collapsed lobe. The silhouette sign helps also in deciding which lobe is collapsed. Collapse of the anteriorly located lobes (the upper and middle) will obliterate portions of the mediastinal and heart outlines, whereas collapse of the lower lobes obscures the outline of the adjacent diaphragm and descending aorta.

When a lobe collapses, the unobstructed lobe(s) on the side of the collapse undergo compensatory

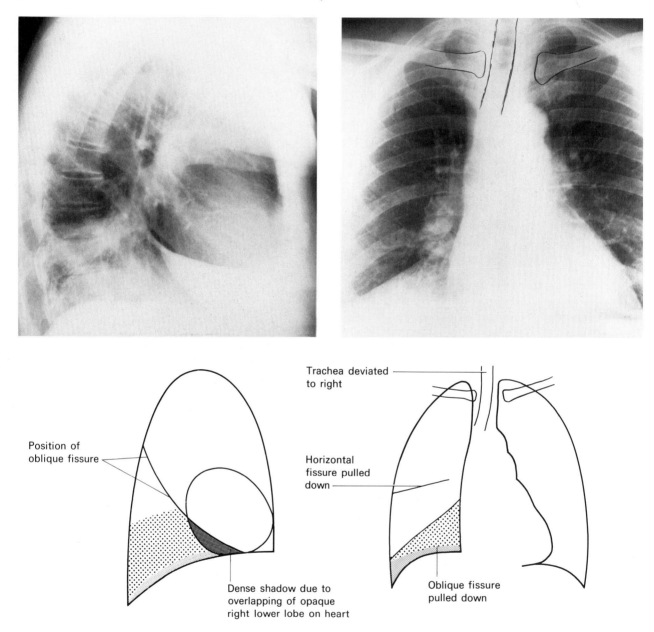

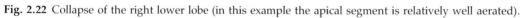

Fig. 2.22 Collapse of the right lower lobe (in this example the apical segment is relatively well aerated).

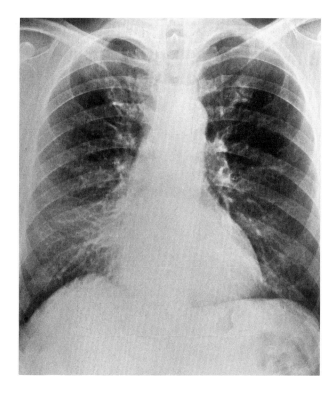

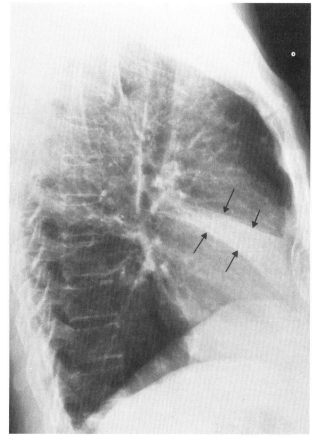

Fig. 2.23 Collapse of the middle lobe. The collapsed lobe is most obvious on the lateral view (arrows). Note the silhouette sign obliterating the lower right heart border.

expansion and the displaced fissures and the movement of the hilum towards the collapsed lobe are then recognisable. The fissure is seen as a well defined boundary to an airless lobe. The mediastinum and diaphragm may move towards the collapsed lobe. Since lobar collapse is such an important diagnosis and one that is often misinterpreted, it is worth devoting time to study the appearance of collapse of each of the lobes (Figs 2.22–2.26). Computed tomography shows lobar collapse very well (Figs 2.26 and 2.27), but is rarely necessary simply to diagnose a collapsed lobe.

In collapse of the whole of one lung, the entire hemithorax is opaque and there is substantial mediastinal and tracheal shift (Fig. 2.28).

Collapse in association with pleural abnormality

The presence of air or fluid in the pleural cavity will allow the lung to collapse. In pneumothorax, the diagnosis is obvious but if there is a large pleural effusion with underlying pulmonary collapse it may be difficult to diagnose the presence of the collapse on a chest radiograph. This problem does not arise with CT where it is usually easy to recognise pulmonary collapse despite the presence of a pleural effusion (Fig. 2.29). Even if the collapsed lobe is identified it can be difficult to tell whether the collapse is due to pleural fluid or whether both the collapse and the effusion are due to the same process, e.g. carcinoma of the bronchus.

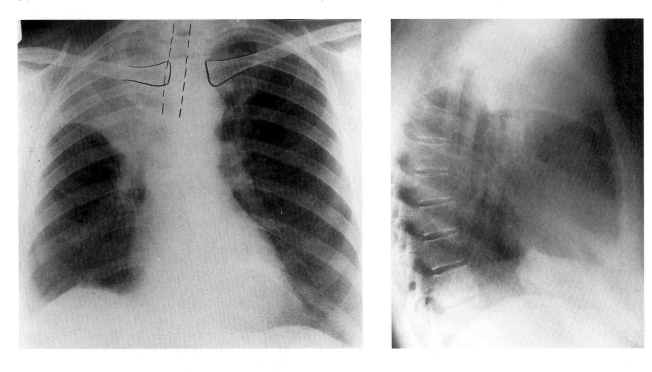

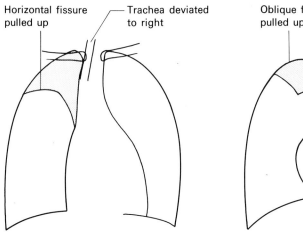

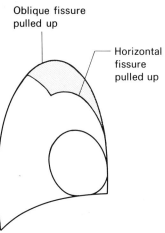

Fig. 2.24 Collapse of the right upper lobe. Note the elevated horizontal fissure.

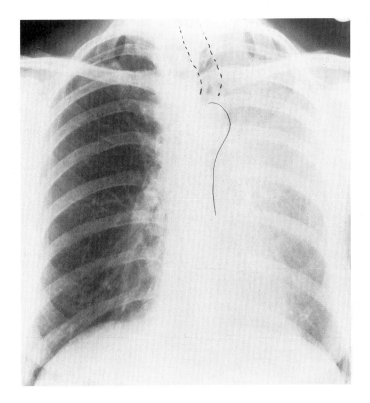

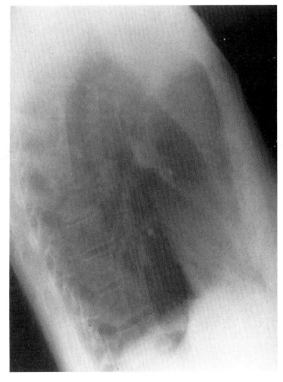

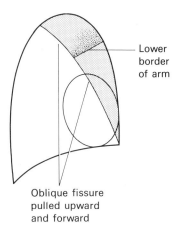

Fig. 2.25 Collapse of the left upper lobe. Note that the lower border of the collapsed lobe is ill-defined on the PA view and that the upper two-thirds of the left mediastinal and heart borders are invisible, but that the aortic knuckle and descending aorta are identifiable. (The visible portions of the aorta have been drawn in for greater clarity.)

Lower border of arm

Oblique fissure pulled upward and forward

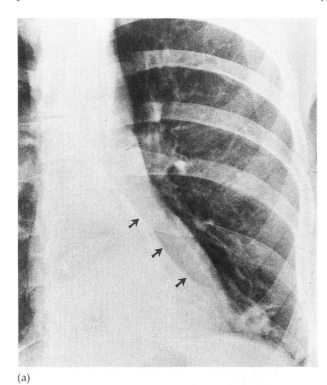

(a)

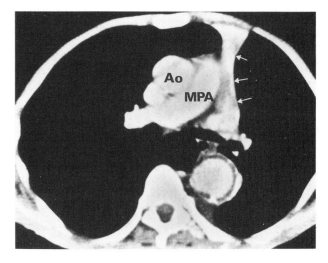

Fig. 2.27 CT scan of a severely collapsed left upper lobe. Note the smooth lateral border of the collapsed lobe formed by the displaced oblique (major) fissure (arrows). The scan shows compensatory over-expansion of the right upper lobe which has crossed the midline anterior to the ascending aorta (Ao) and main pulmonary artery (MPA).

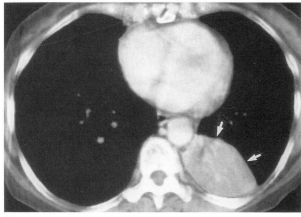

(b)

Fig. 2.26 Collapse of the left lower lobe. (a) Chest radiograph. The triangular shadow of the collapsed lobe is seen through the heart. Its lateral border is formed by the displaced oblique fissure (arrows). (b) CT scan. The collapsed lobe is seen lying posteriorly in the left thorax. The well-defined anterior margin is due to the displaced oblique fissure (arrows).

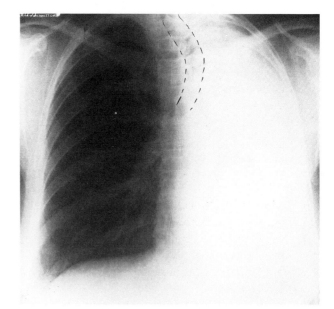

Fig. 2.28 Collapse of left lung showing tracheal and mediastinal displacement.

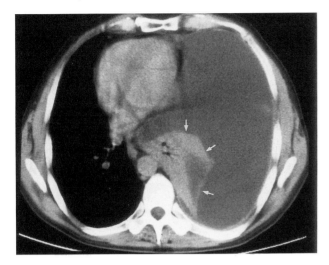

Fig. 2.29 CT showing pleural effusion and pulmonary collapse. The collapsed left lower lobe (arrows) can be clearly seen beneath the large left pleural effusion.

Collapse due to lobar fibrosis or bronchiectasis

In both these states a lobe may be reduced in volume, sometimes very severely, but usually the lobe remains at least partially aerated.

Collapse due to pulmonary embolus

With collapse due to pulmonary embolus the involved lobe, or lobes, usually show a combination of patchy consolidation and loss of volume. The loss of volume is rarely very great.

Spherical shadows (lung mass, lung nodule)

The diagnosis of a solitary spherical shadow in the lung (Fig. 2.30) is a common problem.

The usual causes of a solitary pulmonary nodule are:
- bronchial carcinoma
- benign tumour of the lung, hamartoma being the most common
- infective granuloma, tuberculoma being the most common in the UK, fungal granuloma being the most frequent in the USA

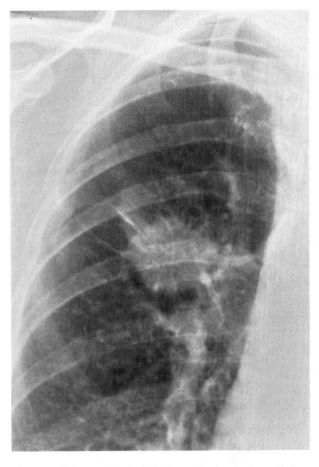

Fig. 2.30 Solitary spherical shadow. The large size and the irregular infiltrating edge are important diagnostic features suggesting primary carcinoma of the lung.

- metastasis
- lung abscess.

With the exception of lung abscess, the lesions in this list rarely cause symptoms, the mass being noted on a routine chest film. When a nodule is discovered in a patient who is over 40 and a smoker, bronchial carcinoma becomes the major consideration. Primary carcinoma is unlikely, particularly in a patient under 30 years of age.

The list of possible diagnoses given above contains

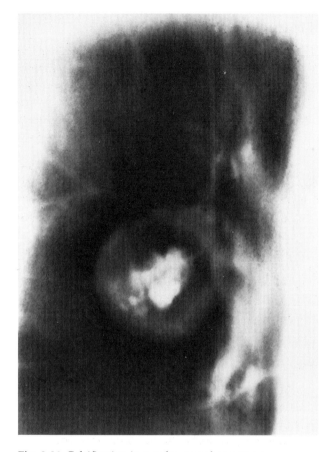

Fig. 2.31 Calcification in a pulmonary hamartoma (tomogram). The central flocculant ('popcorn') calcification is typical of that seen in hamartomas.

lesions requiring totally different forms of management. Hamartomas and granulomas are best left alone, whereas bronchial carcinoma, active tuberculosis and lung abscess require treatment. Careful observation of the following features may help in making the diagnosis.

Comparison with previous films

Being able to assess the rate of growth of a spherical lesion in the lung is one of the most important factors in determining the correct management of the patient.

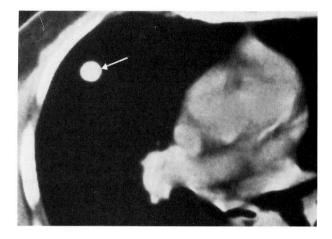

Fig. 2.32 CT of a calcified nodule (arrow). The calcific density of this fungal granuloma is clearly shown by CT. No calcification was evident on plain chest radiographs.

Lack of change over a period of 18 months or more is a strong pointer to either a benign tumour or an inactive granuloma. An enlarging mass is highly likely to be a bronchial carcinoma or a metastasis.

Calcification

The presence of calcification is the other vital observation to make, because substantial calcification virtually rules out the diagnosis of a malignant lesion. Calcification is a common finding in hamartomas, tuberculomas and fungal granulomas. In hamartomas it is often of the 'popcorn' type (Fig. 2.31). CT is of great value in detecting calcification and confirming that the calcification is within the lesion, not just projected over it. Uniform calcification is difficult to recognise on plain chest radiography. With CT, however, uniform calcification can be diagnosed and in such cases carcinoma of the lung can be excluded from the differential diagnosis (Fig. 2.32).

Involvement of the adjacent chest wall

Destruction of the adjacent ribs is virtually diagnostic of invasion by carcinoma. Tumours of the lung apex

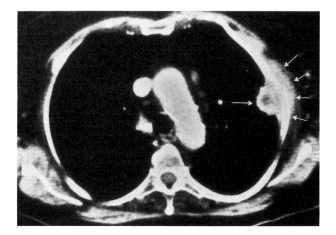

Fig. 2.33 CT showing invasion of chest wall by bronchial carcinoma (single arrow). The soft tissue mass within the chest wall (multiple arrows) is best appreciated by comparison with the normal opposite side.

are particularly liable to invade the chest wall and adjacent bones (Pancoast's tumour). CT or bone scan may be indicated to demonstrate this invasion (Fig. 2.33).

The shape of the shadow

Primary carcinomas nearly always show a lobulated, notched or infiltrating outline (Fig. 2.34). Even if only one small portion of the lesion has an ill-defined edge the diagnosis of primary carcinoma should be seriously considered. If the shadow is perfectly spherical and the edge very well defined it is likely to be a hamartoma a tuberculoma or a metastasis (Fig. 2.35).

The shape may be obvious from plain films but CT (or conventional tomography) can be used to show the edge of a pulmonary nodule to advantage.

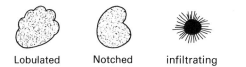

| Lobulated | Notched | infiltrating |

Fig. 2.34 Outline of primary carcinoma of the lung. (See also Fig. 2.105, p. 91)

Cavitation

If the centre of the mass undergoes necrosis and is coughed up, air is seen within the mass. Such air is often accompanied by fluid, in which case an air−fluid level will be visible on erect films. The air, which may be difficult to appreciate, is seen as a translucency within the mass. This feature is particularly well seen at CT.

Cavitation almost always indicates a significant lesion. It is very common in lung abscess (Fig. 2.36), relatively common in primary carcinomas (Fig. 2.37) and occasionally seen with metastases. It does not occur in benign tumours or inactive tuberculomas.

The distinction between cavitating neoplasms and lung abscesses can be very difficult and sometimes impossible, particularly if the walls are smooth. If, however, either the inner or outer walls are irregular the diagnosis of carcinoma is highly likely.

Size

A solitary lesion over 4 cm in diameter which does not contain calcium is nearly always either a primary carcinoma or a lung abscess. Lung abscesses of this size, however, virtually always show cavitation.

Other lesions

The rest of the film should be checked carefully after a lung mass has been found. Finding a second lesion may alter the diagnostic possibilities; finding a metastasis or a small pleural effusion may completely alter the management of the patient.

Multiple lesions

Multiple well-defined spherical shadows in the lungs are virtually diagnostic of metastases (see Fig. 2.112, p. 94). Occasionally, such a pattern is seen with abscesses, or with granulomas due to collagen vascular disorders.

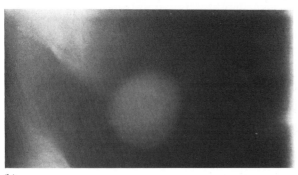

(a)

(b)

The role of CT in solitary pulmonary nodules

The indications for CT in a patient with a solitary pulmonary nodule are to:
• Diagnose the nature of the nodule. The role here is limited since the signs on plain films and knowledge of the rate of growth provide adequate information in most cases. CT is better able to detect calcification in a nodule than conventional films. As mentioned above, extensive calcification of a nodule effectively excludes primary carcinoma of the lung (Fig. 2.32).
• Stage the extent of disease in those cases where the nodule is likely to be a primary carcinoma.
• Localise accurately the nodule prior to bronchoscopic or percutaneous needle biopsy in cases where localisation is difficult from conventional films.
• Establish whether or not the nodule is solitary or multiple when the lesion in question is likely to be a metastasis and when surgical resection of the mass is being considered.

Line shadows

The term 'line shadow' refers to a line, usually no thicker than an ordinary pencil line, traversing the lung. All line shadows except fissures and the walls of the large central bronchi are abnormal. Septal lines are by far the most important.

Septal lines

The pulmonary septa are connective tissue planes containing lymph vessels. They are normally invisible. It is only when they become thickened that they can be

Fig. 2.35 Solitary pulmonary nodule with smooth outline and without calcification or cavitation. (a) Plain film. (b) Tomogram. In this instance the lesion proved to be a hamartoma. The differential diagnosis includes tuberculoma, fungal granuloma and metastasis. Primary carcinoma is unlikely in a spherical, completely smooth, small nodule.

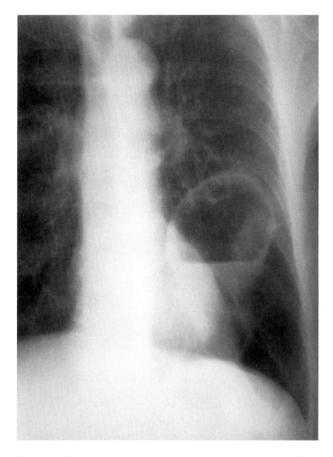

Fig. 2.36 Cavitation in a lung abscess showing a relatively thin, smooth wall and an air–fluid level.

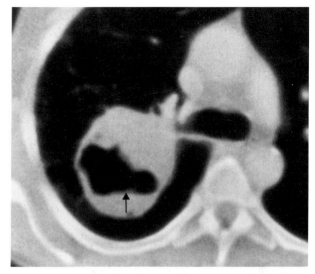

Fig. 2.37 CT of a cavitating primary carcinoma of the lung. The variable thickness of the cavity wall is a striking feature. The air–fluid level is also well seen (arrow).

Pleuropulmonary scars

Scars from previous infection or infarction are a common cause of line shadows. They usually reach the pleura and are often associated with visible pleural thickening. Such scars are of no significance to the patient.

Emphysematous bullae

Bullae (blebs) are often bounded and traversed by thin line shadows. Bullae have few if any normal vessels within them and this makes the interpretation easy (Fig. 2.39).

The pleural edge in a pneumothorax

The pleural edge in a pneumothorax is seen as a line approximately parallel with the chest wall. No lung vessels will be seen beyond the pleural line. Once the line is spotted the diagnosis is rarely in doubt (see Fig. 2.55, p. 54).

seen on the chest film. There are two types of septal lines:

1 Kerley A lines, which radiate towards the hila in the mid and upper zones. These lines are much thinner than the adjacent blood vessels and do not reach the lung edge (Fig. 2.38a).

2 Kerley B lines, which are horizontal, never more than 2 cm in length and are seen best at the periphery of the lung. Unlike the blood vessels they often reach the edge of the lung (Fig. 2.38b).

There are two important causes of septal lines
• pulmonary oedema
• lymphangitis carcinomatosa.

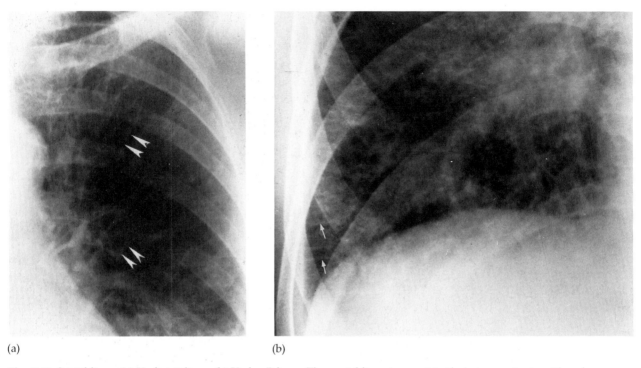

(a)   (b)

Fig. 2.38 Septal lines. (a) Kerley A lines. (b) Kerley B lines. The septal lines (arrows) in these two patients with pulmonary oedema are thinner than the adjacent blood vessels. The B lines are seen in the outer centimetre of lung where blood vessels are invisible or very difficult to identify.

Widespread small shadows

Nodular and reticular shadows

Chest films with widespread small (2–5 mm) pulmonary shadows often present a diagnostic problem. With few exceptions it is only possible to give a differential diagnosis when faced with such a film. A final diagnosis can rarely be made without an intimate knowledge of the patient's symptoms and signs.

Many descriptive terms have been applied to these shadows, the commonest being 'mottling', 'honeycomb', 'fine nodular','reticular' and 'reticulonodular' shadows. In this book we will use two basic terms: 'nodular', to signify discrete small round shadows (Fig. 2.40) and 'reticular' to describe a net-like pattern of small lines. Often there are both nodular and reticular elements and this is called 'reticulonodular' (Fig. 2.41).

All these patterns are due to very small lesions in the lung, no more than 1 or 2 mm in size. Individual lesions of this size are invisible on a chest film. That these very small lesions are seen at all is explained by the phenomenon of superimposition; when myriads of tiny lesions are present in the lungs it is inevitable that many will lie in line with one another. It follows that when very small non-calcified shadows are visible the lung must be diffusely involved by disease. It is worth noting that the size of the multiple small shadows seen on the x-ray film gives no clue to the size of the responsible lesions, except to predict that they are small; nor can the shape of the lung shadows be reliably used to predict the shape of the lesions seen at pathology.

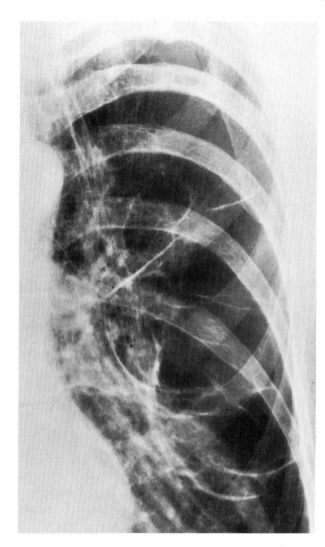

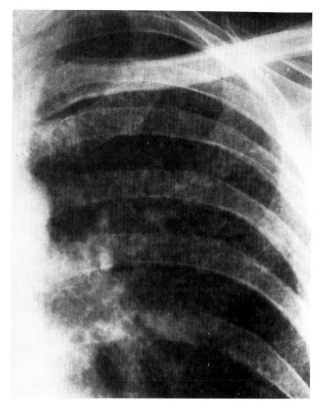

Fig. 2.40 Nodular shadowing in the lung in a patient with miliary tuberculosis.

Fig. 2.39 Line shadows due to walls of bullae (blebs). The bullae are air spaces devoid of blood vessels.

How to decide whether or not multiple small pulmonary shadows are present

Often, the greatest problem is to decide whether widespread abnormal shadowing is present at all, since normal blood vessels can also appear as nodules and interconnecting lines. To be confident involves looking carefully at many hundreds of normal films to establish a normal pattern in one's mind (Fig. 2.42). Look particularly at the areas between the ribs where the lungs are free of overlying shadows. The normal vessel pattern is a branching system which connects up in an orderly way. The vessels are larger centrally and they become smaller as they travel to the periphery. There are no visible vessels in the outer 1–2 cm of the lung. Vessels seen end-on appear as small nodules, but these nodules are no bigger than vessels seen in the immediate vicinity and their number corresponds to the expected number of vessels in that area.

An important sign in questionable cases is that the abnormal shadows obscure the adjacent vessels and, therefore, the borders of the mediastinum and diaphragm may be less sharp than normal.

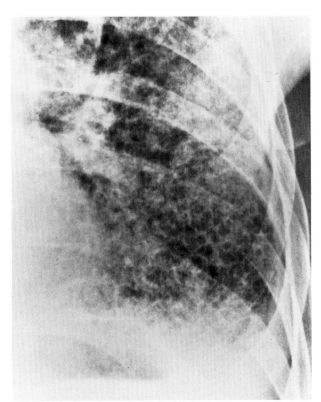

(a)

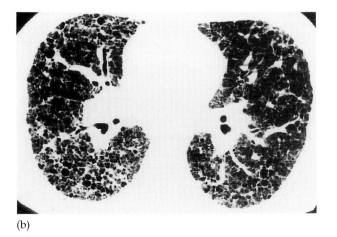

(b)

Fig. 2.41 (a) Reticulonodular shadowing in the lung in a patient with fibrosing alveolitis. (b) Thin-section, high resolution CT scan of a different patient with cryptogenic (idiopathic) fibrosing alveolitis showing the honeycomb pattern to advantage.

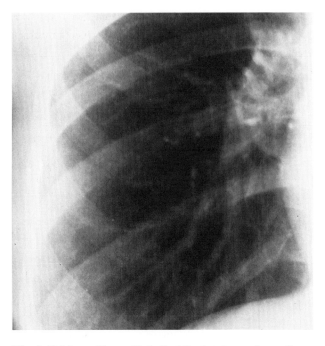

Fig. 2.42 Normal lung. Note that the lung vessels are the only identifiable shadows in those areas which are free of overlying ribs but no vessels are visible in the outer 2 cm of the lung. Vessels seen end-on appear as small nodules.

Having decided that abnormal shadowing is present and determined its pattern, the next step is to decide whether or not the shadows are maximal in one or more zone of the lungs, or whether they are uniformly distributed. Other abnormalities on the film should then be sought.

Inevitably, there will be cases in whom there is doubt, both clinically and radiographically, whether or not there is diffuse lung disease. In these circumstances, thin-section HRCT can be of considerable help, because the evidence of lung disease may be quite convincing with CT, even though the chest radiograph is normal or borderline.

Thin-section high resolution CT can also be of help in defining the character and distribution of the abnormal shadowing (Fig. 2.41b). A few conditions have quite specific appearances. Lymphangitis carcinomatosa (see p. 93) and fibrosing alveolitis, for example, both cause a characteristic appearance, although the precise cause of diffuse pulmonary fibrosis cannot be ascertained by CT scanning.

Having made all these observations, it is possible to provide a differential diagnostic list. The more important and common appearances are given in Table 2.1.

Table 2.1 Commoner causes of nodular and reticular shadowing

Diagnosis	Radiographic pattern	Distribution of shadows	Other features which may be seen	Thin-section high resolution CT (HRCT)
Miliary tuberculosis	Small nodules of uniform size	Uniform	± Mediastinal/hilar lymph nodes One or more patches of consolidation	Not necessary
Sarcoidosis	(a) Fine nodular	Uniform	Hilar and paratracheal lymph nodes	Shows disease well but adds little of diagnostic value
	(b) Reticulonodular	Often predominant in mid and upper zones	Hilar and paratracheal lymph nodes	
Coal miners' pneumoconiosis	Nodular	Predominant in upper zones	Progressive massive fibrosis in the complicated form of the disease Emphysema	Adds little of diagnostic value
Asbestosis	Fine reticulo-nodular	Predominant in lower zones	Pleural thickening and/or calcification	Useful for documenting the severity of fibrosis, and for showing pleural plaques where the diagnosis is in doubt
Fibrosing alveolitis	Reticulonodular	Often predominant in lower zones, but may show a variety of patterns	Diaphragm often high and indistinct	Characteristically shows basal and peripherally predominant reticulo-nodular shadowing
Lymphangitis carcinomatosa	Reticulonodular	No predominant pattern	Septal lines Bronchial wall thickening Hilar adenopathy Other signs of carcinoma	The combination of septal lines and small nodules produces a characteristic pattern
Pulmonary oedema	Ill-defined nodules	Often central predominance with clear zone at periphery of lobes	Cardiac enlargement Left atrial enlargement Septal lines	Not indicated

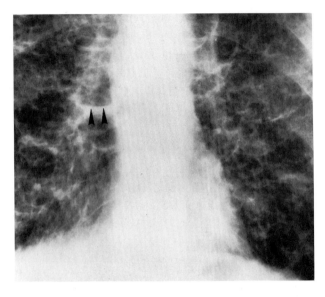

Fig. 2.43 Ring shadows in bronchiectasis. Each ring shadow represents a dilated bronchus. A fluid level in one of the dilated bronchi is arrowed.

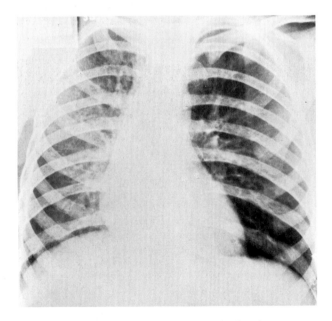

Fig. 2.44 Inhaled foreign body causing check valve obstruction of the left main bronchus. Note the increased transradiancy of the left lung, and the slight displacement of the heart to the right. (The film was exposed in expiration.)

Multiple ring shadows of 1 cm or larger

Such shadows are diagnostic of bronchiectasis (Fig. 2.43). The shadows represent dilated thick-walled bronchi. If they contain air and fluid they will show fluid levels.

Widespread small pulmonary calcifications

Such calcifications may occur following pulmonary infection with tuberculosis, histoplasmosis or chickenpox.

Increased transradiancy of the lungs

Generalised increase in transradiancy

Generalised increased transradiancy of the lungs is one of the signs of emphysema. The other signs outlined on p. 81 must be present for the diagnosis to be made.

Localised increase in transradiancy

When only one hemithorax appears more transradiant than normal the following should be considered:
• *Compensatory emphysema*. This occurs when a lobe or lung is collapsed or has been excised and the remaining lung expands to fill the space.
• *Pneumothorax*. The diagnosis of a pneumothorax depends on visualising the lung edge with air peripheral to it, and checking that the space one believes to be a pneumothorax does not contain any vessels (see Fig. 2.55, p. 54).
• *Reduction in the chest wall soft tissues*, e.g. mastectomy.
• *Air-trapping due to central obstruction* (Fig. 2.44). Most obstructing lesions in a major bronchus lead to lobar collapse. Occasionally, particularly with an inhaled foreign body, a check valve mechanism occurs leading to air-trapping. Inhaled foreign bodies are commonest in children; they usually lodge in a major bronchus. Often, the chest radiograph is normal but

sometimes the affected lung becomes abnormally transradiant and the heart is displaced to the opposite side on expiration. Air-trapping is best appreciated at fluoroscopy when the fixed position of the hemidiaphragm is noted and the mediastinum can be seen to swing away from the obstructed side on expiration.

• *Rare causes* of increased transradiancy of one lung include massive pulmonary embolus and McLeod's syndrome (Swyer–James syndrome), a condition that follows severe pneumonia in childhood.

The pleura

Pleural effusion

The radiological appearances of fluid in the pleural cavity are the same regardless of whether the fluid is a transudate, an exudate, pus or blood. On a plain chest radiograph, a large effusion may hide an abnormality in the underlying lung.

Free pleural fluid—plain radiographic findings (Fig. 2.45)

Free fluid collects in the most dependent portion of the pleural cavity and always fills in the costophrenic angles. Free pleural effusions assume two basic shapes, usually seen in combination with one another:
1 Usually the fluid surrounds the lung, higher laterally than medially. It also runs into the fissures, particularly into the lower end of the oblique fissures. Very large effusions run over the top of the lung.

The smooth edge between the lung and the fluid can be recognised on an adequately penetrated film, providing that the underlying lung is aerated. This smooth edge should always be looked for: it is diagnostic of pleural pathology.

Fig. 2.45 Large right pleural effusion. The shadow of the pleural fluid is entirely homogeneous and lies outside the lung edge. The fluid appears higher laterally than medially, a point that can be useful in differentiating pleural fluid from pulmonary shadows. In this instance the trachea and heart are in normal position but no pulmonary disease was present.

2 Sometimes, even with a large effusion, little or no fluid is seen running up the chest wall. The fluid is then known as a 'subpulmonary effusion' (Fig. 2.46). The upper border of the fluid is much the same shape as the normal diaphragm, and since the true diaphragm shadow is obscured by the fluid it may be very difficult, or even impossible, to tell from the standard erect film if any fluid is present at all.

It is not always possible to distinguish on chest radiographs whether basal shadowing is due to pleural effusion or to pulmonary collapse/consolidation. If there is doubt, a frontal film taken with the patient lying on one side (a lateral decubitus view) can be of help. The fluid, if free to move, will then lie along the dependent lateral chest wall. This technique is particularly valuable when the effusion is largely or wholly subpulmonary.

Since a pleural effusion occupies space in the thorax, compression collapse of the underlying lung is inevitable, the compressed lung being otherwise normal. Alternatively, both the pleural effusion and the

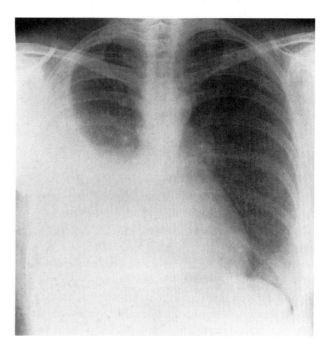

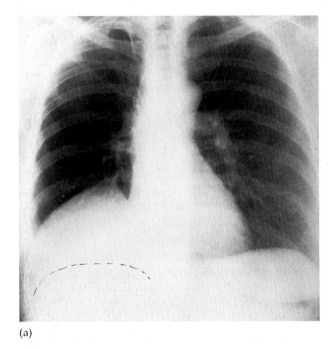

(a)

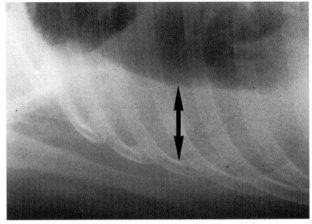

(b)

Fig. 2.46 Large right subpulmonary effusion. Almost all the fluid is between the lung and the diaphragm. The right hemidiaphragm cannot be seen. (a) Its estimated position has been pencilled in (the patient has had right mastectomy). (b) In the lateral decubitus view, the fluid moves to lie between the lateral chest wall and the lung edge (arrows).

pulmonary collapse may be due to the same primary process, e.g. carcinoma of the bronchus.

At *computed tomography*, pleural effusions are seen as homogeneous density between the chest wall and lung (Fig. 2.47). Just as with the plain chest radiograph, it is not possible to distinguish transudate from exudate, nor can one tell whether the shadow is due to fluid, blood or pus. Free pleural fluid will move to the dependent portion of the chest and scans are sometimes taken in the lateral decubitus position to demonstrate this movement.

Surprisingly, it is sometimes difficult to say at CT whether fluid is pleural effusion or ascites. The distinction is made by noting the relationship of the fluid to the diaphragm. Pleural fluid collects outside the diaphragmatic dome and can be seen posterior to the portion of diaphragm that covers the bare area of the liver (Fig. 2.48a).

Distinguishing pleural effusion from pulmonary consolidation or collapse at CT is relatively easy because the pleural fluid is usually lower in density than the collapsed or consolidated lung and the pleural effusion is of homogeneous density and has a smooth interface with the pleura covering the underlying lung. Air bronchograms are particularly well seen at CT and their presence is unequivocal evidence that one is looking at collapsed or consolidated lung (see Figs 2.13 and 2.14).

At ultrasound, pleural fluid can be recognised as a transonic area between the lung and diaphragm (Fig. 2.48b). Since the diaphragm is so well seen there is no confusion with ascites.

Loculated pleural fluid (Fig. 2.49)

Loculated effusions occur when the free flow of fluid within the pleural cavity is prevented by pleural adhesions. Although loculation occurs in all types of effusion, it is a particular feature of empyema. Such loculations may either be at the periphery of the lung or within the fissures between the lobes. Loculated interlobar effusions may closely simulate lung tumours on chest radiographs, particularly in the PA view, but the distinction can be made by noting that on the lateral film the effusion is lens-shaped, lying within the oblique or horizontal fissure. It is not surprising

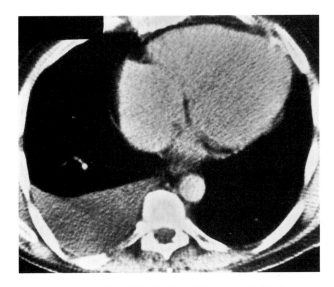

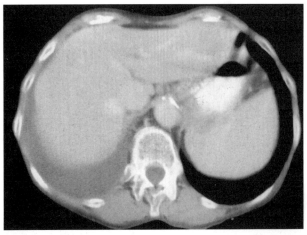

(a)

Fig. 2.47 CT of pleural fluid. The right pleural effusion is of homogeneous density, with a CT number between zero and soft tissue. Its well-defined meniscus shaped border with the lung is typical.

that the lateral view provides the answer since this is the one that best demonstrates the fissures.

Ultrasound can be particularly useful in defining the presence, size and shape of any loculated pleural collection. Pleural aspiration may be performed under ultrasound guidance.

Computed tomography scanning (Figs 2.50 and 2.51) can be utilised to distinguish loculation of pleural fluid from adjacent pulmonary disease, a distinction that is particularly valuable when empyema is suspected. Like ultrasound, CT can be used to direct the placement of drainage tubes.

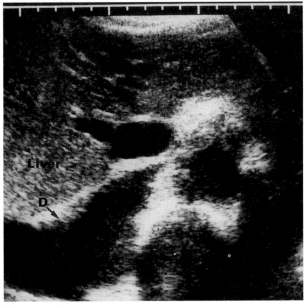

(b)

Causes of pleural effusion

There are many causes for pleural effusion. In some cases the cause is visible on the chest film or CT scan.

● *Infection*. Pleural effusions which are due to pneumonia are on the whole small, and the pneumonia is usually the dominant feature on the chest film. Large

Fig. 2.48 CT and ultrasound of pleural effusion. (a) CT scan. The section is taken through the lowermost portion of the pleural cavity and at this level the distinction from ascites is a potential problem because the diaphragm itself is not visible. Pleural fluid, as here, is not affected by the peritoneal reflections of the bare area (see Fig. 10.1, p. 286).
(b) Ultrasound scan—transverse image. The pleural effusion (PE) is seen as a transonic area behind the diaphragm (D). IVC, inferior vena cava.

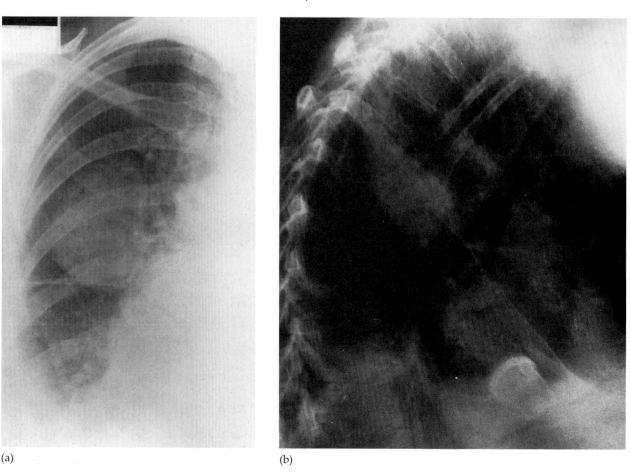

(a)   (b)

Fig. 2.49 Loculated pleural fluid. In this instance the fluid is loculated in the oblique (major) fissure. In the PA view (a) it could be confused with an intrapulmonary mass, but the lateral view (b) shows the characteristic shape of interlobar pleural fluid (arrow).

loculated effusions in association with pneumonia often indicate empyema formation (Fig. 2.50). In some cases of tuberculosis the effusion is the only visible abnormality and the effusion may be large.

Subphrenic abscess nearly always produces a pleural effusion.

• *Malignant neoplasm*. Effusions occur with pleural metastases, but it is unusual to see the pleural deposits themselves on plain chest radiographs. They are occasionally visible at CT as pleural nodules. Such effusions are frequently large. If the effusion is due to bronchogenic carcinoma, other signs of tumour are usually evident.

• *Cardiac failure*. Small bilateral pleural effusions are frequently seen in acute left ventricular failure. Larger pleural effusions may be present in longstanding congestive cardiac failure. The effusions are usually bilateral, often larger on the right than the left. Other evidence of cardiac failure, such as alteration in the size or shape of the heart, pulmonary oedema or the signs of pulmonary venous hypertension, are usually present.

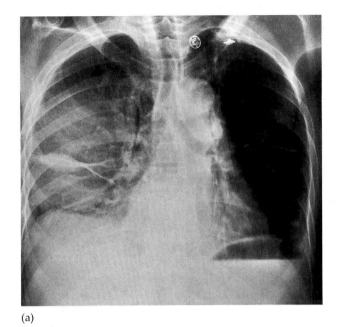

(a)

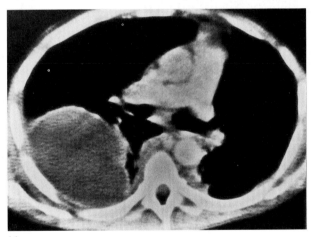

(b)

(c)

Fig. 2.50 Loculated pleural fluid (empyema), showing the value of CT in distinguishing pleural fluid from pulmonary consolidation. The fluid is loculated behind the right lower lobe and in the horizontal (minor) fissure. On the plain chest films (a) and (b) the large posterior collection resembles right lower lobe consolidation. The CT scan (c) clearly shows the characteristic shape and location of loculated pleural fluid.

• *Pulmonary infarction* may cause pleural effusion. Such effusions are usually small and accompanied by a lung shadow which is due to the pulmonary infarct itself.

• *Collagen vascular diseases*. Pleural effusions, either unilateral or bilateral, are relatively common in these conditions. They may be the only abnormal features on a chest film.

• *Nephrotic syndrome, renal failure, ascites and Meig's syndrome* are all associated with pleural effusions, the cause of which cannot be determined from the chest film.

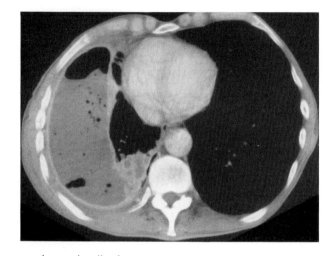

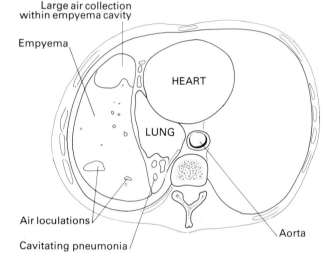

Large air collection
within empyema cavity

Empyema

HEART

LUNG

Air loculations

Cavitating pneumonia

Aorta

Fig. 2.51 Empyema. CT scan showing loculated air–fluid collection in right pleural cavity. Small loculations of air are seen within the pus.

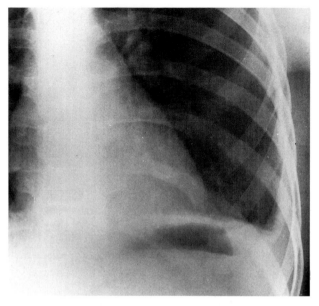

Fig. 2.52 Pleural thickening at the left base. This patient had been treated for a tuberculous pleural effusion, which had resolved leaving pleural thickening, which obliterated the left costophrenic angle.

usually much smaller. It is sometimes impossible to distinguish pleural fluid from pleural thickening on conventional projections, especially if comparison with previous films is not possible. The problem can be resolved by a lateral decubitus view, where free fluid will move to lie along the lateral chest wall, whereas fibrotic thickening is unaltered in appearance.

Localised plaques of pleural thickening along the lateral chest wall commonly indicate asbestos exposure. Such plaques may show irregular calcification.

Pleural thickening (pleural fibrosis) (Fig. 2.52)

Fibrotic pleural thickening, especially in the costophrenic angles, may follow resolution of a pleural effusion, particularly following pleural infection or haemorrhage. The appearances of pleural thickening are similar to pleural fluid but pleural scarring is always smaller than the original pleural effusion,

Pleural tumours (Fig. 2.53)

Pleural tumours produce lobulated masses based on the pleura. Malignant pleural tumours, both primary (malignant mesothelioma) and secondary, frequently cause pleural effusions which may obscure the tumour itself. The commonest pleural tumours are metastatic carcinoma, breast carcinoma being the most frequent

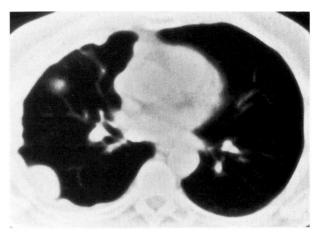

(b)

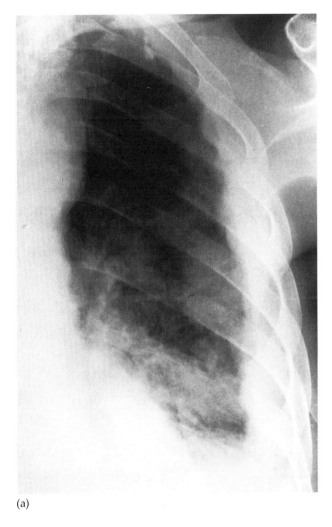

(a)

Fig. 2.53 (a) Lobulated pleural thickening due to malignant neoplasm. The tumour in this instance was a malignant mesothelioma of the pleura. (b) CT scan of mesothelioma of the pleura in the right hemithorax.

primary tumour to spread to the pleura. Primary pleural tumours are relatively uncommon. Since many malignant mesotheliomas are secondary to asbestos exposure the other features of asbestosis (pulmonary fibrosis, pleural plaques and pleural calcification) may be seen.

Pleural calcification (Fig. 2.54)

Irregular plaques of calcium may be seen with or without accompanying pleural thickening. When unilateral they are likely to be due to either an old empyema, usually tuberculous, or an old haemothorax. Bilateral pleural calcification is often related to asbestos exposure (see Fig. 2.88, p. 77). Sometimes no cause for pleural calcification can be found.

Pneumothorax (Fig. 2.55)

The diagnosis of pneumothorax depends on recognising:
• the line of pleura forming the lung edge separated from the chest wall, mediastinum or diaphragm by air
• the absence of vessel shadows outside this line.

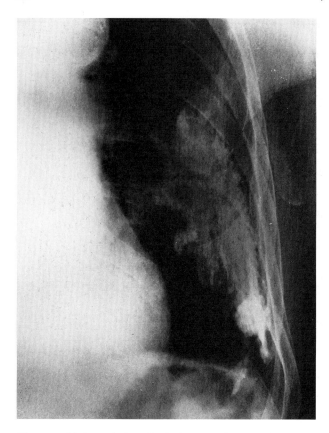

Fig. 2.54 Unilateral pleural calcifications due to old tuberculous empyema.

Lack of vessel shadows alone is insufficient evidence on which to make the diagnosis, since there may be few, or no, visible vessels in emphysematous bullae. One might have expected that the collapsed lung beneath the pneumothorax would be more opaque than normal, but in fact, unless the pneumothorax is very large, there may be no appreciable increase in the density of the lung.

The detection of a small pneumothorax can be very difficult. The cortex of the normal ribs takes a similar course to the line of the pleural edge, so the abnormality may not strike the casual observer. Sometimes a pneumothorax is more obvious on a film taken in expiration.

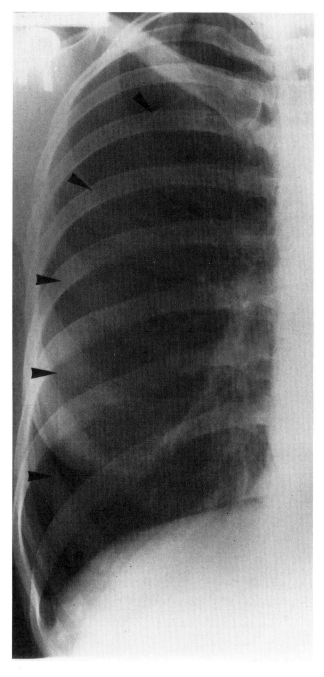

Fig. 2.55 Pneumothorax. The pleural edge is arrowed. The diagnosis of pneumothorax requires the identification of this edge and a clear space beyond it.

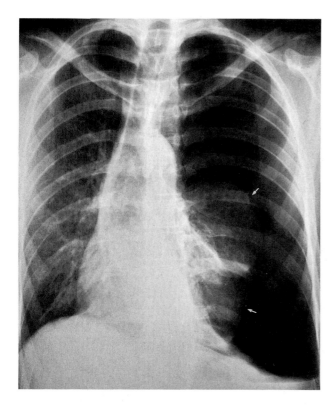

Fig. 2.56 Tension pneumothorax. The left hemidiaphragm is depressed and the mediastinum is shifted to the right. The left lung (arrows) is substantially collapsed.

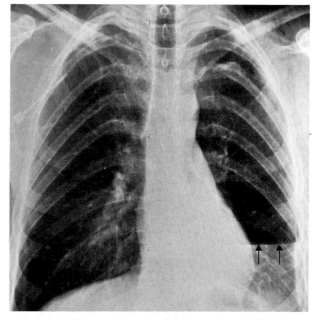

Fig. 2.57 Hydropneumothorax. The arrows point to the air–fluid level in the pleural space. In this case the edge of the lung is difficult to see on the PA view; most of the fluid and air were loculated posteriorly.

Once the presence of a pneumothorax has been noted, the next step is to decide whether or not it is under tension. This depends on detecting mediastinal shift and flattening or inversion of the hemidiaphragm (Fig. 2.56).

It is worth noting that tension pneumothoraces are invariably large because the underlying lung collapses due to increased pressure in the pleural space.

Causes of pneumothorax

Pneumothorax is associated with many underlying disorders of the lung including:
- emphysema
- trauma
- certain forms of pulmonary fibrosis
- tuberculosis
- metastases, rarely.

The majority, however, occur in young people with no recognisable lung disease. These patients have small blebs or bullae at the periphery of their lungs which burst.

Hydropneumothorax, haemopneumothorax and pyopneumothorax

In most cases of pneumothorax, whatever the cause, some fluid is present in the pleural cavity. In spontaneous pneumothorax the amount is usually small.

Fluid in the pleural cavity, whether it be a pleural effusion, blood or pus, assumes a different shape in the presence of a pneumothorax. The diagnostic feature is the air–fluid level (Fig. 2.57).

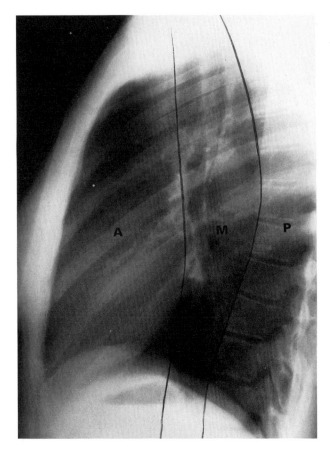

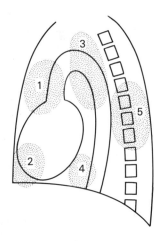

ANTERIOR
1. Thyroid tumour
   Thymic tumour or cyst
   Teratoma/Dermoid cyst
   Lymphadenopathy
   Aortic aneurysm

2. Pericardial cyst
   Fat pad
   Morgagni hernia

MIDDLE
3. Thyroid tumour
   Lymphadenopathy
   Bronchogenic cyst
   Aortic aneurysm

4. Hiatus hernia

POSTERIOR
5. Neurogenic tumours
   Soft tissue mass of vertebral
     infection or neoplasm
   Lymphadenopathy
   Aortic aneurysm

Fig. 2.58 The anterior (A), middle (M) and posterior (P) compartments of the mediastinum. The divisions are arbitrary and do not correspond to those used by anatomists. The anterior mediastinum refers to the structures anterior to the trachea and the major bronchi. The posterior mediastinum refers to structures posterior to a line joining the anterior boundary of the vertebral bodies.

Fig. 2.59 The causes of mediastinal masses divided according to location. Note that both lymphadenopathy and aortic aneurysms occur in all three major compartments.

The mediastinum

The mediastinum is one continuous space between the sternum at the front, the spine and ribs at the back and the lungs on the two sides. The mediastinum is divided into anterior, middle and posterior divisions for descriptive purposes (Fig. 2.58). It should be realised, however, that masses often cross from one compartment to the other. Local or generalised widen-

ing can be due to many different pathological processes. These are usually classified according to their position in the mediastinum (Fig. 2.59); so if a mediastinal mass is identified on the frontal chest radiograph, the next step must be to attempt to localise it in the lateral view. This may be quite easy, but anterior mediastinal masses are sometimes difficult to visualise on the lateral view (Fig. 2.60). Therefore, if no obvious abnormality is seen on the lateral film, the anterior mediastinum should be carefully reviewed. In most people a transradiant area, known as the retrosternal space, can be identified behind the sternum in front of

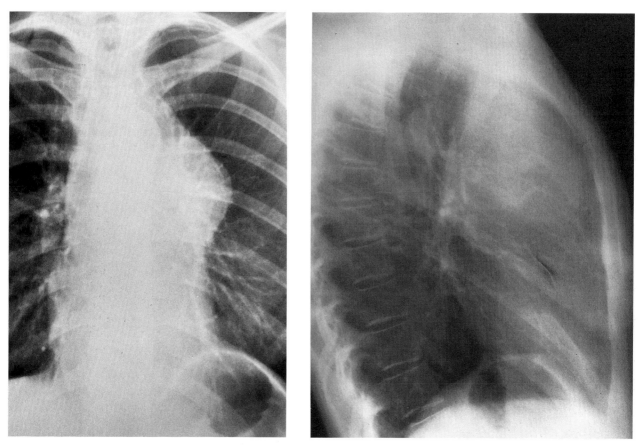

Fig. 2.60 Anterior mediastinal mass. There is a large mass situated anteriorly in the mediastinum projecting to the left side which was due to a mass of lymph nodes involved by malignant lymphoma. Diagnosing the anterior location of the mass depends on noting the density of the retrosternal areas. This area should normally have the same density as the retrocardiac area.

the ascending aorta. If this space is uniformly opaque it is probable that there is anterior mediastinal pathology. It should be realised, however, that this space is sometimes opaque in obese but otherwise normal subjects.

Computed tomography of the normal mediastinum

The greatest impact of CT in chest radiology has been in imaging the mediastinum, where its two major advantages are most apparent: the cross-sectional display of anatomy and the ability to distinguish clearly fat, soft tissue and opacified blood vessels.

The appearances at four levels of the thorax are illustrated in Figure 2.61. The features to note while viewing these images are:

1 The bulk of the mediastinum is due to blood vessels. Blood vessels are easy to recognise as tubular structures retaining a near constant diameter on several adjacent sections. They can be opacified by intravenous contrast medium (in some centres such opacification is used almost routinely).

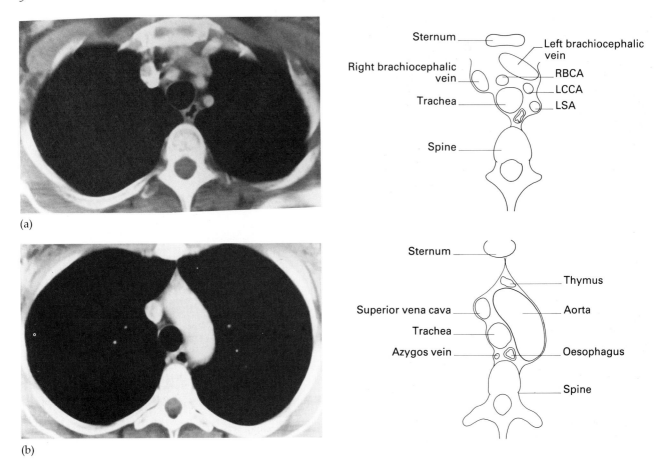

(a)

(b)

Fig. 2.61 CT of normal mediastinum. The levels at which the four selected levels were taken is shown in (e). Intravenous contrast has been given; it is particularly concentrated in the right brachiocephalic vein and superior vena cava. Air is present in the oesophagus; this can be a normal finding. LCCA, left common carotid artery; LMB, left main bronchus; LSA, left subclavian artery; RBCA, right brachiocephalic (innominate) artery; RMB, right main bronchus.

2 The only other normal structures of appreciable size are the thymus, oesophagus, trachea, and bronchi. The thymus is the most difficult to assess because it is so variable in size.

3 Normal lymph nodes are small, usually less than 6 mm in diameter (maximum 10 mm) and most are not visible.

4 The mediastinal structures are surrounded by fat. The sites listed below normally contain nothing but fat or small lymph nodes. They are, therefore, areas in which small masses, particularly enlarged lymph nodes, can be readily recognised:

• between the right tracheal wall and the adjacent lung (with the one exception of the azygos vein which lies in the right tracheobronchial angle)

• between the right wall of the oesophagus and the adjacent lung all the way down the chest, an anatomical region known as the azygo-oesophageal recess

• anterior and to the left of the aorta and main pulmonary artery (other than the thymus and the left brachiocephalic vein).

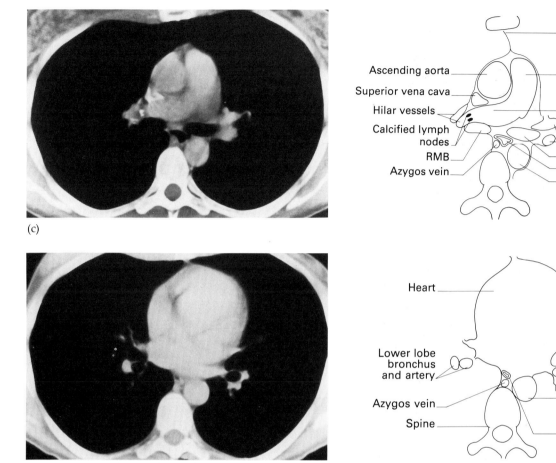

(c)

(d)

Fig. 2.61 (Continued)

Mediastinal masses

Computed tomography scanning provides a much clearer idea of the position, shape and size of any mass than is possible from the plain chest radiograph; occasionally the CT density even enables a specific diagnosis to be made.

Plain chest films in mediastinal masses

• Intrathoracic thyroid masses (goitres) are the most frequent cause of a mediastinal mass (Fig. 2.62). The

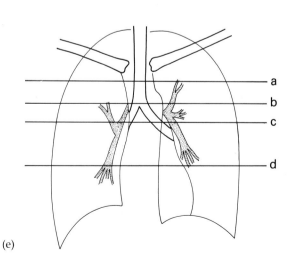

(e)

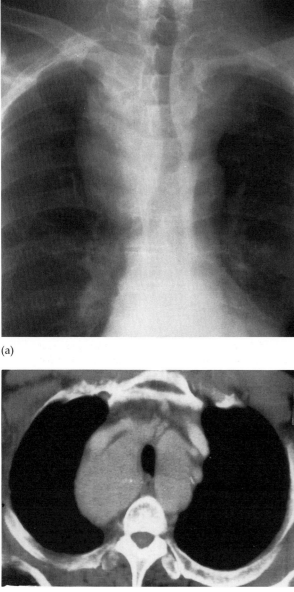

(a)

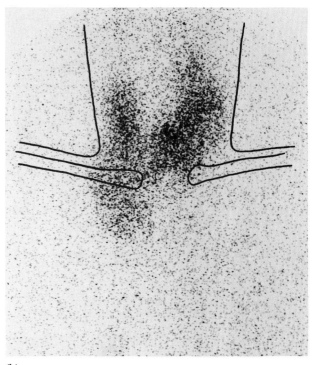

(b)

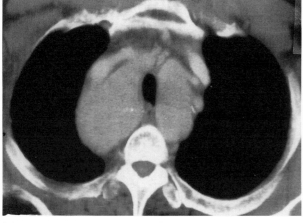

(c)

Fig. 2.62 Retrosternal goitre. (a) The plain chest film shows a large superior mediastinal mass narrowing the trachea. (b) A radionuclide scan in the same patient shows uptake of the ^{123}I below the level of the clavicles on the right, confirming that the mass is due to thyroid tissue. (c) CT scan, in another patient, showing a bilateral superior mediastinal mass that was shown on adjacent sections to be contiguous with the thyroid gland in the neck and to have the same density as thyroid tissue. Note the compression of the trachea.

characteristic feature is that the mass extends from the superior mediastinum into the neck and almost invariably compresses or displaces the trachea.

• Lymphadenopathy is the next most frequent cause of a mediastinal swelling. Lymphadenopathy may occur in any of the three compartments and it is often possible to diagnose enlarged lymph nodes from their lobulated outlines on plain chest radiographs and from the multiplicity of masses on CT scanning (Fig. 2.63).

• Neurogenic tumours are by far the commonest

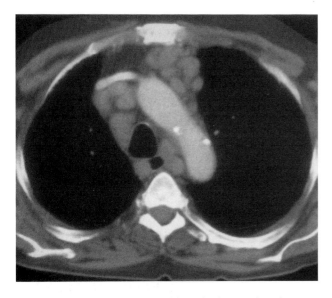

Fig. 2.63 Extensive mediastinal lymphadenopathy (due to lymphoma) shown by CT scanning.

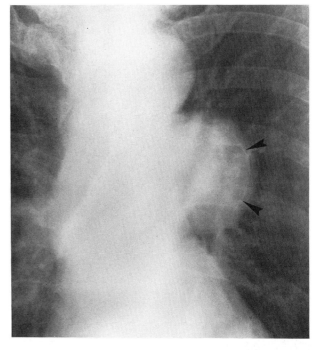

Fig. 2.64 Calcification in an aneurysm arising from the descending aorta. The arrows point to the distinctive curvilinear calcification within the mass, which is in intimate contact with the aorta.

posterior mediastinal lesions. They frequently cause pressure deformity of the adjacent ribs and thoracic spine.

● Certain tumours, such as dermoid cysts and thymomas, are, for practical purposes, confined to the anterior mediastinum.

● Calcification occurs in many conditions but almost never in malignant lymphadenopathy. Occasionally, the calcification is characteristic in appearance, e.g. in aneurysms of the aorta (Fig. 2.64).

● A mediastinal mass due to a hiatus hernia is usually easy to diagnose on plain films because it often contains air and may have a fluid level, best seen on the lateral view (Fig. 2.65). A film taken after a mouthful of barium has been swallowed will easily confirm or exclude the diagnosis of hiatus hernia.

● Masses in the right cardiophrenic angle anteriorly are virtually never of clinical significance. They are nearly all either large fat pads, benign pericardial cysts or hernias through the foramen of Morgagni (Fig. 2.66).

Computed tomography of mediastinal masses

Computed tomography scanning is the best method of assessing mediastinal abnormalities when problems remain unanswered from the plain chest radiographs. It provides additional information because:

1 Abnormalities can be accurately localised. Knowledge of the precise shape, position, and size of the mass frequently narrows the differential diagnosis. For instance, contiguity of the mass with the thyroid in the neck suggests a goitre (Fig. 2.62), and multiple oval-shaped masses suggest lymphadenopathy (Fig. 2.63).

2 Occasionally, the density of the abnormality reveals its nature:

  ● Fat can be recognised as such. This is useful in distinguishing large cardiophrenic angle fat pads

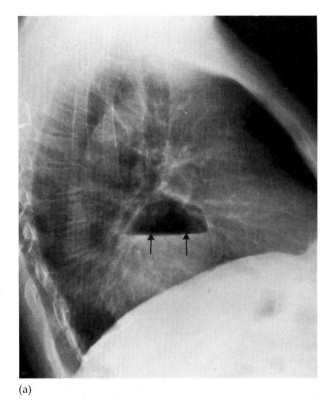

(a)

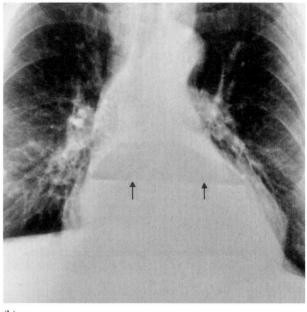

(b)

Fig. 2.65 Hiatus hernia. (a) Lateral and (b) PA chest films show the characteristic retrocardiac density containing an air–fluid level (arrows).

or unusual fat collections from tumours, e.g. in Cushing's disease. Cystic teratomas (dermoid cysts) may contain recognisable fat (Fig. 2.67).

• Thyroid tissue has a characteristic density. Because of its high iodine content, it is of higher attenuation than muscle prior to contrast medium administration. After contrast, it enhances brightly (Fig. 2.62). (A radio-iodine scan is an alternative to CT for confirming that an intrathoracic mass is a goitre—see Fig. 2.62).

• Intravenous contrast enhancement permits ready differentiation of aneurysms (Fig. 2.68) and anomalous blood vessels from other masses.

• Calcification is more readily seen at CT than on plain radiographs (Fig. 2.68). The presence of calcification in a mass excludes malignant neoplastic adenopathy.

• Cysts containing clear fluid e.g. pericardial cysts and some bronchogenic cysts can be recognized as

such by a CT number close to water (0 Hounsfield units).

Magnetic resonance imaging of mediastinal masses

Magnetic resonance imaging gives similar information to CT regarding mediastinal masses. It is, therefore, rarely indicated. MRI does have certain specific advantages. For example, aneurysms and vascular anomalies are readily demonstrable without the need for contrast medium.

Pneumomediastinum

Air in the mediastinum indicates a tear in the oesophagus or an air leak from the bronchi. These may be spontaneous or follow trauma including trauma from endoscopy or swallowed foreign bodies.

Spontaneous leakage from the bronchial tree is most

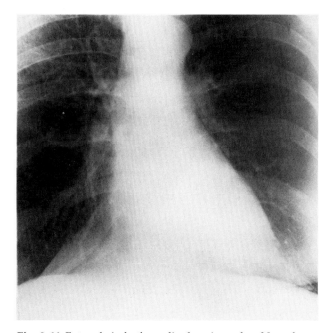

Fig. 2.66 Fat pads in both cardiophrenic angles. Note the loss of clarity of the adjacent cardiac outline—an example of the silhouette sign. The anterior location was confirmed on the lateral view.

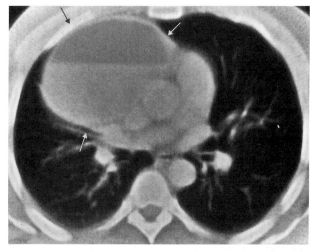

Fig. 2.67 Dermoid cyst (arrows) shown by CT to contain fat. In this cyst the fat can be seen floating in the upper third of the cyst. Note that the density of part of the cyst is the same as subcutaneous fat.

commonly seen in patients with asthma, where the air tracks through the interstitial tissues of the lung into the mediastinum following rupture of a small airway.

The air is seen as fine streaks of transradiancy within the mediastinum, often extending upward into the neck (Fig. 2.69).

Hilar enlargement

The normal hilar shadows are composed of the pulmonary arteries and veins. The hilar lymph nodes cannot be identified as separate shadows. The walls of the central bronchi are too thin to contribute to any extent to the bulk of the hilar shadow. The main lower lobe arteries are the thickness of an adult's little finger (9–16 mm). Any lobulation of the hilum, or any increase in density compared with the opposite side are indications of a mass (Fig. 2.70).

Hilar enlargement presents two main diagnostic

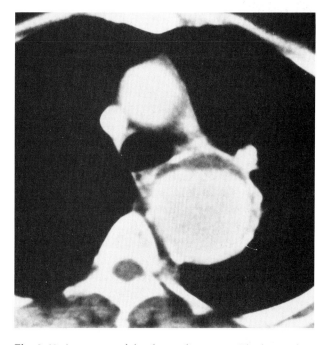

Fig. 2.68 Aneurysm of the descending aorta. The lumen has been opacified by intravenous contrast enhancement. Calcification is seen in the wall of the aneurysm.

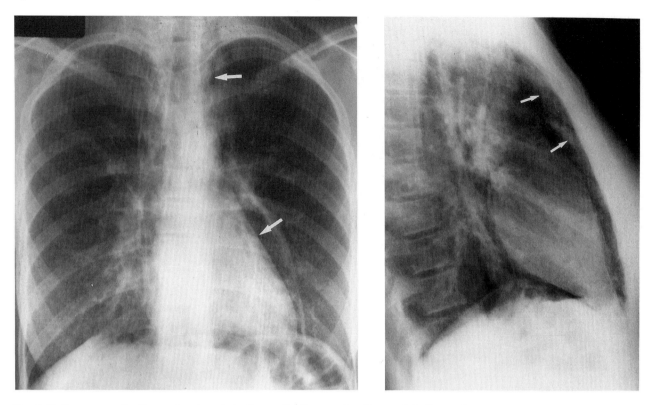

Fig. 2.69 Pneumomediastinum showing air in the mediastinum extending up into the neck.

problems. Firstly, is the enlarged hilum due entirely to large blood vessels or to a mass? Secondly, if a hilar mass is present, what is its nature?

It is usually possible to decide whether hilar enlargement is due to enlargement of the pulmonary arteries from the plain film findings by appreciating the branching nature of the shadows and the fact that vascular enlargement is usually bilateral and accompanied by enlargement of the main pulmonary artery and heart (Fig. 2.71). (The causes of enlargement of the pulmonary artery are discussed on p. 114.) On occasion, it is necessary to employ more sophisticated investigations to distinguish between enlarged blood vessels and a mass. The precise technique employed will depend on the availability of specialised equipment. Computed tomography, particularly with the use of intravenous contrast medium, will usually answer the question. Computed tomography will also demonstrate the mediastinal structures; finding abnormalities within the mediastinum, such as adenopathy, may clarify the nature of the hilar abnormality and may also give important information regarding the extent of disease.

Magnetic resonance imaging is the single best technique for elucidating hilar enlargement. It is rarely required because plain films and computed tomography usually give the necessary information. Its advantage lies in the fact that there is very little signal from the hilar structures in normal individuals using the usual spin-echo sequences; there is no signal from fast-flowing blood in the major hilar vessels and none from the air within the bronchi. Thus, any hilar mass stands out clearly against the low signal background (Fig. 2.72).

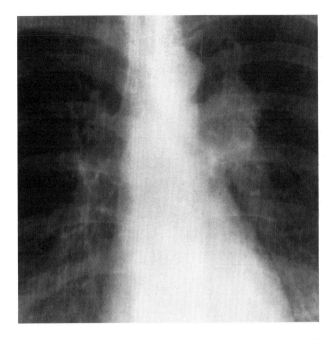

Fig. 2.70 Lobulated mass at left hilum due to enlarged lymph nodes. The right hilum is normal. The lymphadenopathy in this case was due to metastases from a bronchial carcinoma in the left lower lobe.

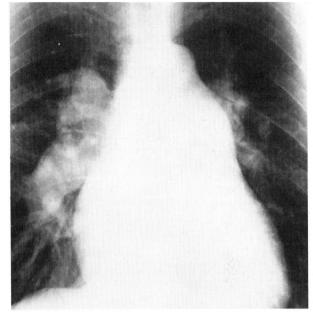

Fig. 2.71 Enlargement of the hilar arteries in a patient with severe pulmonary hypertension. Note that the heart and the main pulmonary artery are also enlarged and that the hilar shadows branch in the manner expected of arteries.

Hilar masses

Hilar masses are nearly always due to either lymph node enlargement or carcinoma of the bronchus.

Lymph node enlargement

Usually more than one lymph node is enlarged, so the hilum appears lobulated in outline. The adjacent bronchi are normal or very slightly narrowed.

Unilateral enlargement of hilar lymph nodes may be due to:
• Metastases from carcinoma of the bronchus (Fig. 2.70), in which case the primary tumour is often visible; metastases from other sites are rare.
• Malignant lymphoma.
• Infections, particularly tuberculosis and histoplasmosis in endemic areas. Hilar adenopathy is

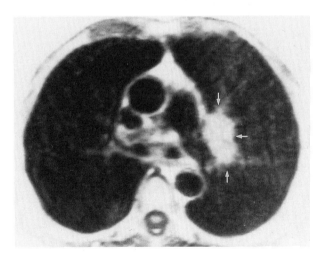

Fig. 2.72 MRI of pulmonary hila. There is a mass (metastatic carcinoma in lymph nodes) at the left hilum (arrows) which stands out clearly, because there is very little signal from normal hilar vessels. The right hilum is normal.

occasionally seen accompanying acute bacterial infections. Tuberculosis is the commonest cause of unilateral hilar adenopathy in children.

Bilateral enlargement of hilar nodes occurs in:
- Sarcoidosis, which is far and away the commonest cause. The diagnosis is almost certain if the hilar enlargement is symmetrical and if the patient is asymptomatic, or has either erythema nodosum or iridocyclitis (see Fig. 2.84, p. 75). Simultaneous enlargement of the right paratracheal nodes is common. Lung changes are sometimes visible (see p. 74).
- Malignant lymphoma (Fig. 2.73).
- Tuberculosis. The African and Asian races show this form of the disease. It is rare to see bilateral hilar enlargement due to tuberculosis in Caucasians.
- Fungus diseases, which are rare causes of bilateral hilar enlargement.

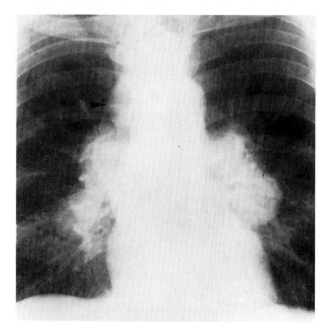

Fig. 2.73 Bilateral hilar adenopathy. The enlarged hila are clearly lobular in outline and there is also enlargement of the right paratracheal nodes (arrow). The diagnosis in this patient was malignant lymphoma.

Neoplasm

Primary carcinoma of the bronchus frequently presents as a hilar mass. If narrowing of the adjacent bronchus is visible or if lobar collapse/consolidation is present, the diagnosis of carcinoma is virtually certain.

The diaphragm

The position of the diaphragm may reflect disease. Both domes of the diaphragm may be pushed up by abdominal distension or they may be high as a result of lung disease. Unilateral elevation of a hemidiaphragm occurs with loss of volume of the ipsilateral lung or it may be due to abdominal pathology, such as an abdominal mass or a subphrenic abscess. In each of these situations, the cause of the elevated hemidiaphragm should be visible, or at least suspected, from the clinical features or from chest or abdominal films. It should always be borne in mind that subpulmonary effusion may mimic elevation of one or both hemidiaphragms (see Fig. 2.46, p. 48). It is also important to realise that minor elevation of a hemidiaphragm is a relatively common incidental finding of no significance. Marked elevation of one hemidiaphragm with no other visible abnormality suggests either paralysis or eventration.

Paralysis of the diaphragm results from disorders of the phrenic nerves, e.g. invasion by carcinoma of the bronchus. The signs are elevation of one hemidiaphragm (see Fig. 2.104, p. 90) which on fluoroscopy or ultrasound shows paradoxical movement, i.e. it moves upward on inspiration.

Eventration of the diaphragm is a congenital condition in which the diaphragm lacks muscle and becomes a thin membranous sheet. Except in the neonatal period it is almost always an incidental finding and does not cause symptoms. When the whole of one hemidiaphragm is involved, almost invariably the left, that hemidiaphragm is markedly elevated. On fluoroscopy or ultrasound, the hemidiaphragm may remain fixed

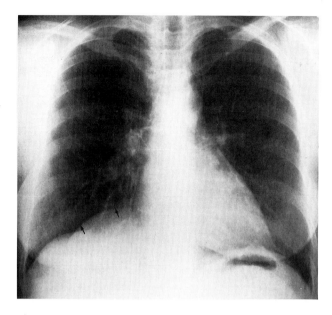

Fig. 2.74 Localised eventration of the diaphragm. There is a smooth localised elevation of the medial half of the right hemidiaphragm (arrows). On the lateral view the eventration involved the anterior half of the right hemidiaphragm.

during inspiration and expiration, but when more severely involved it moves paradoxically and cannot be distinguished from paralysis. The eventration may only involve part of one hemidiaphragm, resulting in a smooth 'hump' (Fig. 2.74).

Rupture of the diaphragm is discussed on page 88.

The chest wall

The chest wall should be examined for evidence of soft tissue swelling or rib abnormality. Because ribs are curved structures, some portions will always be foreshortened on plain chest radiographs. Therefore, if a rib abnormality is suspected, oblique views should be obtained.

Soft tissue swelling occurs with a number of rib lesions: fractures, infections and neoplasms (Fig. 2.75). The soft tissue swelling may be more obvious than the rib lesion on a chest radiograph. If an opacity suggest-

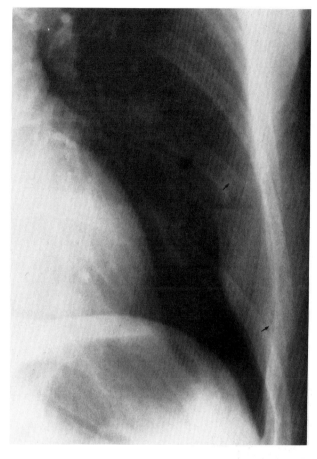

Fig. 2.75 Soft tissue swelling associated with a rib lesion. In this patient with myeloma in a rib, the soft tissue swelling is more obvious than the rib destruction. The bone between the two arrows has been destroyed. This important sign could be easily overlooked unless special attention is paid to identifying rib destruction in the region of soft tissue swelling.

ing soft tissue swelling is seen arising from the chest wall, it is vital to obtain a good view of the underlying ribs using oblique views or tomography where necessary.

Clearly, many diseases of bone such as Paget's disease, myeloma and metastases involve the ribs or sternum in much the same way as elsewhere in the skeleton.

Computed tomography or MRI can be very useful in elucidating chest wall disease. The greatest advantage is in the display of soft tissue masses and bone destruction, particularly chest wall invasion from an underlying carcinoma of the lung (see p. 93).

Congenital abnormalities of the ribs are common but rarely of clinical significance. It is important not to mistake bifid ribs or fused ribs for lung shadows.

Pneumonia and lung abscess

Bacterial pneumonia

The common feature of all pneumonias is a cellular exudate within the alveoli. The damage to the pulmonary parenchyma varies. With pneumococcal pneumonia, for example, complete resolution usually occurs, whereas with certain other infections, notably staphylococci, klebsiella, anaerobic bacteria and tuberculosis, lung destruction with cavitation is common.

Pneumonia may be secondary to obstruction of a major bronchus, carcinoma being a common cause of obstruction. Bronchial obstruction should always be considered in any patient presenting with consolidation of one lobe or of two lobes supplied by a common bronchus (e.g. the right middle and lower lobes), particularly if there is associated loss of volume.

The major purpose of chest radiographs in patients with suspected chest infection is to establish whether or not pneumonia is present. Diagnosing the infective agent on radiological grounds is rarely possible, since there is considerable overlap in the appearance of various bacterial pneumonias and there is even overlap in the appearance of bacterial, fungal and viral pneumonias.

The basic radiological features of pneumonia are one or more areas of consolidation. Cavitation may occur within the consolidated area. Consolidation may be accompanied by loss of volume of the affected lobe, a feature that is particularly common in children. The appearance of consolidation varies from a small ill-defined shadow to a large shadow involving the whole of one or more lobes (lobar pneumonia) (see Fig. 2.17, p. 29); the pattern depends on the infecting organism and the integrity of host defences. The common infecting organism in community acquired lobar pneumonia is *Streptococcus pneumoniae*. In pneumococcal pneumonia there is dense consolidation of one lobe, usually without loss of volume. There may be an associated pleural effusion.

When the consolidation is patchy, involving one or more lobes, it is commonly referred to as bronchopneumonia (Fig. 2.76). The most frequent causes of community acquired bronchopneumonia are *Staphylococcus aureus*, various Gram-negative and anaerobic bacteria, and *Mycoplasma pneumoniae*.

The differentiation between pneumonia and pulmonary oedema or pulmonary infarction may, at times, be difficult or impossible radiographically. The clinical features usually decide the issue.

Viral and mycoplasma pneumonia

Viral pneumonia and pneumonia due to *Mycoplasma pneumoniae* may produce widespread ill-defined consolidation (Fig. 2.77) and loss of clarity of the vascular markings, which on occasion may resemble pulmonary oedema. Alternatively, only a localised area of consolidation may be seen. Pleural effusions are rare. The radiological abnormality may persist for many weeks after clinical recovery.

Lung abscess

A lung abscess is a localised suppurative lesion of the lung parenchyma.

The most frequent causes are:
• Aspiration of food or secretions; such abscesses are usually in the apical (superior) segments of the lower lobes or in the posterior segments of the upper lobes.
• Infection beyond an obstructing lesion in the bronchus.
• Infected emboli, particularly in drug addicts.

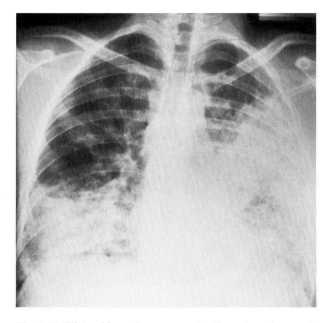

Fig. 2.76 Bilateral bronchopneumonia. There is widespread bilateral patchy consolidation.

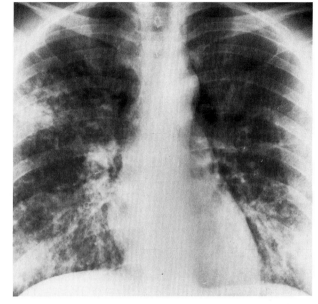

Fig. 2.77 Mycoplasma pneumonia, showing widespread ill-defined consolidation in both lungs.

A lung abscess is usually seen as a spherical shadow containing a central lucency due to air within the cavity. An air–fluid level may be present. It can be difficult or impossible to distinguish an infective lung abscess from a cavitating lung neoplasm or cavitation in Wegener's granulomatosis.

Pulmonary tuberculosis

Pulmonary tuberculosis is usually divided into primary and postprimary forms even though these divisions are not clear cut. Primary tuberculosis is the result of the first infection with *Mycobacterium tuberculosis* and usually occurs in childhood. Postprimary tuberculosis, the usual form in adults, is believed to be re-infection, the patient having developed relative immunity following the primary infection.

Primary tuberculosis

In primary tuberculosis an area of consolidation, known as the Ghon focus, develops in the periphery of the lung—usually in the mid or upper zones. Usually, the pulmonary shadow is small, but it may occasionally involve most of the lobe. Sometimes the pulmonary consolidation is so small that it is nearly invisible. The consolidation is often accompanied by visibly enlarged hilar or mediastinal lymph nodes (Fig. 2.78a). This combination of pulmonary consolidation and lymphadenopathy is known as the *primary complex*. The clinical features of the primary complex vary. The majority of patients have few symptoms and the disease is usually not recognised. The remainder have fever, cough and malaise and occasionally erythema nodosum.

In most cases, whether treated or not, the primary complex heals and often calcifies. A calcified primary complex often remains visible throughout life.

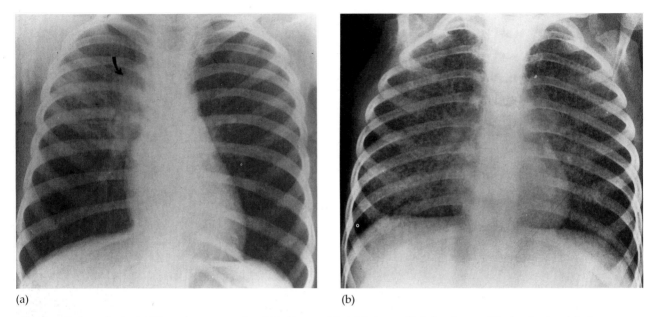

(a)   (b)

Fig. 2.78 Tuberculosis. (a) The primary complex. This 7-year-old child shows ill-defined consolidation in the right lung together with enlargement of the draining lymph nodes (arrow). (b) Miliary tuberculosis. The innumerable small nodular shadows uniformly distributed throughout the lungs in this young child are typical of military tuberculosis. In this instance, no primary focus of infection is visible.

Spread of infection

Spread of infection may occur through:
• The bronchial tree, leading to tuberculous bronchopneumonia which radiologically appears as patchy or lobar consolidation. It often involves more than one lobe, may be bilateral and frequently cavitates.
• The blood stream, resulting in *miliary tuberculosis* (Fig. 2.78b) in which there are innumerable small nodules in the lungs, all of much the same size and fairly evenly distributed. Usually, the nodules are well defined but in severe cases they become relatively confluent so that the individual nodules are difficult to appreciate. The primary focus may be visible and a pleural effusion may be present. It is important to note that early in the course of the illness the chest film may be normal.

Primary tuberculosis may present with a pleural effusion. Occasionally the primary complex is also visible, but more often the effusion is an isolated abnormality.

Postprimary tuberculosis

Postprimary tuberculosis usually presents as cough, haemoptysis, weight loss, night sweats or malaise. Occasionally, the disease is discovered on a routine chest film. Postprimary tuberculosis is usually confined to the upper posterior portions of the chest, namely the apical and posterior segments of the upper lobes and the apical segments of the lower lobes. The initial lesions are multiple small areas of consolidation (Fig. 2.79a) and are often bilateral. Occasionally, the disease takes the form of lower or middle lobe bronchopneumonia. If the infection progresses the consolidations enlarge and frequently cavitate. Cavities are seen as rounded air spaces (translucencies) completely surrounded by pulmonary shadowing (Fig. 2.79b). The diagnosis of cavitation can be difficult and may require tomography.

The infection may undergo partial or complete healing at any stage. Healing occurs by fibrosis, often with

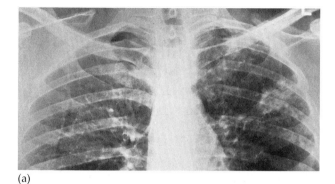

(a)

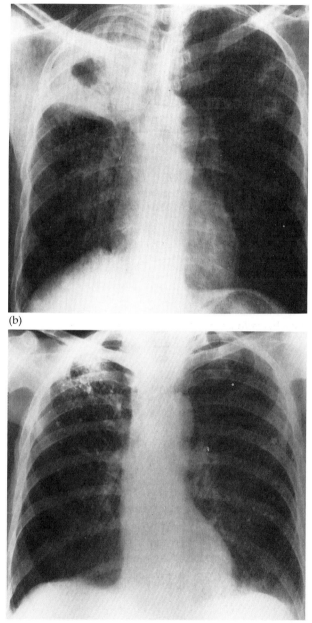

(b)

Fig. 2.79 Postprimary tuberculosis. (a) There are ill-defined consolidations scattered in both upper lobes; their size and distribution should suggest the diagnosis of postprimary tuberculosis. (b) The right upper lobe is consolidated and contains a large central cavity. Patchy consolidation due to tuberculous bronchopneumonia is seen in the right mid and lower zones and in the left upper zone.

calcification (Fig. 2.80), but both fibrosis and calcification may be seen in the presence of continuing activity.

In some cases, the predominant or sole feature is mediastinal and/or hilar adenopathy. It is not clear whether these cases are primary or postprimary tuberculosis; this form is commonest in non-Caucasians (Fig. 2.81).

As with the primary form, postprimary tuberculosis may spread to give widespread bronchopneumonia or miliary tuberculosis.

Pleural effusions are frequent. When they resolve they often leave permanent pleural thickening which may calcify.

Tuberculoma refers to a tuberculous granuloma in the form of a spherical mass, usually less than 3 cm in diameter. The edge is usually sharply defined and these lesions are often partly calcified. Conventional or computed tomography may be needed to demonstrate the calcification. Most tuberculomas are inactive but viable tubercle bacilli may be present even in the calcified lesions.

Fig. 2.80 Old calcified tuberculous disease. There are numerous foci of calcification in both lungs. The right upper lobe shows extensive fibrosis and bullae. There was no evidence in this patient that active infection was present. However, given this film in isolation, active disease could not be excluded.

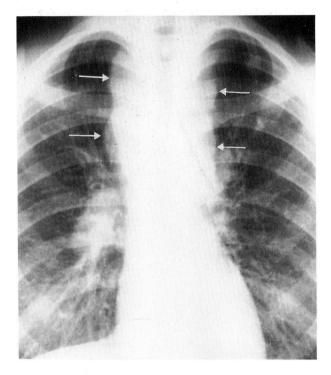

Fig. 2.81 Mediastinal lymphadenopathy (arrows) due to tuberculosis.

Mycetoma (Fig. 2.82). The fungus *Aspergillus fumigatus* may colonise old tuberculous cavities to produce a ball of fungus (mycetoma) lying free within the cavity. Since the fungus ball usually occupies only a portion of the available space, air is seen between the mycetoma and the wall of the cavity. The shape and position of this rim varies with the position of the patient. Cavities containing mycetomas are usually surrounded by other evidence of old tuberculous infection, particularly fibrosis and calcification of the adjacent lung.

Is the disease active?

An important role for radiology in patients with pulmonary tuberculosis is to try and determine whether the disease is active or inactive. This can be very difficult and is sometimes impossible. It is important to realise that there is no way of excluding activity unless serial films over a prolonged period are available. Valuable diagnostic signs of activity are:
- development of new lesions on serial films
- demonstration of cavities.

Lack of change over a period of years is useful evidence against activity, but the change in serial chest films may be subtle, even with active disease. It should be remembered that the presence of calcification does not exclude activity.

Many routine chest films in asymptomatic patients show evidence of tuberculosis. In a few, the diagnosis of active disease will be readily apparent by the presence of cavities or by comparison with previous films. In the remainder it can be a considerable problem to decide which patients to investigate further and which to accept as having old inactive infection. The better defined the shadows and the greater the calcification, the less the likelihood of activity. The presence of ill-defined shadows, even if partially calcified, is suggestive of active disease. However, the decision is often largely based on the clinical findings and the results of sputum examination for tubercle bacilli.

Fungal and parasitic diseases

When fungi are inhaled they may produce lung infection. The radiological appearances vary with the particular fungus, but two broad divisions can be made:
- Infection of the otherwise normal patient by such organisms as those causing histoplasmosis, coccidioidomycosis and blastomycosis (Fig. 2.83). These organisms, which are found chiefly on the continent of North America, produce lesions in the lung that are very similar and often identical to tuberculosis. Cavitation is a particular feature. Healing by fibrosis and calcification is frequent.
- Infection in the compromised host. With impaired immunity of the host, fungi such as *Candida albicans* and *Aspergillus fumigatus*, as well as several of the fungi native to North America, may cause widespread pneumonia. It is not possible to predict the infecting organism from the chest film. Indeed, it is usually not

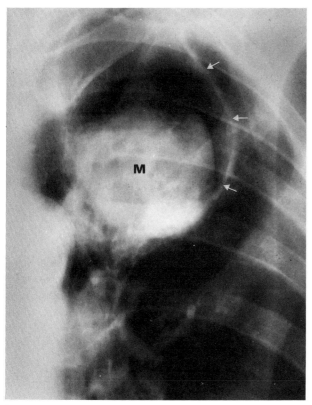

(a)

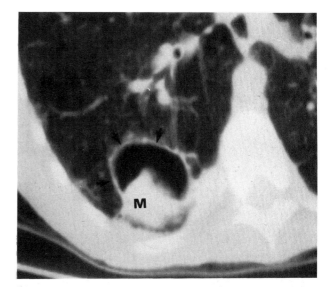

(b)

Fig. 2.82 Mycetoma (M) in pre-existing, old tuberculous cavity, the wall of which is arrowed. (a) Plain film. The fungus ball moved around the cavity when the patient was placed on his side. (b) CT scan of a different patient showing a mycetoma in a pre-existing old tuberculous cavity.

possible to distinguish fungal infection from infection with bacteria, viruses and parasites, particularly *Pneumocystis carinii*, in these patients.

Aspergillus fumigatus is a fungus that affects the lung in three ways: it may colonise a pre-existing cavity forming a fungus ball or mycetoma (see p. 72); it may infect the lung in an immunocompromised patient causing a severe pneumonia (see below), or it may be responsible for allergic bronchopulmonary aspergillosis, a condition discussed on page 80.

Hydatid disease. Pulmonary infection with *Echinococcus granulosus* may result in cysts in the lung or pleural cavity. These cysts may be solitary or multiple and are seen as spherical shadows with very well-defined borders.

Pneumonia in the immunocompromised host

Patients who are immunocompromised are not only more susceptible to pulmonary infection, often with unusual organisms, but the pattern of the resulting pneumonia frequently shows an atypical radiographic appearance. Pneumonia in these patients may be due to the usual pathogens, but often it is due to fungi, tuberculosis or *Pneumocystis carinii*. *Pneumocystis carinii* pneumonia is a particular scourge in patients with AIDS (acquired immunodeficiency syndrome).

Pneumonia in immunocomprised patients usually causes widespread non-specific pulmonary shadowing. It may not even be possible to say whether the shadowing is due to infection or to such conditions as pulmonary oedema or pulmonary haemorrhage.

The prediliction of patients with AIDS to develop

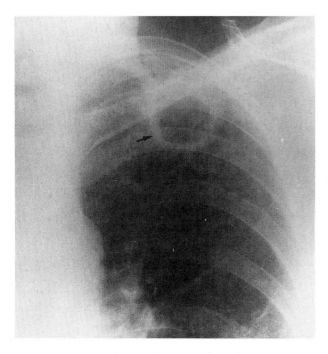

Fig. 2.83 Fungus infection. The cavity (arrow) in this patient from southeast USA was due to North American blastomycosis. Note the similarity to tuberculosis. Other fungi, e.g. histoplasmosis, can give an identical appearance.

Pneumocystis carinii pneumonia means that widespread, uniformly distributed pulmonary shadowing in a patient with AIDS is usually due to this organism, though AIDS patients are also prone to widespread tuberculous infection and the development of widespread Kaposi's sarcoma, both of which can appear similar to *Pneumocystis carinii* pneumonia on plain chest radiography.

Sarcoidosis

Sarcoidosis is characterised pathologically by non-caseating granulomas in many organs including lung, liver, spleen, lymph nodes, skin and bone. The aetiology is obscure and the diagnosis depends on a correlation of the clinical, pathological and radiological manifestations.

The radiological manifestations are largely confined to the chest (the bone lesions are described on p. 327). Nephrocalcinosis is a rare finding.

The features on plain chest radiograph and CT are:
• Hilar and paratracheal lymphadenopathy. When hilar lymphadenopathy is present it is almost invariably bilateral and usually symmetrical (Fig. 2.84). Mediastinal adenopathy is common and the nodes are large enough to be visible on a plain chest radiograph in about half the patients. The mediastinal lymphadenopathy is most readily recognised in the right paratracheal region. On chest CT, the widespread distribution of the lymphadenopathy is apparent. Unlike lymphoma, the lymph node enlargement is never predominant in the anterior mediastinum.
• Reticulonodular shadowing in the lung. The pattern varies from uniform small nodular shadows, which may clear on steroid therapy, to the coarse reticular shadows maximal in the mid and upper zones, which represent gross pulmonary fibrosis (Fig. 2.85). At this stage the pulmonary disease is often irreversible.

The majority of patients with sarcoidosis of the chest have lymphadenopathy only, which clears without treatment and the disease does not progress to pulmonary involvement. Such patients usually do not have chest symptoms, though they may show non-caseating granulomas on transbronchial biopsy. Some present with iridocyclitis, some with erythema nodosum and fever. A few have, in addition, polyarthritis. Many are discovered on routine chest x-ray and have no symptoms or signs.

Approximately 10% develop lung involvement; some of these patients still have visibly enlarged lymph nodes at this stage. Often the lymph nodes get smaller and may return to normal, even though the lung changes persist.

Computed tomography, which can demonstrate the hilar/mediastinal adenopathy and the lung shadowing to advantage, does not provide useful extra information and is not indicated in sarcoidosis.

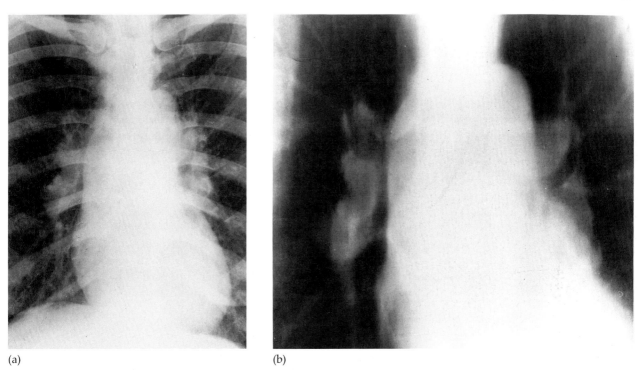

(a)   (b)

Fig. 2.84 Sarcoidosis. (a) Plain film; (b) Tomogram. The lobular outline to the hila is characteristic of lymph node enlargement. In this case the paratracheal nodes are not visibly enlarged. This patient had no symptoms or signs, the abnormality being discovered on a routine chest film.

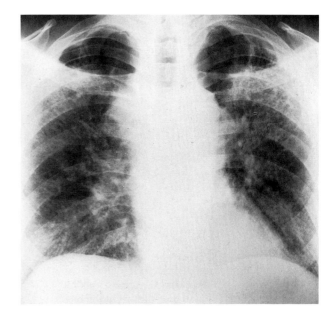

Fig. 2.85 Late fibrotic stage of sarcoidosis. The dense reticulonodular shadowing radiates outwards from the hila, maximally in the mid and upper zones. Enlarged lymph nodes are still visible at the hila and in the right paratracheal region. Many patients with this degree of pulmonary fibrosis, due to sarcoidosis, will not have visibly enlarged lymph nodes.

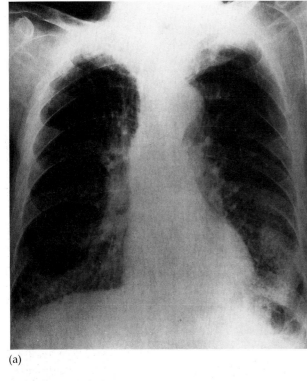

(a)

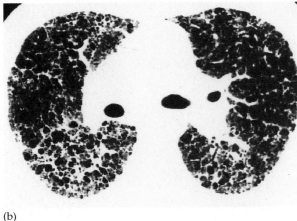

(b)

Fig. 2.86 Idiopathic (cryptogenic) fibrosing alveolitis.
(a) In this example there is reticulonodular shadowing
(honeycomb lung) with basal predominance. Scleroderma
gives a similar picture. Notice that the diaphragm is
indistinct because of the changes in the adjacent lungs.
(b) Thin-section high resolution CT scan of a different
patient showing the honeycomb pattern in the lungs.

Diffuse pulmonary fibrosis (fibrosing alveolitis)

The known causes of diffuse pulmonary fibrosis (synonym usual interstitial pneumonia — UIP) include: extrinsic allergic alveolitis, collagen vascular diseases (including rheumatoid arthritis), pneumoconiosis and sarcoidosis, but a substantial proportion of cases are idiopathic in origin.

Idiopathic pulmonary fibrosis (cryptogenic fibrosing alveolitis)

In cryptogenic fibrosing alveolitis there is thickening of the alveolar walls with fibrosis and desquamation. As the disease progresses the alveolar walls break down and rounded air spaces develop. At this stage the lung is known by the descriptive term 'honeycomb lung'. Fibrosing alveolitis causes a restrictive ventilation defect with severe reduction in gas transfer across the alveolar walls.

The radiological features are:
• Hazy shadowing at the lung bases leading to a lack of clarity of the vessel outlines. Later, ill-defined nodules with connecting lines become discernible.
• Decreased lung volume, often marked, and circular translucencies are seen producing the pattern known as honeycomb lung (Fig. 2.86). Eventually, the heart and pulmonary arteries enlarge due to increasingly severe pulmonary hypertension.

These signs are seen on both plain chest radiographs and CT. Computed tomography, particularly if performed with thin-section HRCT technique, is more sensitive for detecting the changes and demonstrates the distribution and severity of disease to advantage (Fig. 2.86b). However, CT — even HRCT — is of limited clinical value in most cases.

Determining the cause of diffuse pulmonary fibrosis

The distribution of the pulmonary shadowing may give a clue to its aetiology. In idiopathic pulmonary fibrosis, the lung shadowing is often maximal at the bases and at the lung periphery, though it may be

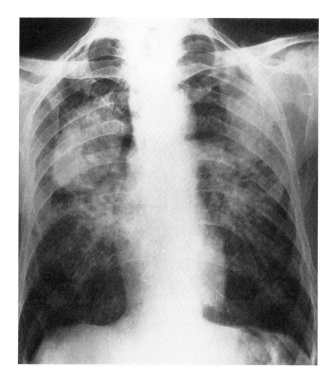

Fig. 2.87 Progressive massive fibrosis (PMF). Note the large oval shadows in the upper halves of both lungs. A nodular pattern is present elsewhere in the lung fields.

fairly uniformly distributed in advanced cases (Fig. 2.86). Scleroderma and rheumatoid arthritis give an identical picture. In sarcoidosis, the abnormal shadowing is usually maximal in the mid and upper zones (Fig. 2.85), whereas in extrinsic allergic alveolitis it is often maximal in the upper zones.

The combination of pulmonary fibrosis with certain other signs may lead to a specific diagnosis:

• Substantial past or present hilar/mediastinal adenopathy suggests sarcoidosis (Fig. 2.85).
• Coexistent conglomerate masses in the mid and upper zones are virtually diagnostic of silicosis or coal miners' pneumoconiosis (Fig. 2.87).
• Coexistent bilateral pleural thickening and calcification are diagnostic of asbestosis (Fig. 2.88).
• Past or present pleural effusions are highly suggestive of rheumatoid arthritis.

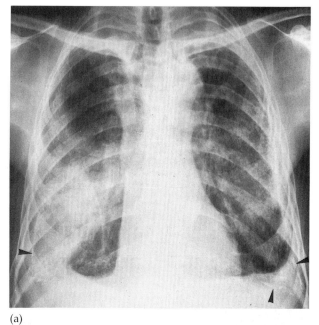

(a)

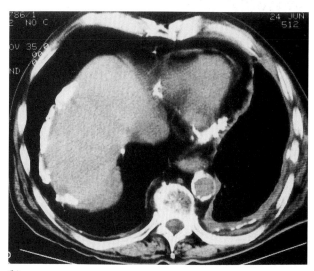

(b)

Fig. 2.88 Asbestos-related pleural disease. (a) There is extensive bilateral pleural thickening and pleural calcification (arrows) best appreciated along the lateral chest wall. (b) CT scan showing numerous calcified pleural plaques, predominantly over the right hemidiaphragm, but also along the left posterolateral chest wall.

Radiation pneumonitis (Fig. 2.89)

Radiation pneumonitis may occur following x-ray therapy for intrathoracic neoplasms and breast carcinoma. The response of the lung to radiation varies from patient to patient. Initially, there is no radiological change, but within a few weeks ill-defined small shadows, indistinguishable from infective consolidation, are seen in the radiation field. If the inflammatory change goes on to fibrosis, there is dense coarse shadowing which may be sharply demarcated from the normal lung in a geometric fashion, conforming to the field of radiation but ignoring the lobar boundaries of the lung. There is loss of volume of the

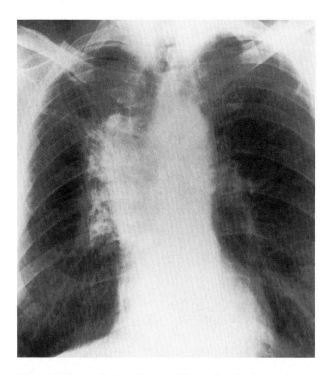

Fig. 2.89 Postradiation fibrosis. The patient had a carcinoma in the right upper lobe centrally, for which he had received radiation therapy. Notice the geometric outline to the shadowing corresponding to the radiation field. There has been contraction of the irradiated lung resulting in mediastinal deviation and distortion of the pulmonary vessels.

fibrosed areas. Extensive pleural thickening is also sometimes seen.

Collagen vascular diseases

This group of diseases includes rheumatoid arthritis, systemic lupus erythematosus, polyarteritis nodosa, systemic sclerosis, dermatomyositis and Wegener's granulomatosis. All affect the chest directly to varying degrees, but often the effects are secondary to involvement of other organs, e.g. the heart and kidneys with resultant heart failure, pulmonary oedema and pericardial effusion. Various radiological signs occur.

Rheumatoid lung

The most common finding in the chest is pleural effusion. Pulmonary fibrosis, often indistinguishable from that seen in idiopathic fibrosing alveolitis, is another important finding.

An interesting feature of pulmonary involvement in rheumatoid arthritis is the development of rounded granulomas in the periphery of the lung, histologically similar to the subcutaneous nodules seen in this disease. These spherical nodules, which may be single or multiple, rarely exceed 3 cm in size. Eventually, many cavitate and resolve.

Coal miners with rheumatoid arthritis may suffer from *Caplan's syndrome*, in which numerous discrete, round granulomas are seen in the lung.

Systemic lupus erythematosus

The chest radiograph is usually normal. The commonest abnormalities are pleural effusion and cardiac enlargement due to pericardial effusion. Patchy consolidation in the lungs is occasionally seen.

Scleroderma and dermatomyositis

The cardinal feature is basal reticulonodular shadows due to pulmonary fibrosis, similar to that seen in cryptogenic fibrosing alveolitis. Usually, the fibrosis appears confined to the bases but, occasionally, it is more widespread. Pleural effusion is rare.

Polyarteritis nodosa

Patchy consolidations, which may be fleeting and repetitive, and pleural effusions are occasionally seen in patients with polyarteritis nodosa.

Wegener's granulomatosis

The lungs may show one or more well-defined consolidations or masses, usually in the mid zones, which may cavitate. These lesions are often difficult to distinguish from bronchogenic carcinoma or metastases on radiographic grounds alone.

Pneumoconiosis

The pneumoconioses include a group of conditions caused by the inhalation of a variety of dusts. Some of these dusts are inert and although they may give rise to widespread small nodules on the chest film the dust causes no symptoms, e.g. siderosis in iron foundry workers due to the inhalation of iron or iron oxide. Other pneumoconioses, notably silicosis and coal workers' pneumoconiosis, are much more serious because the inhaled dust can cause fibrosis in the lungs. Significant pulmonary fibrosis can occur with asbestos exposure.

Coal workers' pneumoconiosis

Simple pneumoconiosis is due to dust retention in the lungs with minor fibrosis. It is recognised radiologically by many small nodules, initially in the mid and upper zones, eventually involving the whole of the lung fields (Fig. 2.90). Simple pneumoconiosis does not give rise to symptoms and the diagnosis is made on the basis of the chest x-ray appearances.

For reasons that are not entirely clear, progressive massive fibrosis (PMF) may supervene. It can be recognised by homogeneous shadows, which are often ovoid in shape, in the upper halves of the lungs. The shadows may be unilateral or bilateral and there is usually nodular shadowing in the rest of the lungs (Fig. 2.87). Progressive massive fibrosis may be associated with breathlessness and it may result in cor pulmonale.

Asbestos-related disease

Inhalation of asbestos fibres may lead to:

1 *Pleural fibrosis and calcification.* Localised plaques of pleural thickening, some of which are calcified, are seen along the lateral chest wall (Fig. 2.88). The plaques in themselves are harmless, but they are a useful pointer to previous asbestos exposure.

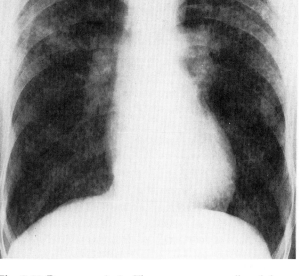

Fig. 2.90 Pneumoconiosis. There are many small nodules involving the whole of the lung fields. The patient was a coal miner.

The differential diagnosis from post-inflammatory and post-traumatic pleural thickening and calcification is made by noting the extent of the pleural disease: usually, it is bilateral in asbestos-related pleural disease whereas it is frequently unilateral in the other conditions. If the costophrenic angles are sharp, healed inflammatory disease or old haemothorax is very unlikely, whereas in asbestos-related pleural disease the costophrenic angles may be clear.

2 *Pulmonary fibrosis*. Pulmonary fibrosis in asbestosis is symmetrically bilateral and maximal at the bases. It produces very fine reticulonodular shadowing. Sometimes the shadowing is so fine that only a haze over the lung bases can be appreciated.

Each of these signs may exist in isolation, but when all are seen together the diagnosis of asbestos-related disease is certain.

Diseases of the airways

Asthma

The chest film in asthma is usually normal or shows only a low flat diaphragm due to air trapping. Bronchial wall thickening may be seen. The main purpose of the chest x-ray in asthma is:
- to determine complications, e.g. atelectasis, pneumothorax, etc.
- to detect underlying pneumonia
- to exclude other causes of acute dyspnoea, e.g. pulmonary oedema or, rarely, tracheal obstruction.

A chest x-ray should only be undertaken when one or more of the above is a realistic possibility.

Allergic bronchopulmonary aspergillosis results from hypersensitivity to *Aspergillus fumigatus*. Asthma is the cardinal clinical feature of this disease. The radiological signs are allergic consolidations in the lung and bronchiectasis, particularly in the mid and upper zones. The thickened walls of the dilated bronchi may be visible on a plain chest film.

Bronchiolitis

Severe bronchiolitis in young children, even when life-threatening, may show surprisingly little change on the chest film. The major sign is overinflation of the lungs leading to a low position of the diaphragm. Some children show widespread small ill-defined areas of consolidation, but in many the lungs are clear.

Acute bronchitis

Acute bronchitis in adults and older children does not produce any radiological abnormality unless complicated by pneumonia.

Chronic obstructive pulmonary disease

Chronic obstructive pulmonary disease is an imprecise but convenient term which covers several common diseases, including chronic bronchitis, emphysema and bronchiectasis.

Chronic bronchitis and emphysema

Chronic bronchitis is a clinical diagnosis based on productive cough for at least three consecutive months in two successive years. Pathologically, there is hypertrophy of the mucous glands throughout the bronchial tree with a great increase in the number of goblet cells. There is thickening of the mucous membranes and airways obstruction occurs. Bronchopneumonia is a common complication.

Emphysema is defined pathologically as 'a condition of the lung characterised by increase beyond normal size of air spaces distal to the terminal bronchiole with destructive changes in their walls'. Two types are recognised—centrilobular and panacinar, depending on the extent of acinar destruction. Chronic bronchitis and emphysema often coexist though pure forms of each are seen.

Chest radiograph in chronic bronchitis. The chest film in uncomplicated chronic bronchitis is normal. Indeed, patients may die from respiratory failure due to chronic bronchitis and have a normal chest film. If the film is abnormal, a complication such as emphysema, pneumonia or cor pulmonale has occurred, and the radiological features are then those of the complication in question.

Chest radiograph in emphysema. Centrilobular emphysema cannot be recognised radiologically. Its presence can be deduced when the signs of pulmonary hypertension and congestive heart failure are seen in a patient known to have chronic bronchitis. The precise significance of the centrilobular emphysema is still under debate.

The signs of panacinar emphysema are (Fig. 2.91):
• Increased lung volume. The lungs increase in volume because of the combined effect of airways obstruction on abnormally compliant lungs. The diaphragm is pushed down and becomes low and flat. The heart is elongated and narrowed. The ribs are widely spaced and more lung lies in front of the heart and mediastinum. (Overinflation of the lungs can be said to be present if the hemidiaphragms at their midpoint are below the seventh rib anteriorly or the twelfth rib posteriorly.)
• Attenuation of the vessels. The reduction in size and number of the blood vessels can be generalised or localised. If severe, the involved area is called a bulla. The edge of a bulla may be indistinct or may be quite sharply limited by a line shadow. In some cases the normal lung adjacent to the bulla is compressed and appears opaque.

Bronchiectasis

Bronchiectasis is defined as irreversible dilatation of the bronchi. Depending on the extent and location of the disease there may be impairment of drainage of bronchial secretions leading to persistent infection.

The conditions which cause bronchiectasis include pulmonary infection in childhood, cystic fibrosis and longstanding bronchial obstruction.

Pulmonary tuberculosis is a common cause but since

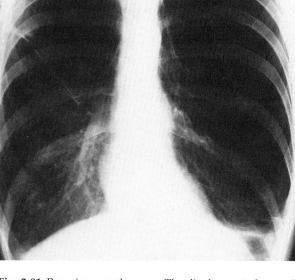

Fig. 2.91 Panacinar emphysema. The diaphragm is low and flat and the ribs are widely spaced, indicating overinflation of the lungs. The peripheral vessels in most of the left lung and the upper half of the right lung are small and attenuated, indicating lung destruction.

it usually affects the upper lobes, the drainage of secretions is good and such patients rarely have symptoms due to their bronchiectasis.

The radiological features are (Fig. 2.92):
• Visibly dilated bronchi. If these contain air, the thickened walls of the dilated bronchi may be seen as tubular or ring shadows. If filled with fluid, the dilated bronchi will be opaque or air–fluid levels will be present. Since these fluid levels are very short they have to be looked for very carefully.
• Persistent consolidation, often containing dilated bronchi.
• Loss of volume of the affected lobe or lobes is almost invariable.

A proportion of patients with symptomatic bronchiectasis have normal plain chest films.

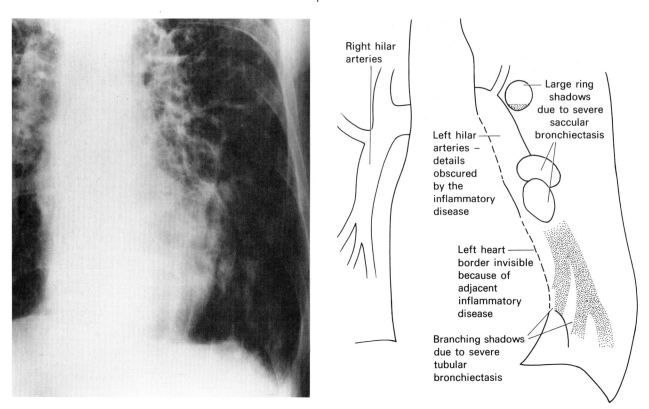

Right hilar arteries

Left hilar arteries – details obscured by the inflammatory disease

Large ring shadows due to severe saccular bronchiectasis

Left heart border invisible because of adjacent inflammatory disease

Branching shadows due to severe tubular bronchiectasis

Fig. 2.92 Bronchiectasis. Plain film showing a mixture of saccular and tubular bronchiectasis. The branching ectatic bronchi resemble large blood vessels but should not be confused with them.

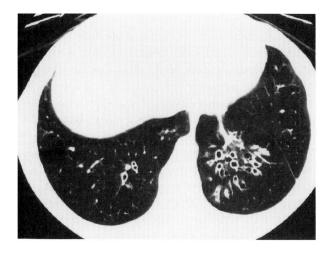

Fig. 2.93 Bronchiectasis. Thin-section high resolution CT scan showing thick walled, dilated bronchi crowded together in the left lower lobe. The normal appearance is seen in the right lower lobe.

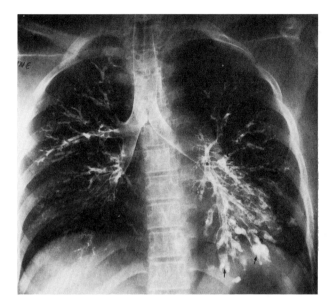

Fig. 2.94 Bronchiectasis. Bronchogram showing bronchiectasis in the left lower lobe. Note that the affected bronchi (arrowed) are occluded as well as dilated. The remaining bronchi in the left upper lobe and right lung are normal.

Computed tomography has now replaced bronchography as the method of determining the presence of bronchiectasis, where this is in doubt, and the extent of disease. A specialised thin-section technique is employed in order to obtain high resolution images (Fig. 2.93).

Bronchography, which outlines the lumen of the bronchi with contrast media, is the definitive method of making the diagnosis of bronchiectasis (Fig. 2.94). Bronchography is rarely performed nowadays; the only remaining indication is establishing the extent of bronchiectasis prior to surgical resection, a role that is gradually being taken over by HRCT.

Cystic fibrosis

Cystic fibrosis is an inherited disorder of exocrine glands resulting in secretion of viscid mucus. In cystic

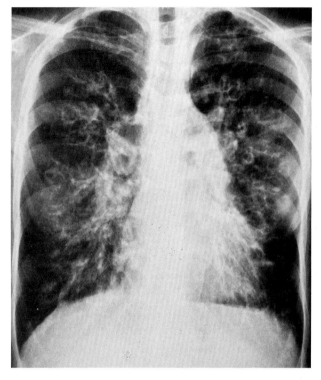

Fig. 2.95 Cystic fibrosis in a 14-year-old child. There is bronchial wall thickening, ring shadows of bronchiectasis and widespread ill-defined shadowing. All these phenomena tend to be maximal in the mid and upper zones. The diaphragm is somewhat low due to obstructive airways disease.

fibrosis the small airways become blocked and secondary infections supervene. The finding of a high sodium chloride concentration in the sweat is diagnostic of the condition.

The radiological findings are (Fig. 2.95):
• Small ill-defined consolidations, maximal in the upper zones, some of which show cavitation.
• Bronchial wall thickening and the signs of bronchiectasis; both usually maximal in the upper zones.
• Evidence of airway obstruction. The diaphragm is low and flat and the heart is narrow and vertical, until cor pulmonale develops when cardiac enlargement may occur.

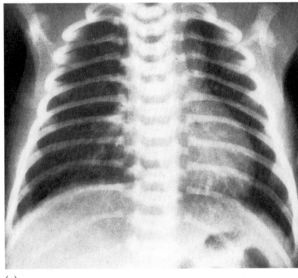

(a)

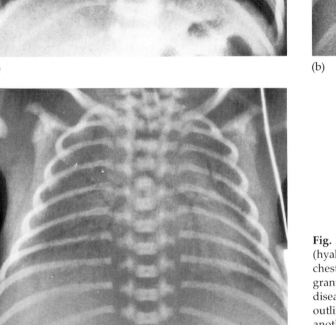

(b)

(c)

Fig. 2.96 The neonatal respiratory distress syndrome (hyaline membrane disease). (a) Normal premature neonatal chest film for comparison. (b) This film shows the general granular opacity of the lungs typical of hyaline membrane disease. The vessels, the heart borders and the diaphragm outlines are indistinct. (c) The air bronchogram sign in another baby with hyaline membrane disease. Note the uniformity of distribution of the changes in the lungs—an important diagnostic feature of hyaline membrane disease.

Respiratory distress in the newborn

There are many causes of respiratory distress in the first few days of life. Abnormalities are visible on the chest x-ray in the majority; only two conditions are discussed here.

Hyaline membrane disease is one of the commonest abnormalities. It is a disease of the premature infant and is due to deficiency of surfactant in the lungs. Consequently the alveoli collapse, so preventing gas exchange. The chest radiographic appearance is one of the most important criteria in making the diagnosis.

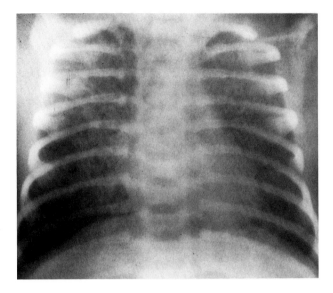

Fig. 2.97 Meconium aspiration. This baby born at term had fetal distress during delivery and was born through meconium-stained liquor. The film shows patchy consolidations rather than the uniform changes seen in hyaline membrane disease. The diaphragm is lower than normal in position, which is another differentiation from hyaline membrane disease.

The basic signs are widespread very small pulmonary opacities and visible air bronchograms (Fig. 2.96). The air bronchograms are visible because the bronchi are surrounded by airless alveoli. The changes are nearly always uniform in distribution. In the milder forms, the nodules are small and the air bronchograms may be the most obvious and easily recognised sign. In the more severe forms, the pulmonary opacities become more obvious and may be confluent; the lungs then appear almost opaque, except for air bronchograms.

Meconium aspiration (Fig. 2.97). In meconium aspiration the pulmonary shadowing is usually patchy and distinctly streaky. Air bronchograms are not an obvious feature. In meconium aspiration the diaphragm is often lower than normal due to the airways obstruction associated with sticky meconium in the bronchi.

Complications of therapy

In addition to establishing the initial diagnosis in neonates with various causes of respiratory distress, the plain chest film is vital in detecting complications of therapy. These include lobar collapse, pneumomediastinum and pneumothorax.

Adult respiratory distress syndrome

Adult respiratory distress syndrome (ARDS) is the name given to a syndrome in which the pulmonary capillaries become leaky and proteinaceous fluid escapes from the vascular lumen into the surrounding pulmonary interstitium and alveoli. The condition is also known as 'non-cardiogenic pulmonary oedema'. There are many precipitating causes including severe trauma, significant hypotension, septicaemia and fat embolism. It is believed that these insults produce a cascade of events, the nature of which still needs to be elucidated, leading to capillary damage and hence to increased capillary permeability.

The patients become increasingly short of breath and hypoxic, requiring mechanical ventilation to stay alive. The mortality, even with intense therapy and assisted ventilation, can be very high. There is no specific treatment.

Radiologically (Fig. 2.98), the chest x-ray shows widespread pulmonary shadowing resembling cardiogenic pulmonary oedema at first, but becoming more widespread and more uniform over the ensuing 24–48 hours. The radiological abnormality may only develop 12–24 hours after the onset of tachypnoea, dyspnoea or hypoxaemia. Since such patients with ARDS require assisted ventilation, the chest film is used to detect the complications of ventilator therapy, notably pneumothorax and pneumomediastinum.

Pulmonary embolism and infarction

Pulmonary embolism from thrombi originating in the veins of the legs and pelvis is very common in patients confined to bed, particularly those with heart disease

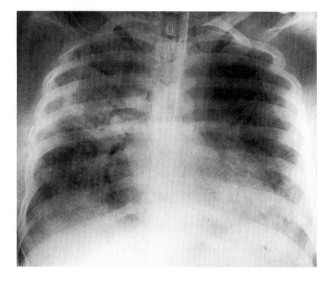

Fig. 2.98 Adult respiratory distress syndrome (ARDS). There is widespread consolidation of the lungs. This patient had suffered extensive trauma to the limbs.

and those who have had major surgery. The clinical and radiological manifestations depend on the size and number of the emboli.

Plain film abnormalities

Massive embolism. In most cases the chest film in massive pulmonary embolism is unremarkable. There may be a visible reduction in the size of the arteries beyond the occlusion, but this is a very difficult sign to recognise and it is usually not possible to be sure that the smallness of the vessels is due to embolism rather than to pre-existing pulmonary disease, such as emphysema or old infection.

Large emboli. In many cases there is no infarction, even with large emboli, and therefore the chest film is normal. However, in some patients, particularly those with heart disease, infarction does occur. Radiologically, an infarct appears as an area of consolidation based on the pleura, indistinguishable from pneumonia. Infarcts often involve both lung bases and

cause elevation of the diaphragm and pleural effusion. The differentiation between pneumonia and pulmonary infarction depends on clinical factors and, if necessary, a radionuclide lung scan (see below).

Small emboli. Small emboli do not produce any radiological abnormality unless they occur over a long period of time and cause pulmonary hypertension. (See page 116 for the signs of pulmonary hypertension.)

Radionuclide lung scans

The diagnosis of pulmonary embolism on radionuclide lung scanning depends on observing the distribution of radionuclide particles in the lungs following intravenous injection. The radionuclide particles do not reach the under-perfused portions of the lungs and, therefore, one or more defects are seen in the perfusion scan. A normal perfusion scan for practical purposes excludes pulmonary embolism.

A ventilation scan is also required in patients with perfusion defects in order to differentiate between the various other causes of perfusion defects which include pneumonia, pulmonary oedema, tumours, bronchiectasis and emphysema.

The ventilation and perfusion scans are compared. If similar sized defects are present on both scans, they are regarded as matched; if not, the defects are mismatched.

The major patterns that may be seen when comparing the perfusion and ventilation scans with the chest radiographs are:

1 Mismatched ventilation/perfusion defects (Fig. 2.99).
- Perfusion defects in areas with normal ventilation are highly suggestive of pulmonary embolism without infarction.
- Perfusion defects which are larger than the corresponding ventilation defects suggest pulmonary infarction. Such cases will often show consolidation on plain chest radiograph.

2 Matched ventilation/perfusion defects (Fig. 2.100) are usually due to pneumonia, pulmonary oedema or

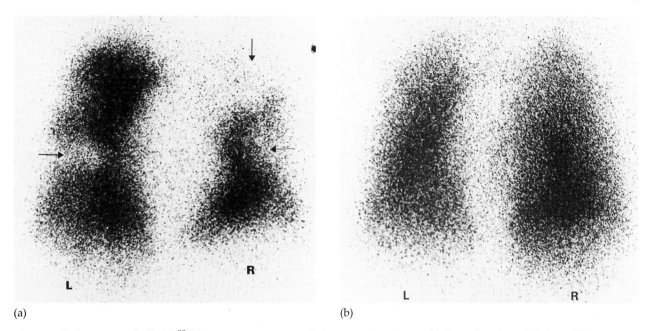

(a)　　　　　　　　　　　　　　　　　　　　(b)

Fig. 2.99 Pulmonary emboli. (a) ⁹⁹ᵐTc macroaggregate perfusion scan showing multiple wedge-shaped defects. The more obvious ones have been arrowed. (b) The ventilation scan, using ⁸¹ᵐKr, is normal.

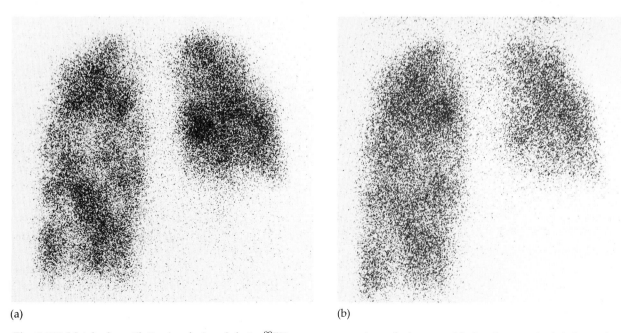

(a)　　　　　　　　　　　　　　　　　　　　(b)

Fig. 2.100 Matched ventilation/perfusion defects. ⁹⁹ᵐTc macroaggregate perfusion scan (a) showing matched defects when compared to the ⁸¹ᵐKr ventilation scan (b). Both are anterior scans. The patient had widespread emphysema.

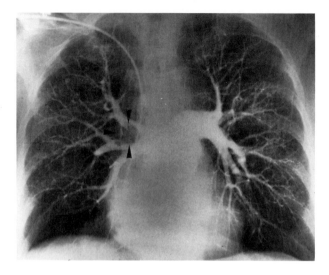

Fig. 2.101 Pulmonary arteriogram in pulmonary embolism. There is a large embolus causing a filling defect at the bifurcation of the right pulmonary artery (arrows). Note also the reduction in branches of the lower lobe arteries due to obstruction by emboli. (The catheter can be seen passing from the right arm into the heart.)

airways disease. However, they may sometimes be seen with pulmonary infarction and are, therefore, classified as 'indeterminate'.

Pulmonary angiography (Fig. 2.101)

Pulmonary angiography is the most accurate method of diagnosing pulmonary emboli. It requires definite indications, e.g. to confirm massive embolism prior to surgical intervention, or when there is significant doubt about the presence or absence of pulmonary emboli after viewing the chest radiograph and radio-nuclide lung scans.

Trauma to the chest

Rib fracture can be diagnosed by noting a break or step in the cortex of a rib. Special views of the ribs may be necessary, since rib fractures are often invisible in the standard projections, particularly if the fracture lies below the diaphragm. Extrapleural soft tissue swelling due to bruising, or frank haematoma may be visible and guide the observer toward the site of the fracture.

Rib fractures are frequently multiple and may result in a flail segment.

Pleural effusion often accompanies rib fractures, the fluid frequently being blood.

Pneumothorax may occur if the lung is punctured by direct injury or by the sharp edge of a rib fracture. An air–fluid level in the pleural cavity is common in such situations, due to the associated haemorrhage.

Surgical emphysema of the chest wall may indicate the escape of air from the lungs. The presence of mediastinal emphysema may indicate the unusual phenomenon of rupture of a bronchus.

Pulmonary contusion. Localised traumatic alveolar haemorrhage and oedema (Fig. 2.102) may be seen whether or not a rib fracture can be identified. The resulting pulmonary shadow is indistinguishable from other forms of pulmonary consolidation, the relationship to the injury being important in establishing the diagnosis.

Adult respiratory distress syndrome (ARDS) may follow severe trauma to any part of the body. *Fat embolism* is a specific subtype of ARDS, but its radiographic manifestations are identical to those of the other causes of ARDS (see p. 85).

Rupture of the diaphragm due to penetrating injury or compression of the abdomen may permit herniation of the stomach or intestines into the chest. Such herniation is much commoner on the left than the right. There is usually a pleural effusion and the 'diaphragm' outline becomes indistinct during the acute stage. Gas shadows of the stomach or intestines are seen above the presumed position of the diaphragm, the diaphragm itself often being invisible. Barium meal and

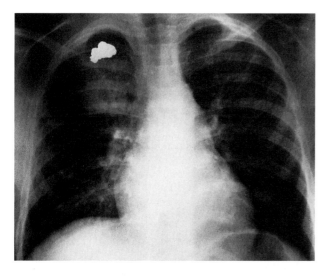

Fig. 2.102 Pulmonary contusion from a gunshot wound. The ill-defined consolidation represents haemorrhage and oedema in the right upper lobe. The deformed metallic fragments of the bullet are clearly visible.

follow-through may be indicated to establish the diagnosis.

Rupture of the aorta is a particularly serious consequence of rapid deceleration injuries. In patients that survive, the injury to the aorta is usually at the level of the ligamentum arteriosum. Bleeding into the mediastinum may cause visible mediastinal widening, and bleeding into the pleural cavity may occur.

Aortography is usually indicated in patients with unexplained mediastinal widening following trauma to establish the diagnosis of aortic rupture, since venous bleeding which does not require emergency surgery can cause similar signs. Widening of the mediastinum can be a very difficult sign to assess, particularly on the portable AP films that are often the only films that can be taken in these severely injured patients. Computed tomography scanning may be used to exclude blood in the mediastinum in those cases where the nature of mediastinal widening is uncertain from plain film observations.

Aortic rupture can occur with surprisingly mild trauma, and though fractures of the ribs or sternum are usually present there are many cases on record without visible damage to the thoracic cage.

In some patients the diagnosis of aortic rupture is only made several months or years after the injury when the development of an aneurysm is noted.

Rupture of the tracheobronchial tree only occurs with major chest trauma. The cardinal signs are pneumomediastinum, or pneumothorax that does not respond to chest tube suction. The main complication is subsequent bronchostenosis.

Neoplastic disease

Carcinoma of the bronchus

Carcinoma of the bronchus is a very common primary malignant tumour. It is commoner in men than women and has a clear association with cigarette smoking. With the exception of some squamous cell carcinomas and the rare alveolar cell carcinoma, it is not possible to predict the cell type with any certainty from the chest x-ray appearances.

The majority of bronchial carcinomas arise in larger bronchi at, or close to, the hilum. These tumours are usually suspected on radiological grounds and confirmed or excluded by bronchoscopy and transbronchial biopsy. The remainder arise peripherally. It is convenient to consider the radiological features of central and peripheral tumours separately.

Signs of a central tumour

• The tumour itself may present as a hilar mass (Fig. 2.103) and/or narrowing of a major bronchus. The narrowing may be irregular or smooth.
• The effect of obstruction by the tumour (Fig. 2.104) is usually a combination of collapse and consolidation. The alveoli collapse because air is absorbed beyond the obstructed bronchus and cannot be replaced, whereas consolidation is the consequence of retained secretions and secondary infection.

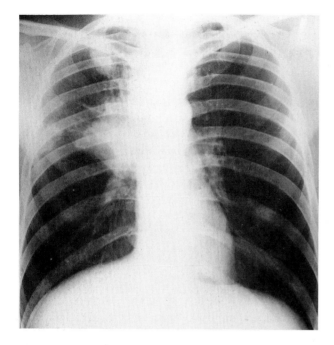

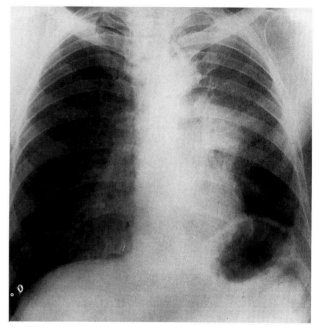

Fig. 2.103 Right hilar mass due to carcinoma of the bronchus. There is also a patch of consolidation in the right upper lobe laterally, due to the central obstruction.

Fig. 2.104 Carcinoma of the bronchus at the left hilum causing collapse of the left upper lobe and paralysis of the left phrenic nerve. The elevated left hemidiaphragm is too high to be due to the lobar collapse; it is due to phrenic nerve involvement by the tumour at the left hilum.

Signs of a peripheral tumour

A peripheral tumour usually presents as a solitary pulmonary mass. There are several causes for such a mass and these are discussed on p. 37.

The signs of a peripheral primary carcinoma are:
• A rounded shadow with an irregular border; lobulation, notching and infiltrating edges are the common patterns (Fig. 2.105).
• Cavitation within the mass (Fig. 2.37). Peripheral squamous cell carcinomas show a particular tendency for cavitation. The walls of the cavity are classically thick and irregular, but thin-walled smooth cavities due to carcinoma do occur.

Signs of spread of bronchial carcinoma

The signs of spread of bronchial carcinoma may be visible on plain chest radiography. Computed tomo-graphy has made a major contribution to the staging of lung cancer, because it may show mediastinal involvement of lymph nodes or direct invasion of the mediastinum by tumour that is either not visible or is questionable on the plain chest film — information that may save the patient an unnecessary thoracotomy.
• *Hilar and mediastinal lymph node enlargement due to lymphatic spread of tumour.* Only greatly enlarged lymph nodes can be recognised on plain chest radiograph. The sites in which nodes are most readily identified are at the hilum and in the right paratracheal area (Fig. 2.106). Nodes in the subcarinal region have to be massive if they are to be visible on a plain chest film. Computed tomography, on the other hand, has the ability to show even mildly enlarged nodes, nodes that are completely invisible on plain film. However, enlargement of lymph nodes does not necessarily mean

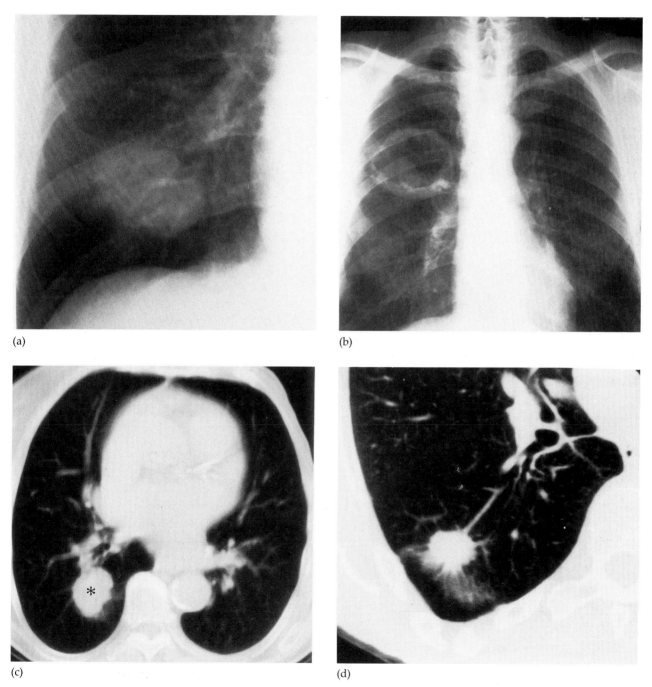

(a)

(b)

(c)

(d)

Fig. 2.105 Appearance of peripheral lung carcinoma. (a) A lobulated and (b) a cavitating mass are shown on plain films. (c) A lobulated (∗) and (d) a spiculated mass are shown on CT.

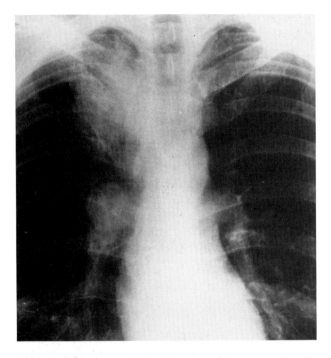

Fig. 2.106 Carcinoma of the right upper lobe (arrowed) with large lymph node metastases at the right hilum.

metastatic involvement, since reactive hyperplasia to the tumour or associated infection can be responsible for nodal enlargement as can existing disease such as previous granulomatous infection, sarcoidosis or coal-workers' pneumoconiosis. In practice, the role of CT is to decide which patients need mediastinoscopy or mediastinotomy prior to thoracotomy, and to tell the surgeon which nodes to biopsy. Nodes below 1 cm in diameter can be considered as normal in size and need not be biopsied. Nodes above 1 cm in diameter should be biopsied prior to surgical resection of the primary tumour, though it should be borne in mind that nodes of 2 cm or greater (Fig. 2.107) in a patient with a bronchial carcinoma almost invariably contain metastatic neoplasm.

- *Pleural effusion* in a patient with lung cancer is usually due to malignant involvement of the pleura, but it may be secondary to associated infection of the lung or coincidental, as in heart failure.

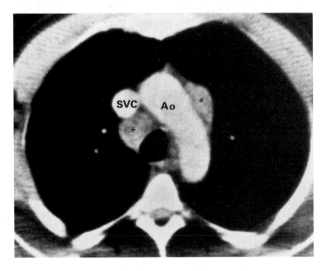

Fig. 2.107 Mediastinal adenopathy. CT scan shows two greatly enlarged lymph nodes (*). Ao, aorta; SVC, superior vena cava.

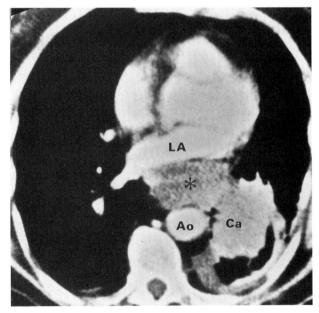

Fig. 2.108 Mediastinal invasion. CT scan showing bronchial carcinoma (Ca) in left lower lobe invading the mediastinum (*). Ao, aorta; LA, left atrium.

• *Invasion of the mediastinum.* On plain films the signs are widening of the mediastinal shadow and elevation of a hemidiaphragm suggesting involvement of the phrenic nerve by tumour (Fig. 2.104).

Mediastinal widening can be a difficult sign to evaluate, particularly in older people with aortic unfolding. Computed tomography is a much more sensitive and accurate method of assessing mediastinal invasion by tumour because the neoplasm can be directly visualised (Fig. 2.108).

• *Invasion of the chest wall* (Fig. 2.109). Destruction of a rib immediately adjacent to a pulmonary shadow is virtually diagnostic of bronchial carcinoma with chest wall invasion. Recognising the rib destruction can be difficult, one has, therefore, to make a conscious effort to look at the ribs directly. Oblique views may be helpful in detecting bone destruction. Computed tomography scanning can demonstrate soft tissue invasion when the bone is not visibly eroded on plain

films (Fig. 2.33, p. 39). Imaging techniques, even CT and MRI, may not always be reliable at excluding chest wall invasion and local chest wall pain remains the most important indication that the tumour has crossed the pleura.

• *Rib metastases.* Carcinoma of the lung frequently metastasises to the ribs where it produces bone destruction. Sclerotic secondary deposits from lung carcinoma are rare.

• *Pulmonary metastases.* Primary lung carcinoma occasionally metastasises to other parts of the lungs. The rounded shadows that result are similar to secondary deposits from other primary tumours.

• *Lymphangitis carcinomatosa* (Fig. 2.110) is the term applied to blockage of the pulmonary lymphatics by carcinomatous tissue. Lymphangitis carcinomatosa

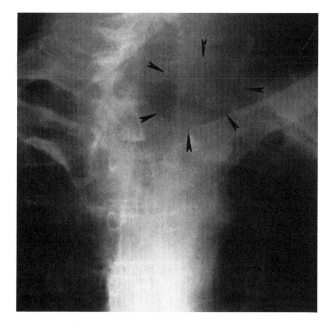

Fig. 2.109 Pancoast's tumour. The carcinoma arising at the apex of the left lung has invaded and destroyed the adjacent ribs and spine. Note that no bone is visible within the area indicated by the arrows.

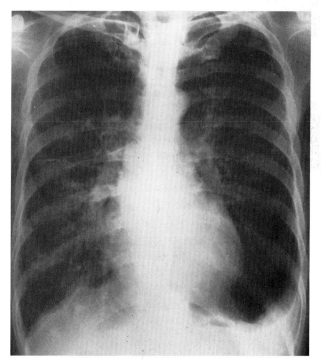

Fig. 2.110 Lymphangitis carcinomatosa. There is widespread ill-defined pulmonary shadowing with numerous septal lines. A small left pleural effusion is also present. The patient had a carcinoma of the stomach.

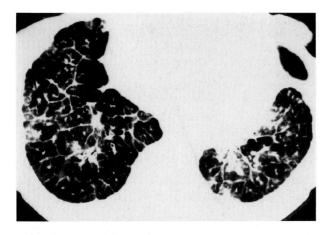

Fig. 2.111 Lymphangitis carcinomatosa. The combination of ill-defined shadows and widespread connecting lines representing thickened interlobular septa is very well shown by thin-section high resolution CT.

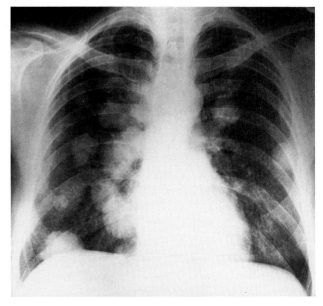

Fig. 2.112 Pulmonary metastases. There are numerous rounded shadows of varying sizes in both lungs.

can be due to spread from abdominal and breast cancers as well as from carcinoma of the lung. The lymphatic vessels become grossly distended and the lungs become oedematous. The signs can be identical to those seen in interstitial pulmonary oedema (septal lines, loss of vessel clarity and peribronchial thickening), but if the heart is normal in size and there is hilar adenopathy and/or lobar consolidation, the diagnosis of lymphangitis carcinomatosa becomes more certain. The clinical story is very helpful, since if the changes are due to pulmonary oedema, the patient will usually complain of sudden onset of breathlessness, whereas the patient with lymphangitis carcinomatosa will give a story of slowly increasing dyspnoea over the preceding weeks or months. Computed tomography, particularly thin-section HRCT has proved very valuable in demonstrating lymphangitis carcinomatosa, because the appearances, in the correct clinical circumstances, are specific enough to obviate the need for biopsy (Fig. 2.111).

Metastatic neoplasms

Metastases from extrathoracic primary tumours may be seen in the lungs, the pleura or the bones of the thoracic cage. Hilar and mediastinal lymph node enlargement due to metastases is uncommon, other than from carcinoma of the bronchus.

Pulmonary metastases produce one or more rounded shadows within the lung (Figs 2.112 and 2.113). Typically, metastases are spherical and well defined, although irregular borders are occasionally seen. Usually, they are multiple and vary in size. As with primary tumours, metastases have to be almost a centimetre in diameter or larger to be visible on plain chest radiographs or conventional tomograms. Computed tomography scanning can demonstrate metastases as small as 3–6 mm. There is, however, a disadvantage attached to the excellent sensitivity of CT. Some small nodules are not metastases, but benign processes such as tuberculomas or fungal granulomas. This is a major diagnostic problem in many parts of the United States where fungal granulomas are very common.

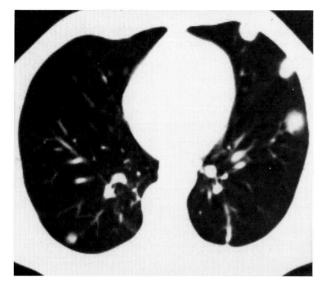

Fig. 2.113 CT scan of pulmonary metastases (malignant teratoma of testis). The peripheral location shown here is typical.

Pleural metastases usually give rise to pleural effusion. The individual pleural metastases are rarely seen.

Metastases to ribs are common with those primary tumours that metastasise to bone, namely bronchus, breast, kidney, thyroid and prostate. All except prostatic and breast cancers produce mainly or exclusively lytic metastases. Sclerotic metastases in an elderly man suggest a prostatic primary cancer. Sclerotic or mixed lytic and sclerotic deposits in a woman suggest that the primary carcinoma is in the breast.

   With lytic metastases the best sign is destruction of the cortex, particularly of the upper border of the rib. One should be wary of diagnosing destruction of the lower borders of the posterior portions of the ribs, since these regions are indefinite even in the normal. When in doubt it is always wise to compare with the opposite side. Another pitfall in the diagnosis of rib metastases is that blood vessels in the lungs may cause confusing shadows. This cannot arise at the edges of the chest where there is no lung over the ribs, so that

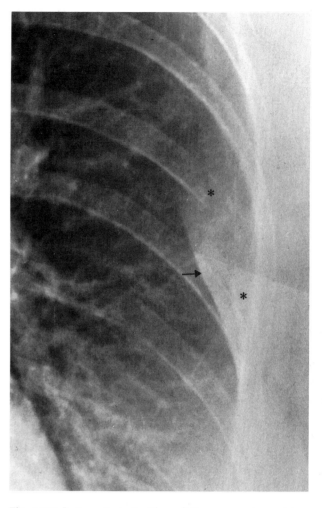

Fig. 2.114 Lytic metastasis. The soft tissue mass (arrow) is more obvious than the underlying bone destruction shown between the two asterisks.

is a useful place to look for bone destruction. Soft tissue swelling is frequently seen adjacent to the rib deposit, so it is a good rule to look at the outer margin of the lung for soft tissue swelling as a clue to the presence of rib metastases (Fig. 2.114).

   When sclerotic metastases are suspected the best place to look is in the medulla of the ribs, particularly where the lung does not overlie the ribs.

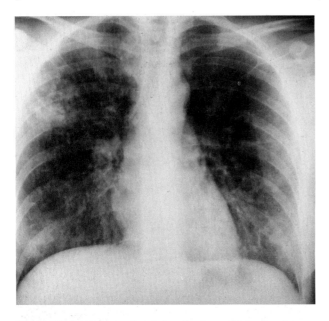

Fig. 2.115 Lymphoma involving the lung. The extensive pulmonary consolidations were due to neoplastic involvement. Pneumonia can give a similar appearance.

Lymphoma

The common manifestations of intrathoracic malignant lymphoma are mediastinal and hilar adenopathy and pleural effusion. These features can often be seen on plain films and conventional tomography but CT scanning is much the best method of confirming or excluding intrathoracic lymph node enlargement. Pulmonary involvement by lymphoma is unusual (Fig. 2.115). It may take the form of large areas of infiltration of the lung parenchyma, resembling pulmonary consolidation, or occasionally it is seen as one or more mass lesions, which may cavitate. Pleural masses are a rare feature.

Since pulmonary infection is a common complication in patients with malignant lymphoma it may be impossible to decide on radiological grounds whether the pulmonary consolidation is due to lymphomatous tissue or due to infection.

MAMMOGRAPHY

X-ray examination of the breast is carried out with dedicated equipment which produces low kilovoltage x-rays in the range 28–32 kV which demonstrate the soft tissues of the breast to advantage. The normal breast tissue on a mammogram shows the glandular, ductal and connective tissue against a background of fat, the appearances changing with the age of the patient. With increasing age, involution of the breast occurs so that the glandular tissue atrophies. The mammographic appearances of the normal breast vary greatly from one patient to another.

The main purpose of mammography is to detect breast carcinoma. It is now used to screen women for breast cancer, and can also be helpful in patients presenting with a lump or lumpy areas in the breast.

Mammographic signs

The cardinal mammographic sign of carcinoma is a mass with ill-defined or spiculated borders (Fig. 2.116). An important sign suggesting malignancy is clustered, fine linear or irregular calcifications—so-called malignant microcalcifications (Fig. 2.117), which can on occasion be a sign of breast cancer even in the absence of a visible mass. Other signs that may point to the diagnosis of carcinoma are distortion of adjacent breast stroma and skin thickening.

Benign masses tend to be spherical with well-defined borders (Fig. 2.118) and not infrequently contain calcification. The calcifications differ from malignant microcalcification in that they are larger, coarser and often ring-like in configuration (Fig. 2.119).

Ultrasound can be very helpful in determing whether a mass is a simple cyst (Fig. 2.118b), and therefore benign, or solid and, therefore, possibly a carcinoma.

Breast screening

Mammography can detect breast cancer in asymptomatic women even before the tumour is palpable. There is evidence from large scale trials that early detection

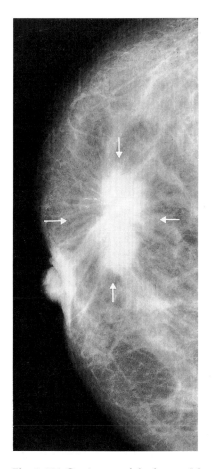

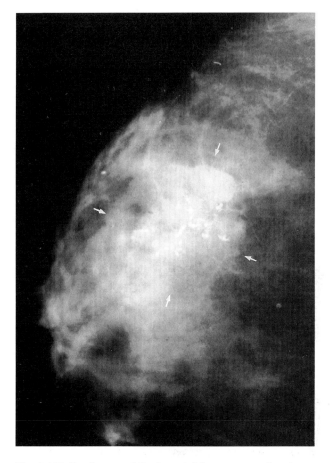

Fig. 2.116 Carcinoma of the breast. Mammogram showing irregular soft tissue mass (arrows) behind the nipple. Microcalcifications are present but difficult to see in reproduction.

Fig. 2.117 Carcinoma of the breast. Mammogram showing ill-defined mass (arrows) containing numerous malignant linear and branching microcalcifications.

by mammography can reduce the mortality from breast cancer in women over the age of 50. Though the precise degree of improved survival is still not certain, reductions in mortality have been found to be as high as 30% of those screened in some series.

Breast cancer is the most frequent cancer in women, affecting one woman in 12. In an attempt to reduce the mortality, the UK government has decided to invite all women aged 50–64 years to attend a screening programme consisting of a mammogram every 3 years. It is expected that at least 50 cancers will be detected by mammography for every 10 000 women screened. Inevitably, a number of breast carcinomas will escape detection by screening mammography.

As with all screening tests there will inevitably be false-positive interpretations. For this reason, all patients with an abnormal mammogram are asked to attend an assessment clinic at which they are given a physical examination, and further mammographic views, ultrasound, or needle biopsy as necessary. In some instances follow-up mammography after a short interval will be advised.

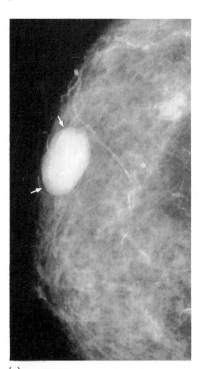

(a)

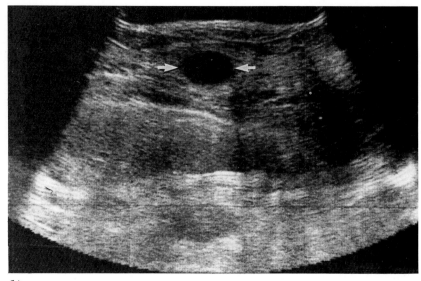

(b)

Fig. 2.118 Benign cyst of breast. (a) Mammogram showing oval, very well defined mass without calcifications (arrows). (b) The mass (arrows) was shown to be cystic on ultrasound; cyst aspiration was undertaken.

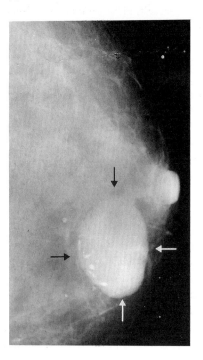

Fig. 2.119 Benign mass in breast (fibroadenoma). Mammogram showing mass (arrows) with very well defined borders and coarse structured calcification.

3

Cardiovascular System

Echocardiography, radionuclide examinations and plain films are the standard non-invasive imaging investigations used in cardiac disease. Echocardiography provides morphological as well as functional information. It is excellent for looking at the heart valves, assessing chamber morphology and volume, determining the thickness of the ventricular wall and diagnosing intraluminal masses. Doppler ultrasound is an extremely useful tool for determining the velocity and direction of blood flow through the heart valves and within cardiac chambers. Radionuclide examinations reflect physiological parameters such as myocardial blood flow and ventricular contractility but provide little anatomical detail, whereas plain radiographs are useful for looking at the effects of cardiac disease on the lungs and pleural cavities, but provide only limited information about the heart itself. Cardiac fluoroscopy (screening) is occasionally used to look at the movement of prosthetic valves and to demonstrate cardiac calcifications. MRI provides both functional and anatomical information but is only available in specialised centres and is only used for specific reasons.

Techniques

Plain radiography

The standard plain films for the evaluation of cardiac disease are the posteroanterior (PA) view and a lateral chest film (Fig. 3.1). The PA view must be sufficiently penetrated to see the shadows within the heart, e.g. the double contour of the left atrium and valve calcification.

When looking at plain films in patients with possible cardiac disorders, the heart and great vessels should be assessed for size and shape. A potential pitfall is falsely diagnosing heart disease in a patient with a severely *depressed sternum* (pectus excavatum) in whom the cardiac outline appears altered simply due to rotation and displacement (Fig. 3.2). Normally, there are no visible calcifications within the heart and, therefore, any cardiac or pericardial calcifications should be noted and their positions established. Before leaving the mediastinum, the aortic arch should be examined to exclude signs of coarctation and to ensure that it is normally located to the left of the trachea. The lungs should then be examined for evidence of heart failure or alteration in blood flow.

Echocardiography

Three basic techniques are used in cardiac ultrasound: M-mode, two-dimensional sector scanning (sometimes called 'real time' echocardiography) and Doppler echocardiography. Because ultrasound is absorbed by the bones of the thorax and by air in the lungs, the views of the heart are necessarily limited.

M-mode

M-mode is a continuous scan recorded over a period of time using a pencil-beam of sound directed towards the structure of interest. The distance between the various structures and their movement towards and away from the transducer are recorded for short periods, usually 5–10 seconds, allowing measurements of chamber dimensions and wall thickness to be made.

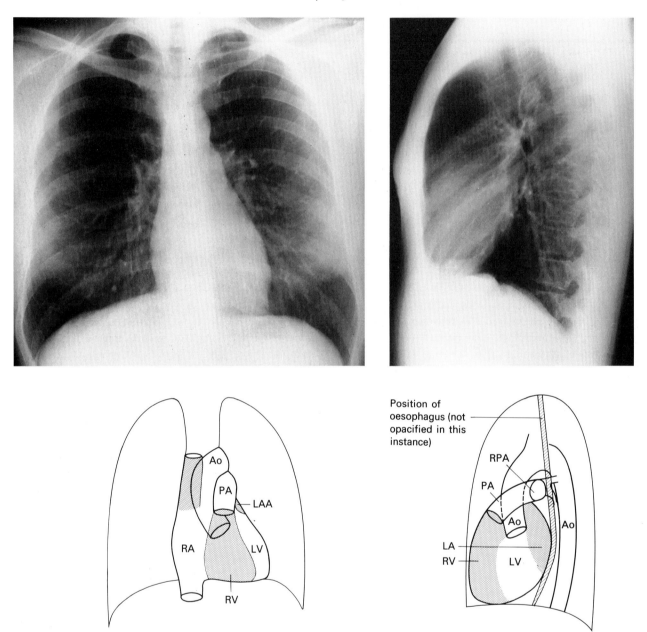

Fig. 3.1 Outline of heart in PA and lateral views. Ao, aorta; LAA, left atrial appendage; LA, left atrium; LV, left ventricle; PA, pulmonary artery; RA, right atrium; RPA, right pulmonary artery; RV, right ventricle.

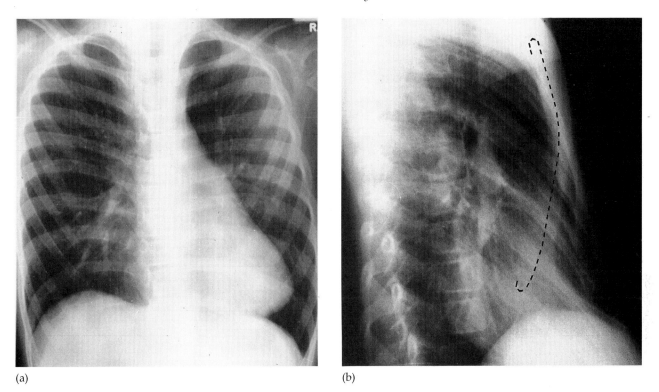

(a)   (b)

Fig. 3.2 Pectus excavatum. (a) PA view. Note how the heart is displaced and altered in shape by the depressed sternum. (b) Lateral film. The edge of the sternum has been traced in on this film. There was no cardiac disease in this patient.

Also, the pattern of movement of a structure, e.g. valve leaflets, may allow an abnormality to be diagnosed and may also provide an indication of its severity. The normal appearance of selected M-mode images is illustrated in Figure 3.3. M-mode examinations have been largely replaced by two-dimensional sector scanning, but they are still used for certain specific measurements such as the dimensions of the left ventricle in systole and diastole.

Two-dimensional sector scanning

Two-dimensional echocardiography demonstrates a fan-shaped slice of the heart in motion, which can be recorded on video tape, or still photographs can be made when necessary. By angling the transducer, the 'slice' can be moved through the heart to allow the observer to build up a mental picture of a three-dimensional image. Since tiny bubbles of air accompany the injection of almost any liquid and because ultrasound reliably detects even tiny gas bubbles within the blood stream, injections of saline can be used as a harmless intravascular 'contrast agent'.

The standard examination consists of a combination of short- and long-axis views, together with the so-called four chamber view (Figs 3.4, 3.5). The short- and long-axis views show a cross-section of the left ventricle and mitral and aortic valves. These views are obtained by placing the transducer in an intercostal space just to the left of the sternum (or, in some individuals, in a subcostal position). The four chamber view, which shows both ventricles and both atria together with the mitral and tricuspid valves, is obtained by placing the transducer over the cardiac

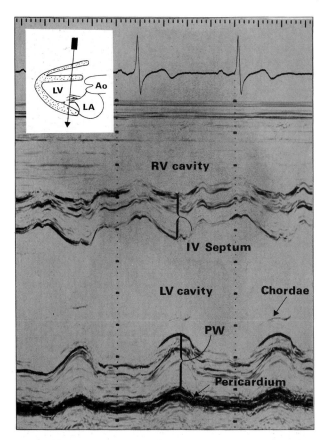

Fig. 3.3 M-mode scan. Parasternal long axis view through the mid left ventricular (LV) cavity. The thickness and movement of the interventricular septum (IV Septum) and the posterior wall (PW) of the left ventricle are well demonstrated and can be correlated with the ECG at the top of the trace. RV, right ventricular. © *1986 Andrew A. McLeod and Mark J. Monaghan.*

apex and aiming upward and medially. A newly introduced device is the oesophageal ultrasound probe, which looks at the cardiac structures from within the oesophagus from behind the heart.

Doppler echocardiography

As discussed on page 6, when sound waves are reflected from a moving object, the frequency of the

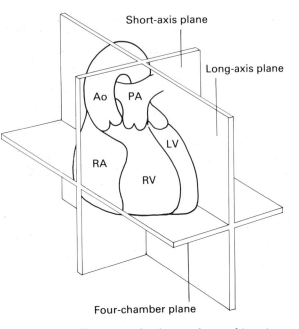

Fig. 3.4 Diagram illustrating the three orthogonal imaging planes used to demonstrate the heart with two-dimensional echocardiography. Ao, aorta; PA, pulmonary artery; RA, right atrium; RV, right ventricle; LV, left ventricle.

reflected waves is altered, depending on the velocity of the reflecting surface. When using Doppler techniques, red blood cells can be used as reflecting surfaces and the velocity of blood flow in a given direction can be calculated (Fig. 3.6). The accuracy of the technique depends on the angle of flow with respect to the ultrasound beam, flow directly in line with the beam being the most accurately measured.

Doppler flow measurements are used to: quantify pressure gradients across stenotic valves; quantify flow; measure cardiac output or left to right shunts; and detect and quantify valvular regurgitation (see Plate 3b, opposite p. 126). Pressure gradients are derived mathematically from formulae that convert velocity across a valve into a pressure gradient. Flow measurements depend on measuring the velocity by Doppler methods and then using standard ultrasound techniques to calculate the cross-sectional areas of the structure through which the blood is flowing.

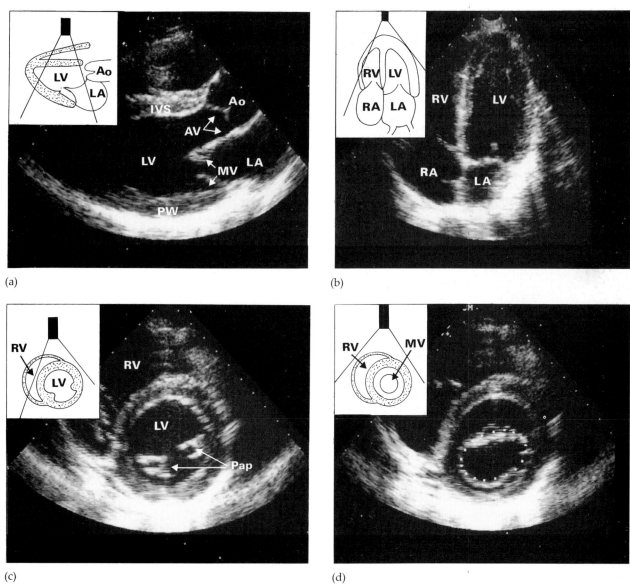

Fig. 3.5 Normal two-dimensional echocardiogram. (a) Parasternal long axis view. (b) Apical four chamber view. (c) Parasternal short axis view at level of papillary muscles. (d) Similar view to (c) but at level of mitral valve. The dots indicate the area of the open valve. Ao, aorta; AV, aortic valve; IVS, interventricular septum; LA, left atrium; LV, left ventricle; MV, mitral valve; Pap, papillary muscles; PW, posterior wall of LV; RA, right atrium; RV, right ventricle. © *1986 Andrew A. McLeod and Mark J. Monaghan.*

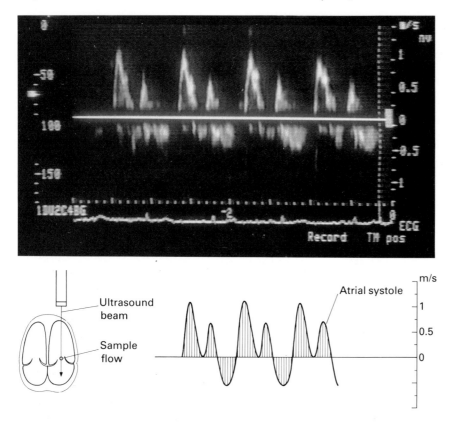

Fig. 3.6 Doppler ultrasound through normal mitral valve in the four-chamber view. Note the rapid initial velocity at 1 m/second, the rapid decline and then a second smaller peak caused by atrial systole.

A relatively newly-introduced technique is colour Doppler, where the direction and velocity of flow are colour-coded to allow the observer to appreciate the direction and magnitude of flow in specific anatomical sites (see Plate 3, opposite p. 126). Colour Doppler is particularly useful in complex congenital heart disease, e.g. finding multiple or unusually situated ventricular septal defects.

Radionuclide studies

Nuclear medicine techniques are simpler to perform than angiocardiography, are non-invasive and can be readily repeated. They give information on cardiac function but provide only limited anatomical detail.

The two most frequently used radionuclide investigations in cardiology are myocardial perfusion scintigraphy and radionuclide angiocardiography. Myocardial infarct imaging is discussed on page 125.

Myocardial perfusion scintigraphy

Myocardial perfusion scintigraphy makes use of the radionuclide thallium-201 (^{201}Tl) which is handled by the myocardial cells similarly to potassium. It is taken up in proportion to blood flow, so regions of reduced myocardial perfusion appear as areas of reduced uptake.

Thallium-201 myocardial imaging is used in the diagnosis of ischaemic heart disease and is particularly useful in patients with chest pain, in whom it is uncertain whether the pain is cardiac in origin. As many patients only show impaired myocardial perfusion on exercise, the patient exercises on a bicycle or on a treadmill. Just prior to maximal exercise, an intravenous injection of ^{201}Tl is given and the cardiac uptake of the radionuclide is then imaged in various projections using a gamma camera. The images are repeated after the patient has rested for 3—4 hours. The sites and sizes of ischaemic areas can be assessed and a distinction between ischaemic and infarcted regions can be made by comparing peak exercise and resting images (see p. 125).

The exercise examination should only be done under medical supervision with full resuscitation equipment available.

Radionuclide angiography

Radionuclide angiocardiography is also known as 'multiple gated equilibrium blood pool imaging', sometimes abbreviated to MUGA (multiple gated) scanning. It uses technetium-99m (^{99m}Tc) attached to red blood cells to image the blood pool. A convenient method of labelling is to inject stannous pyrophosphate intravenously, which acts as a reducing agent. Fifteen minutes later ^{99m}Tc-pertechnetate is injected intravenously, which enters and binds to the red blood cells for several hours.

As an alternative to this so called *in vivo* labelling, an *in vitro* technique can be used whereby 10 ml of blood are withdrawn; the red cells are separated by centrifuging, labelled with ^{99m}Tc, resuspended and then injected into the patient. After about 15 minutes to allow for complete mixing of the radionuclide tagged cells with the remainder of the patient's blood, the heart is imaged using a gamma camera.

Because insufficient radioactive counts are collected from each cardiac cycle, images from successive cardiac cycles are combined using electronic gating. Starting from the R wave of the ECG, each cardiac cycle is divided into a number of equal intervals. Data from each interval in each successive cardiac cycle are summed to give a representative cycle which is then displayed as a moving image on a TV monitor or cine loop. It is usually necessary to record data from about 400—500 cardiac cycles to obtain an adequate image.

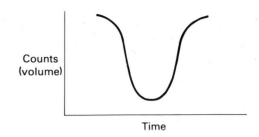

Fig. 3.7 Radionuclide angiocardiography. Graph of counts (ventricular volume) against time.

Radionuclide angiograms are used to calculate *ventricular ejection fractions* in patients with valvular disease and myocardial disorders, and for *wall motion analysis* in patients with ischaemic heart disease.

Since there is uniform mixing of the radionuclide with the blood, the radioactivity is proportional to the amount of blood in the ventricles. Individual frames from the summed cardiac cycles can be displayed on a television monitor. The boundaries of either ventricle in systole and diastole are drawn in by light pen or other electronic device and the computer can then construct curves of ventricular volume against time (Fig. 3.7).

After correcting for background activity, the values of the maximum (end diastole) and minimum (end systole) counts can be obtained and the ejection fraction can then be calculated:

$$\text{ejection fraction} = \frac{\text{end diastolic vol} - \text{end systolic vol}}{\text{end diastolic vol}}$$

Normally, the left ventricular ejection fraction should be greater than 50% and all parts of the ventricular outline should show equal movement. Segments of the wall with reduced movement or aneurysm formation can be demonstrated.

Computed tomography

Computed tomography, using conventional equipment, plays little or no part in the management of

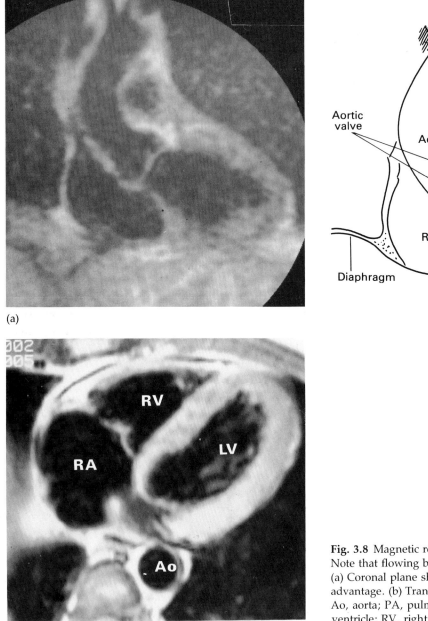

(a)

(b)

Fig. 3.8 Magnetic resonance imaging of the normal heart. Note that flowing blood has no signal and appears black. (a) Coronal plane showing aortic valve and left ventricle to advantage. (b) Transaxial plane (similar to that used for CT). Ao, aorta; PA, pulmonary artery; RA, right atrium; LV, left ventricle; RV, right ventricle.

intracardiac disorders, mainly because of the long scanning times required to image the heart. Pericardial effusions (see Fig. 3.15b, p. 114) and cardiac tumours are recognisable, but they are usually equally well or better seen at ultrasound. Specialised ultrafast CT scanners suitable for cardiac imaging are available in a few centres.

Magnetic resonance imaging

Electronic gating of the standard MRI sequences using the electrocardiogram provides separate images of the heart at various times in the cardiac cycle. With this particular technique, fast flowing blood produces no signal and, therefore, provides a natural contrast medium (Fig. 3.8). An alternative and more recently introduced technique is so-called 'fast imaging', a technique in which the images are obtained in much shorter times than with the standard techniques. The images are viewed as cine-images and are the equivalent of a tomographic cine-angiogram, usually displayed with the blood white and the heart muscle as darker signal.

Magnetic resonance imaging is capable of providing an immense amount of information, but currently its role is relatively limited because the technique is expensive and the specialised equipment and expertise to obtain high-quality cardiac images are only available in a few centres. Also, the other non-invasive diagnostic techniques, notably ultrasound and radionuclide imaging, provide so much information. MRI does, however, provide unique information. It can show:
- Details of complex congenital heart disease.
- Details of myocardial thickness and disease.
- Details of the great vessels, e.g. dissecting aneurysm. This is of particular value because ultrasound is, in general, very poor at showing structures outside the pericardial sac.
- Pericardial disease.
- Intracardiac tumours, which can be shown with great precision, better in many cases than with ultrasound.

Cardiac catheterisation and angiography

Catheters can be introduced under fluoroscopic control into the various chambers of the heart and into vessels that lead in and out of these chambers. Contrast injected through such catheters will provide images of the heart and great vessels. Cardiac angiography is a specialised topic which will not be discussed further.

Coronary angiography, which provides detailed information about coronary artery stenoses, occlusions and collateral or anomalous vessels, is widely practised in patients being considered for cardiac surgery, particularly for coronary artery revascularisation. Catheters are introduced into the femoral artery by the Seldinger technique (see p. 427), or into the brachial artery, usually by cut down, and passed selectively into the orifices of each coronary artery. With transfemoral techniques, separate catheters are usually needed for the left and right sides; 4–7 ml of contrast medium are injected and observed fluoroscopically with video and cine recordings being made simultaneously.

SIGNS OF HEART DISEASE

The heart

Valve movement, deformity and calcification

Information regarding valve movement and deformity is best obtained by echocardiography. The mitral valve is particularly well demonstrated. Normally, the leaflets of all the valves are thin and give rise to clearly defined echoes. The anterior leaflet of the mitral valve moves rapidly towards the transducer as it opens at the beginning of diastole. It then wafts backwards to a half-closed position before being pushed forward again by atrial contraction. With the commencement of systole it closes rapidly. The movements of the posterior leaflet mirror those of the anterior leaflet, but the amplitude is less.

The motion of the aortic valve leaflets is less complex. They open abruptly, stay maximally open

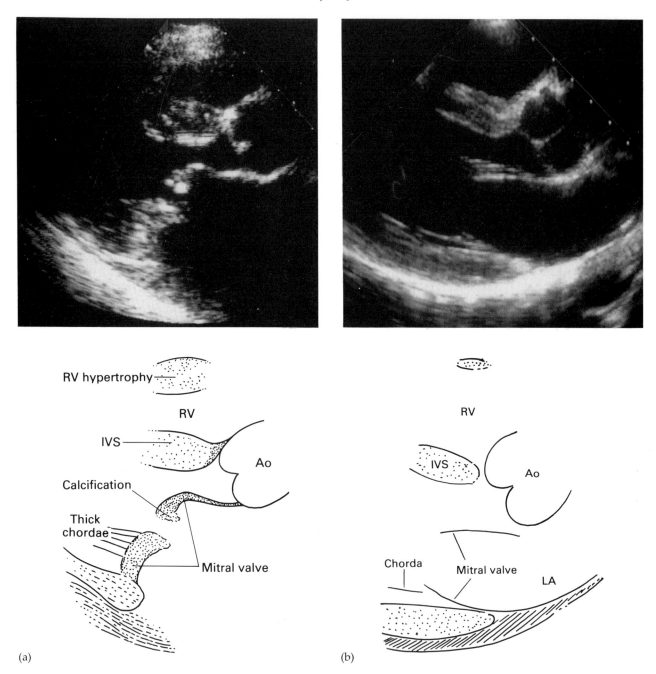

Fig. 3.9 Mitral stenosis. Two-dimensional echocardiogram—parasternal long axis view. (a) The mitral valve is markedly thickened and shows calcification. The image is during diastole when the valve should be open, but in this case the orifice is narrowed and opening is impaired. (b) Normal image for comparison. Ao, aorta; IVS, interventricular septum; LA, left atrium; RV, right ventricle. © *1986 Andrew A. McLeod and Mark J. Monaghan.*

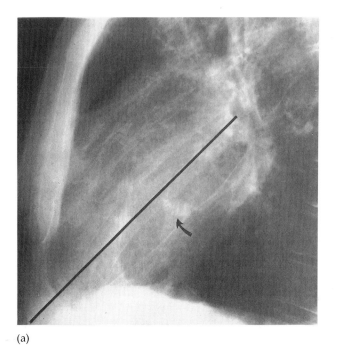

(a)

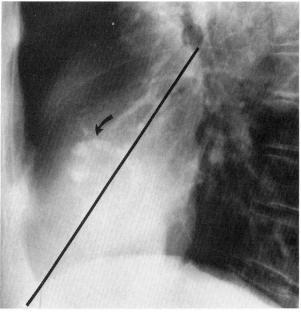

(b)

Fig. 3.10 Valvular calcification. A line is drawn from the sternodiaphragmatic junction to the left main bronchus. (a) Mitral valve calcification. The calcification lies below this line. (b) Aortic valve calcification. The calcification lies above this line.

during the remainder of systole and then close abruptly. The pulmonary and tricuspid valves are more difficult to image — their movements resemble those of the aortic and mitral valves respectively.

Echocardiography is especially valuable in evaluating mitral (Fig. 3.9) and aortic valve disease. Valve stenosis causes thickening of the valve leaflets, restriction of movement and narrowing of the orifice. Calcification, which is often present, is seen as a multiplicity of bright echoes arising within the leaflets (Fig. 3.9a). Valve gradients can be calculated using Doppler estimates for blood velocity and Doppler techniques can also be used to grade the severity of any regurgitation.

The only plain film information directly relating to the morphology of the valves is calcification. Calcification is better seen at fluoroscopy than on plain films. It occurs in the mitral and/or aortic valves in rheumatic heart disease and in the aortic valve alone in adults with congenital aortic stenosis. Valve calcification is easiest to identify on the lateral view. A line at approximately 45 degrees to the horizontal can be drawn from the junction of the diaphragm and sternum obliquely upwards and backwards to the left main bronchus (Fig. 3.10). Calcification in the mitral valve lies behind and below the line, whereas aortic valve calcification lies in front of and above it. Should the line pass through the calcification the smaller portion is ignored, but should it bisect the calcification, serious consideration should be given to the possibility that both valves are calcified. Calcification of the mitral valve ring is occasionally seen in the elderly, and is often associated with mild mitral regurgitation.

Heart size

Overall heart size is most easily assessed on plain chest radiographs. The cardiothoracic ratio (CTR) is a widely used but crude method of measurement; in normal people the transverse diameter of the heart is usually less than half the internal diameter of the chest (Fig. 3.11). Knowing whether or not the heart has increased in size compared with previous films is often more useful than the CTR in isolation. It should, however, be realised that the transverse cardiac diameter varies with the phase of respiration and, to some extent, with the cardiac cycle. Thus changes in transverse diameter of less than 1.5 cm should be interpreted with caution. An overall increase in heart size may be due to dilatation of one or more cardiac chambers and/or to pericardial effusion.

Chamber hypertrophy and dilatation

The causes of chamber enlargement are given in Table 3.1.

Echocardiography

Echocardiography is the most widely used method of diagnosing dilatation and hypertrophy of individual cardiac chambers. The dimensions of each chamber can be readily assessed. For example, the internal diameter of the left ventricle should not exceed 5.7 cm, and that of the left atrium in the parasternal view should be less than 4.0 cm. Echocardiography also provides accurate estimates of wall thickness, e.g. the left ventricular wall and interventricular septum should be between 0.6 and 1.1 cm.

Plain films

Diagnosing ventricular enlargement on plain films is fraught with problems. Only one, or at most two, of the borders of either ventricle are visible (Fig. 3.1). Also, it is difficult to distinguish ventricular hypertrophy from dilatation when looking at the external contours on the heart. In 'pressure overload' conditions such as systemic hypertension and aortic or pulmonary stenosis, the hypertrophied wall encroaches on the ventricular cavity and there is little change in the external contour of the heart until the ventricle fails.

'Volume overload' conditions such as valvular incompetence, left to right shunts, and damaged heart muscle result in dilatation of the relevant ventricles, which is recognised only as an overall increase in transverse cardiac diameter. A further problem is that enlargement of one ventricle affects the shape of the other and it is therefore only occasionally possible to recognise the classic features of left or right ventricular enlargement (Figs 3.12 and 3.13).

Assessment of atrial size on the plain chest radiographs, particularly left atrial enlargement, is easier: the right border of an enlarged left atrium is visible as a double contour adjacent to the right heart border, usually within the main cardiac shadow (Fig. 3.14). The left border is rarely visible though the left atrial appendage, when dilated, is seen as a bulge below the main pulmonary artery on the PA view. With massive enlargement, the left main bronchus is pushed upwards. The posterior margin of the left atrium is best

Table 3.1 Common causes of chamber enlargement

Left atrial enlargement
- Mitral stenosis
- Mitral incompetence
- Left atrial tumour, e.g. myxoma

Right atrial enlargement
- Right ventricular failure
- Tricuspid stenosis
- Tricuspid incompetence

Left ventricular enlargement
- Aortic and mitral incompetence
- Aortic stenosis and systemic hypertension only *after* left ventricular decompensation has occurred
- Ischaemic heart disease and cardiomyopathy of many types, once substantial muscle damage has occurred
- Patent ductus arteriosus and ventricular septal defect in cases with large left to right shunts

Right ventricular enlargement
- Atrial septal defect
- Tricuspid regurgitation
- Pulmonary stenosis and pulmonary hypertension only *after* right ventricular decompensation has occurred

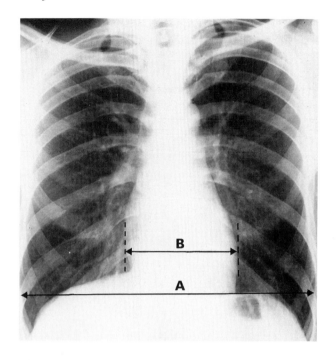

Fig. 3.11 Measurement of heart size. The transverse diameter of the heart is the distance between the two vertical tangents to the heart outline. When calculating the cardiothoracic ratio (CTR) the transverse diameter of the heart (B) is divided by the maximum internal diameter of the chest (A).

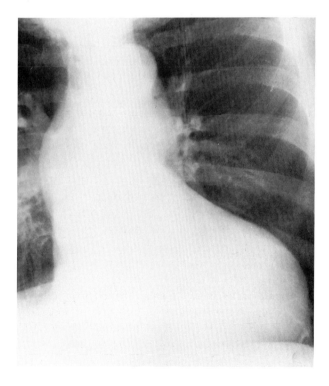

Fig. 3.12 Left ventricular enlargment in a patient with aortic incompetence. The cardiac apex is displaced downwards and to the left. Note also that the ascending aorta causes a bulge of the right mediastinal border — a feature that is almost always seen in significant aortic valve disease.

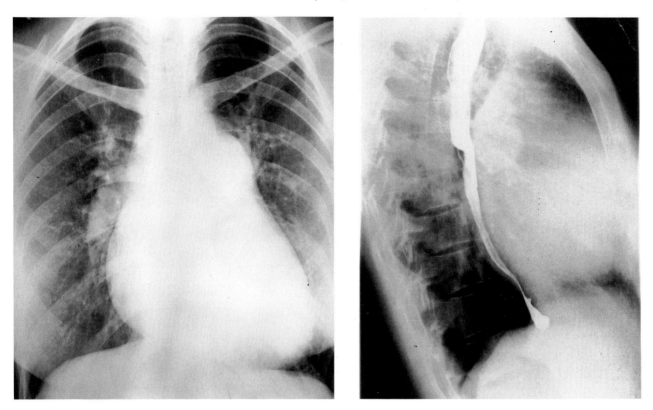

Fig. 3.13 Right ventricular enlargement in an adult with primary pulmonary hypertension. The heart is enlarged with the apex of the heart somewhat lifted off the diaphragm. On the lateral view the enlargement is all anterior, with no displacement of the lower oesophagus and more of the right ventricle than normal in contact with the sternum. Note also the features of pulmonary arterial hypertension — enlargement of the main pulmonary artery and hilar arteries with normal vessels within the lungs.

evaluated on the lateral view. Right atrial enlargement causes an increase in the curvature of the right heart border and is often accompanied by enlargement of the superior vena cava.

Ventricular contractility

Real time echocardiography, radionuclide angiocardiography and cine-MRI are all good non-invasive methods of assessing ventricular wall motion. Two major patterns of *decreased* contractility (hypokinesis) are seen:

- Generalised uniform reduction in contractility, which is usually due to valvular disorder or congestive cardiomyopathy. The ventricles in these conditions are usually dilated. Occasionally, multivessel coronary artery disease can cause a similar pattern.
- Focal reduction in contractility, which may or may not be accompanied by dilatation, is seen with ischaemic heart disease.

Increased contractility of the left ventricle indicates hypertrophy, which can be primary (hypertrophic cardiomyopathy) or secondary to other conditions such as aortic stenosis or systemic hypertension.

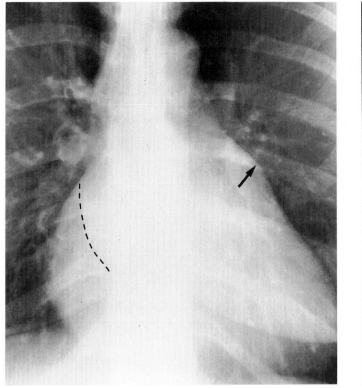
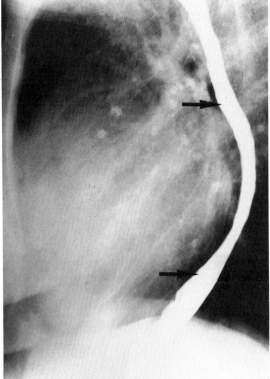

(a)

(b)

Fig. 3.14 (a) Left atrial enlargement in a patient with mitral valve disease showing the 'double contour sign' (the left atrial border has been drawn in) and dilatation of the left atrial appendage (LAA) (arrow). The enlarged LAA should not be confused with dilatation of the main pulmonary artery. The main pulmonary artery is the segment immediately below the aortic knuckle. The LAA is separated from the aortic knuckle by the main pulmonary artery (compare with Fig. 3.18). (b) The lateral view shows how the enlarged left atrium displaces the barium-filled oesophagus between the two arrows.

Pericardial disease

Echocardiography is ideally suited to detect pericardial fluid (Fig. 3.15a). Since patients are examined supine, fluid in the pericardial space tends to flow behind the left ventricle and is recognised as an echo-free space between the wall of the left ventricle and the pericardium. A smaller amount of fluid can usually be seen anterior to the right ventricle. Even quantities as small as 20–50 ml of pericardial fluid can be diagnosed by ultrasound. The nature of the fluid cannot usually be ascertained, and needle aspiration of the fluid may be necessary; such aspiration is best performed under ultrasound control. Pericardial effusion can also be recognised at CT (Fig. 3.15b) and MRI, although they are rarely performed primarily for this purpose. CT and MRI are particularly useful for assessing thickening of the pericardium, whereas echocardiography is poor in this regard.

It is unusual to be able to diagnose a pericardial effusion from the plain chest radiograph. Indeed, a patient may have sufficient pericardial fluid to cause life-threatening tamponade, but only have mild cardiac enlargement with an otherwise normal contour. A marked increase or decrease in the transverse cardiac diameter within a week or two, particularly if no

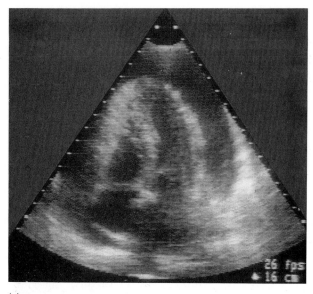

(a)

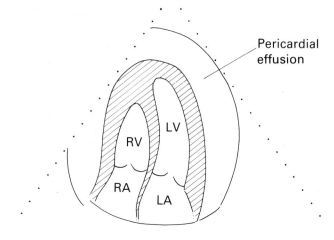

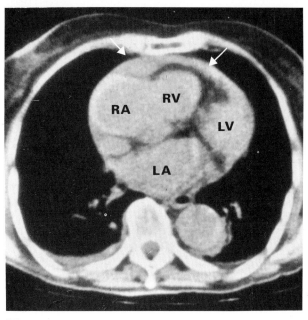

(b)

Fig. 3.15 (a) Large pericardial effusion on an apical four-chamber view echocardiogram. (b) CT scan showing fluid density (arrows) in pericardium.

pulmonary oedema occurs, is virtually diagnostic of the condition. Pericardial effusion should also be considered when the heart is greatly enlarged and there are no features to suggest specific chamber enlargement (Fig. 3.16).

Pericardial calcification is seen in up to 50% of patients with constrictive pericarditis (Fig. 3.17). Calcific constrictive pericarditis is usually postinfective in aetiology, tuberculosis and Coxsackie infections being the common known causes. In many cases no infecting agent can be identified. The calcification occurs patchily in the pericardium, even though the pericardium is thickened and rigid all over the heart. It may be difficult or even impossible to see the calcification on the frontal view. On the lateral film, it is usually maximal along the anterior and inferior pericardial borders. Widespread pericardial calcification is an important sign, because it makes the diagnosis of constrictive pericarditis certain.

Pulmonary vessels

The plain chest film provides a simple method of assessing the pulmonary vasculature. Even though it is not possible to measure the true diameter of the main pulmonary artery on plain film, there are degrees of bulging that permit one to say that it is indeed enlarged (Fig. 3.18). Conversely, the pulmonary artery may be recognisably small. The assessment of the hilar vessels can be more objective since the diameter of the right lower lobe artery can be measured: the diameter at its midpoint is normally between 9 and 16 mm. The size of the vessels within the lungs reflects pulmonary blood flow. There are no generally accepted measurements of normality, so the diagnosis is based on experience with normal films.

By observing the size of these various vessels it may be possible to diagnose one of the following haemodynamic patterns.

Increased pulmonary blood flow (Fig. 3.19)

Atrial septal defect, ventricular septal defect and patent ductus arteriosus are the common anomalies in which there is shunting of blood from the systemic to the pulmonary circuits (so-called left to right shunts), thereby increasing pulmonary blood flow. The severity of the shunt varies greatly. In patients with a haemodynamically significant left to right shunt (2 : 1 or more), all the vessels from the main pulmonary artery to the periphery of the lungs are large. This radiographic appearance is sometimes called *pulmonary*

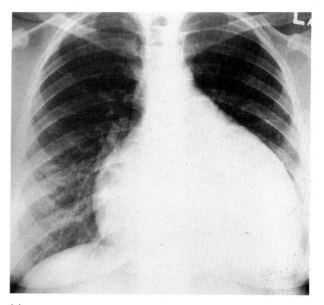

(a)

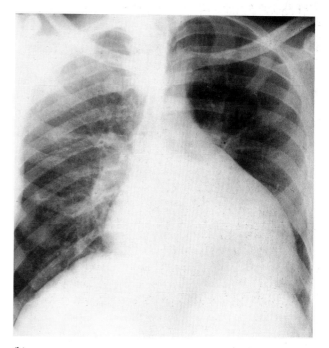

Fig. 3.16 (a) Pericardial effusion. The heart is greatly enlarged. (Three weeks before, the heart had been normal in shape and size.) The outline is well defined and the shape globular. The lungs are normal. The cause in this case was a viral pericarditis. This appearance of the heart, though highly suggestive of, is not specific to pericardial effusion. (Compare with (b).) (b) Congestive cardiomyopathy causing generalised cardiac dilatation. This appearance can easily be confused radiologically with a pericardial effusion.

(b)

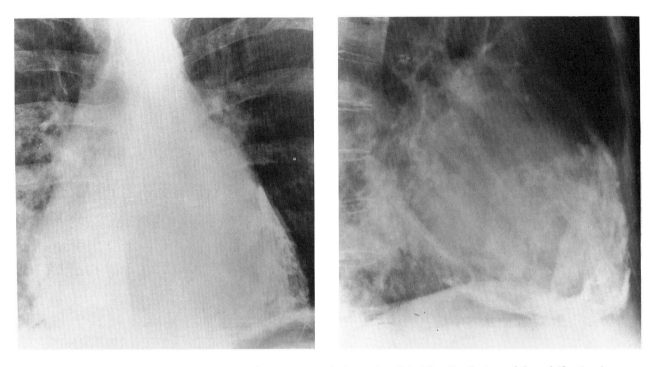

Fig. 3.17 Pericardial calcification in a patient with severe constrictive pericarditis. The distribution of the calcification is typical. It follows the contour of the heart and is maximal anteriorly and inferiorly. As always, it is more difficult to see the calcification on the PA film. (This patient also had pneumonia in the right lower lobe.)

plethora. There is reasonably good correlation between the size of the vessels on the chest film and the degree of shunting.

Decreased pulmonary blood flow

To be recognisable radiologically, the reduction in pulmonary blood flow must be substantial. The pulmonary vessels are all small, an appearance known as *pulmonary oligaemia*. The commonest cause is the tetralogy of Fallot (see Fig. 3.36, p. 131), where there is obstruction to the right ventricular outflow and a ventricular septal defect which allows right to left shunting of the blood.

Pulmonary valve stenosis only causes oligaemia in extremely severe cases in babies and very young children.

Pulmonary arterial hypertension (Figs 3.13 and 3.20)

The pressure in the pulmonary artery is dependent on cardiac output and pulmonary vascular resistance. The conditions that cause significant pulmonary arterial hypertension all increase the resistance of blood flow through the lungs. There are many such conditions including: various lung diseases (cor pulmonale); pulmonary emboli; pulmonary arterial narrowing in response to mitral valve disease or left to right shunts; and idiopathic pulmonary hypertension.

Pulmonary arterial hypertension has to be severe before it can be diagnosed on plain films and it is difficult to quantify in most cases. The plain chest film features are enlargement of the pulmonary artery and hilar arteries, the vessels within the lung being normal or small. When the pulmonary hypertension is part of

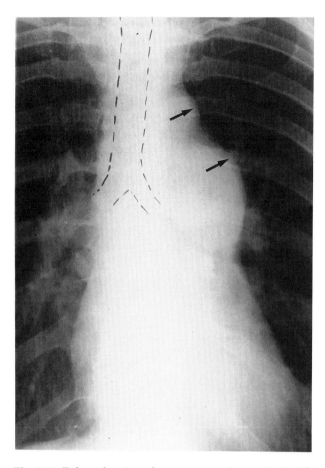

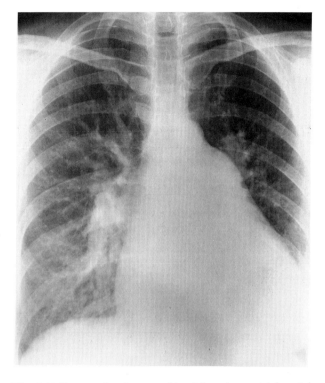

Fig. 3.19 Increased pulmonary blood flow in an atrial septal defect. Note the large heart and enlargement of the pulmonary vessels from the main pulmonary artery to the periphery of the lungs.

Fig. 3.18 Enlarged main pulmonary artery in a patient with pulmonary valve stenosis. The bulge of the main pulmonary artery (lower arrow) is clearly greater than normal and at first glance one might be deceived into diagnosing enlargement of the aorta. However, the aortic knuckle is the first 'bump' on the left mediastinal border (upper arrow). It projects 2.5–3 cm lateral to the trachea. The pulmonary artery forms the segment immediately below the aortic knuckle.

The reason for pulmonary arterial hypertension may be visible on the chest film, e.g. in cor pulmonale the lung disease is often radiologically obvious, and in mitral valve disease the other features described on page 121 will be seen.

Pulmonary venous hypertension (Fig. 3.21)

Mitral valve disease and left ventricular failure are the common causes of elevated pulmonary venous pressure. In the normal upright person, the lower zone vessels are larger than those in the upper zones. In raised pulmonary venous pressure, the upper zone vessels enlarge and in severe cases become larger than those in the lower zones. Eventually, pulmonary

Eisenmenger's syndrome (greatly raised pulmonary arterial resistance in association with atrial septal defect, ventricular septal defect or patent ductus arteriosus, leading to reversal of the shunt so that it becomes right to left), the vessels within the lungs may also be large, but there is still disproportionate enlargement of the central vessels (Fig. 3.20).

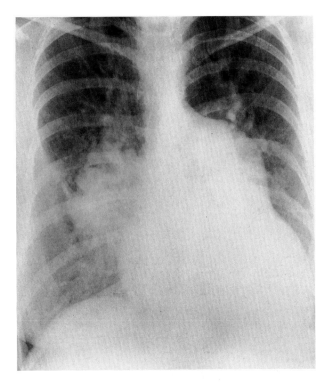

Fig. 3.20 Pulmonary arterial hypertension due, in this case, to an atrial septal defect with Eisenmenger's syndrome. The main pulmonary artery and hilar arteries are massive with an abrupt change in calibre of the vessels at the level of the segmental arteries. Note that the heart is also large.

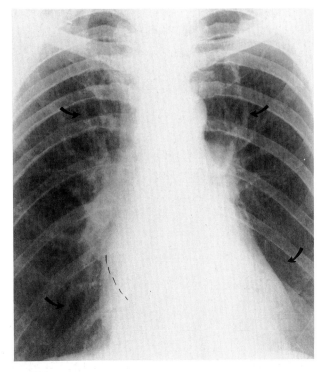

Fig. 3.21 Pulmonary venous hypertension in a patient with mitral valve disease. The upper zone vessels (arrowed) are larger than the equivalent vessels in the lower zones (arrowed). This is the reverse of the normal situation. (The left atrial border has been drawn in.)

oedema will supervene and may obscure the blood vessels.

Pulmonary oedema

The common cardiac conditions causing pulmonary oedema are left ventricular failure and mitral stenosis. Cardiogenic pulmonary oedema occurs when the pulmonary venous pressure rises above 24–25 mmHg (the osmotic pressure of plasma). Initially, the oedema is confined to the interstitial tissues of the lung, but if it becomes more severe fluid will also collect in the alveoli. Both interstitial and alveolar pulmonary oedema are recognisable on plain chest films.

Interstitial oedema (Fig. 3.22)

There are many septa in the lungs which are invisible in the normal chest film because they consist of little more than a sheet of connective tissue containing very small blood and lymph vessels. When thickened by oedema, the peripherally located septa may be seen as line shadows. These lines, known as Kerley B lines, named after the radiologist who first described them, are horizontal lines never more than 2 cm long seen laterally in the lower zones. They reach the lung edge and are, therefore, readily distinguished from blood vessels, which never extend into the outer centimetre of the lung. Other septa radiate towards the hila in the mid and upper zones (Kerley A lines). These are much

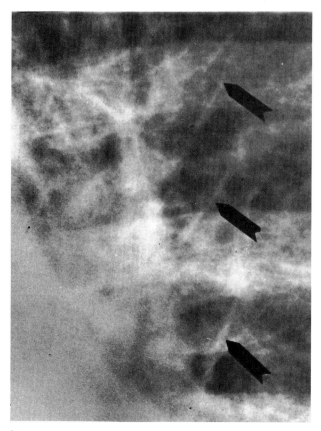

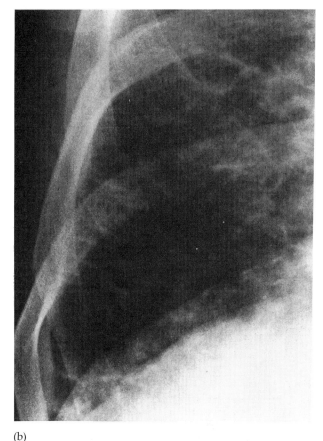

(a)   (b)

Fig. 3.22 Septal lines in interstitial pulmonary oedema. (a) Left upper zone showing the septal lines known as Kerley A lines (arrowed) in a patient with acute left ventricular failure following a myocardial infarction. Note that these lines are narrower and sharper than the adjacent blood vessels. (b) Right costophrenic angle showing the septal lines known as Kerley B lines in a patient with mitral stenosis. Note that these oedematous septa are horizontal non-branching lines which reach the pleura.

thinner than the adjacent blood vessels and are 3–4 cm in length. Another sign of interstitial oedema is that the outline of the blood vessels may become indistinct due to oedema collecting around them. This loss of clarity is a difficult sign to evaluate and it may only be recognised by looking at follow-up films after the oedema has cleared. Because oedema may collect against the fissures, they may appear thickened.

Alveolar oedema (Fig. 3.23)

Alveolar oedema is a more severe form of oedema in which the fluid collects in the alveoli. It is almost always bilateral, involving all the lobes. The pulmonary shadowing is usually maximal close to the hila and fades out peripherally leaving a relatively clear zone, which may contain septal lines, around the edge of the lobes. This pattern of oedema is sometimes referred to as the 'butterfly' or 'bat's wing' pattern.

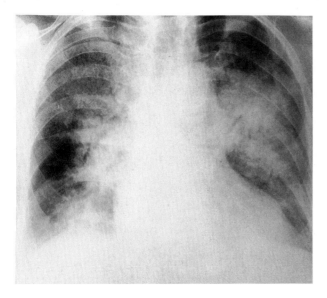

Fig. 3.23 Alveolar oedema in a patient with acute left ventricular failure following a myocardial infarction. The oedema fluid is concentrated in the more central portion of the lungs leaving a relatively clear zone peripherally. Note that all the lobes are fairly equally involved.

The aorta

With increasing age the aorta elongates. Elongation necessarily involves unfolding, because the aorta is fixed at the aortic valve and at the diaphragm. This unfolding results in the ascending aorta deviating to the right and the descending aorta to the left. Aortic unfolding can easily be confused with aortic dilatation.

True dilatation of the ascending aorta may be due to aneurysm formation or secondary to aortic regurgitation, aortic stenosis (Fig. 3.12, p. 111) or systemic hypertension.

The two common causes of *aneurysm* of the descending aorta are atheroma and aortic dissection. A rarer cause is previous trauma, usually following a severe deceleration injury. The diagnosis of aortic aneurysm may be obvious on plain film but it should be realised that substantial dilatation is needed before a bulge of the right mediastinal border can be recognised. Atheromatous aneurysms invariably show calcification in their walls and this calcification is usually recognisable on plain film. Computed tomography with intravenous contrast enhancement is very useful when assessing aortic aneurysms, particularly when diagnosing and showing the extent of aortic dissection. Echocardiography only shows aneurysms of the aortic root. When precise details of an aneurysm or aortic dissection are needed prior to surgery an aortogram may be indicated, but if the only information needed is the presence and/or size of an aneurysm then non-invasive tests such as CT, MRI or ultrasound are preferred (Fig. 3.24).

Two *congenital anomalies* of the aorta may be visible on plain films of the chest: coarctation (see p. 129) and right sided aortic arch, a condition that is sometimes seen in association with intracardiac malformations, notably tetralogy of Fallot, pulmonary atresia and truncus arteriosus. It can also be an isolated and clinically insignificant abnormality. In right aortic arch, the soft tissue shadow of the arch is seen to the right, instead of to the left, of the lower trachea.

Specific cardiac disorders

Heart failure

One or more of the following signs of heart failure may be seen on plain chest radiographs (Fig. 3.25) (these may coexist with the specific disorders described in the remainder of the chapter):

• Cardiac enlargement, with or without specific chamber enlargement.
• Evidence of raised pulmonary venous pressure, namely enlargement of the vessels in the upper zones of the lung.
• Evidence of pulmonary oedema.
• Pleural effusions, which are usually bilateral, often larger on the right than the left, and if unilateral are almost always right sided. In acute left ventricular failure small effusions are seen in the costophrenic angles running up the lateral chest wall. This fluid may, in fact, be oedema in the lungs rather than true pleural effusions.

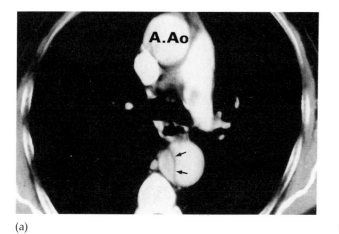

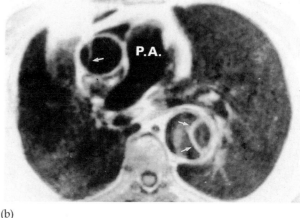

(a)   (b)

Fig. 3.24 Aortic dissection. (a) CT scan showing the displaced intima (arrows) separating the true and false lumina of the descending aorta. (b) MRI scan of a different patient, showing the displaced intima in the ascending and descending aorta (arrows). AAo, ascending aorta; PA, pulmonary artery.

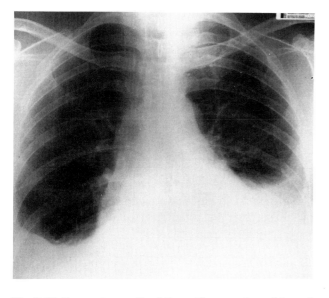

Fig. 3.25 Congestive cardiac failure. There are large bilateral pleural effusions. The heart is enlarged although it is difficult to measure it precisely because the pleural fluid obscures its borders.

Valvular heart disease

Valve stenosis and incompetence often coexist. It is, however, convenient to describe each separately.

Mitral stenosis

At *echocardiography*, the important features of mitral stenosis are enlargement of the left atrium, thickening of the valve leaflets and restriction of valve movement (Fig. 3.26a). The left atrial cavity should be routinely examined for thrombi. Calcifications of the valve appear as intensely echoreflective areas. The ability to measure the orifice of the mitral valve during diastole is a major advantage of two-dimensional echocardiography; a valve area of less than $1\,cm^2$ is classified as 'severe stenosis'. Right ventricular hypertrophy and dilatation may be present in patients whose mitral stenosis has resulted in pulmonary arterial hypertension. With Doppler techniques it is possible to measure the blood flow through the valve and so predict the gradient across the mitral valve. Left atrial myxoma, which can mimic mitral stenosis clinically, can be readily excluded by echocardiography.

The *plain chest radiograph* (Fig. 3.26b) will reveal left atrial enlargement, but the size of the left atrium

(a)

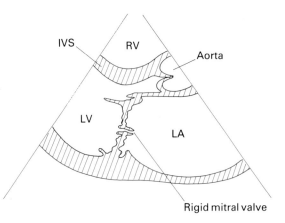

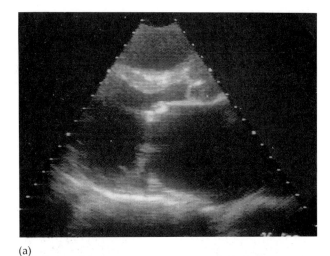

(b)

Fig. 3.26 Mitral stenosis. (a) Parasternal long axis view echocardiogram. Note the thickened mitral valve, which has hardly opened during diastole. (b) Plain film showing enlarged left atrium as a double contour at the right heart border (curved arrow). The left atrial appendage is also enlarged (straight arrow). Note how the upper zone vessels are larger than those in the lower zones. The overall size of the heart is not increased. IVS, interventricular septum.

correlates poorly with the severity of the stenosis. Apart from calcification of the valve (see Fig. 3.10, p. 109), there is little other useful information regarding the heart itself. The chief use of plain films is to show evidence of raised pulmonary venous pressure and pulmonary oedema—features that are not recognisable at echocardiography but which correlate well with the severity of the mitral stenosis.

Unless pulmonary hypertension develops, the transverse cardiac diameter is often normal. Pulmonary hypertension leads to several additional abnormalities: dilatation of the central pulmonary arteries, right ventricular enlargement and, if there is functional tricuspid incompetence, enlargement of the right atrium.

Widespread fine nodules may be seen in the lungs on chest films in patients who develop secondary haemosiderosis.

Mitral regurgitation

At *echocardiography*, the size of the left atrium and left ventricle are readily measured and Doppler techniques can be used to grade the severity of regurgitation. The appearance of a regurgitant valve depends on the cause. In cases of rheumatic valvular regurgitation, there is thickening of the valve cusps, whereas in conditions such as regurgitation secondary to left ventricular dilatation or rupture of the papilla, the valve cusps show no thickening. The abnormal motion seen in mitral valve prolapse, a condition in which there is myxomatous degeneration of the mitral valve, is readily detected with two-dimensional echocardiography and any associated regurgitation can be graded with Doppler techniques.

As with mitral stenosis, left atrial enlargement and evidence of raised pulmonary venous pressure are the important signs of mitral regurgitation on the *plain chest radiograph*. In most cases of mitral regurgitation, the size of the left atrium correlates reasonably well with the severity of the disease. An important difference from mitral stenosis is the presence of left ventricular enlargement.

Aortic stenosis

The *echocardiographic* hallmark of aortic stenosis is thickening of the aortic valve leaflets with narrowing of the orifice. The orifice can be measured; a valve area of less than $1\,cm^2$ indicates 'severe' stenosis. Again, Doppler ultrasound can be used to quantify the gradient.

The major features of aortic stenosis on *plain chest radiograph* are aortic valve calcification and poststenotic dilatation of the ascending aorta (Fig. 3.27). It is rare for an adult patient to have a severe gradient across the aortic valve unless aortic valve calcification is present. Recognisable left ventricular enlargement and raised pulmonary venous pressure are late signs indicating left ventricular failure.

Aortic regurgitation

Echocardiography can demonstrate the regurgitant jet (Plate 3a) and it is possible to grade the severity of regurgitation using Doppler techniques (Plate 3b). Diastolic fluttering of the mitral valve secondary to the regurgitant jet can be seen and is an indirect sign of the condition. An additional major use of echocardiography in aortic regurgitation is to show left ventricular volume and contraction.

On *plain film* the ascending aorta is dilated and

Fig. 3.27 Aortic stenosis showing poststenotic dilatation of the aorta (arrows). Despite the presence of a severe gradient there is little, if any, cardiac enlargement. The lateral view (see Fig. 3.10b) showed heavy calcification of the aortic valve—a feature not visible on the frontal view in this instance.

aortic regurgitation, when severe, leads to enlargement of the left ventricle which can be recognised early in the course of the disease (Fig. 3.12, p. 111). As the severity of the aortic regurgitation increases, the left atrium enlarges and changes due to raised pulmonary venous pressure develop.

Pulmonary stenosis

This condition is discussed under congenital heart disease on page 128.

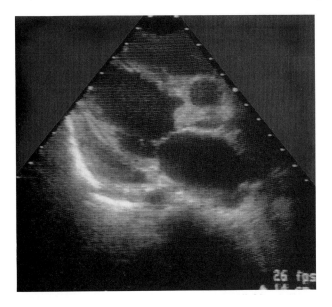

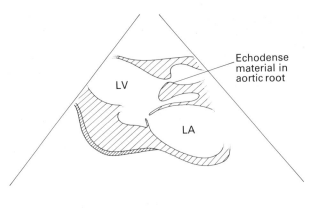

Fig. 3.28 Aortic root abscess and pericardial effusion: parasternal long axis view echocardiogram. Note the echodense material in the aortic root.

Tricuspid stenosis and regurgitation

Both of these conditions give rise to enlargement of the right atrium and superior vena cava. They are almost never seen as isolated abnormalities and the features of coexistent mitral valve disease or pulmonary hypertension often dominate the picture. The echocardiographic features are similar in principle to those seen in mitral valve disease.

Subacute bacterial endocarditis

The only imaging techniques that are capable of diagnosing the infection itself, as opposed to the accompanying valvular regurgitation, are echocardiography and MRI. They can demonstrate the infective vegetations of the endocardial surfaces, particularly on the valves, as well as any adjacent abscess formation (Fig. 3.28). The resolution of the techniques, however, is insufficient to exclude small vegetations. Vegetations on prosthetic valves are extremely difficult to identify.

Left atrial myxoma and other intracardiac masses

Intracardiac tumours are rare: left atrial myxoma is the most frequently encountered. It is a benign tumour which usually arises in the interatrial septum or in the wall of the left atrium. As it enlarges, it becomes pedunculated to float in the left atrial cavity. The myxoma may, therefore, interfere with the function of the mitral valve and mimic mitral stenosis or regurgitation both clinically and on plain chest radiographs. Echocardiography has proved to be an excellent tool for its diagnosis. A mass of echoes is seen in the cavity of the left atrium just behind the mitral valve (Fig. 3.29). The mass usually prolapses into the mitral valve orifice during diastole. The only differential diagnosis is left atrial thrombus in patients with rheumatic mitral stenosis. MRI has also proved to be an excellent method of demonstrating left atrial myxoma and other intracardiac tumours.

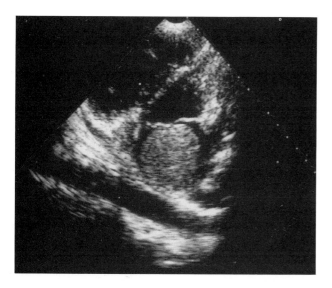

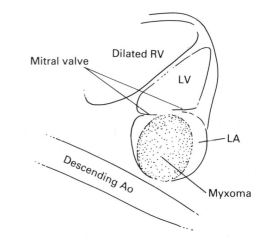

Fig. 3.29 Left atrial myxoma shown by two-dimensional echocardiography — modified apical four-chamber view. © *1986 Andrew A. McLeod and Mark J. Monaghan.*

Ischaemic heart disease

Most patients with angina or myocardial infarction have a normal plain chest film and a normal echocardiogram. The signs which may be present on *plain chest radiograph* include:

- Signs of raised pulmonary venous pressure and pulmonary oedema. The chest radiograph is a sensitive method of detecting these phenomena; indeed it is often more reliable than the physical examination.
- Cardiac enlargement and aneurysm formation. It is only when there is substantial muscle damage that cardiac enlargement occurs. Usually, there are no specific features to the cardiac contour, but an aneurysm may occasionally be recognised on plain film (Fig. 3.30a). Myocardial infarcts occasionally calcify, usually in association with aneurysm formation.
- Atheromatous calcification may be seen in the coronary arteries but, as elsewhere in the body, arterial calcification, though indicating the presence of atheroma, is a poor indicator of its severity.

Two-dimensional *echocardiography* allows one to observe the volume of the left ventricle and the motion of the various segments of its wall. Areas of diminished movement due to infarction can be demonstrated. A major use of echocardiography is to show aneurysms which appear as outwardly bulging thin areas of the myocardium (Fig. 3.30b). They most commonly involve the anterior wall and upper septum of the left ventricle. Blood clot contained within an aneurysm can be recognised as numerous constant echoes in the cavity of the aneurysm.

Thallium-201 *myocardial scintigraphy* allows one to determine areas of myocardial ischaemia and from their location it is sometimes possible to predict which of the coronary arteries is compromised (Fig. 3.31). Thallium scanning not only enables a diagnosis of ischaemia to be made but it can also help distinguish ischaemic muscle from scar due to infarction. Ischaemic areas seen on the exercise scan may show normal activity on the resting scan. Infarcted areas in which there is little, if any, remaining viable myocardium will show a persisting defect on the resting scan. This ability to distinguish ischaemia and infarction may be useful when planning cardiac surgery.

Radionuclide gated blood pool studies are sometimes performed as an alternative to ^{201}Tl scintigraphy in order to diagnose myocardial ischaemia. Ischaemic but viable areas may move normally at rest but not on exercise, whereas infarcted areas move poorly both at

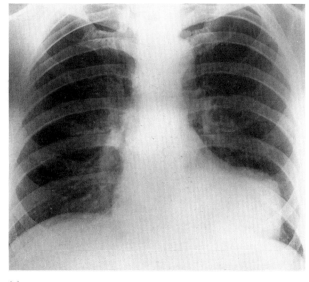

(a)

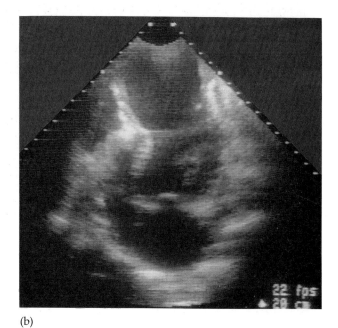

(b)

Fig. 3.30 Left ventricular aneurysm. (a) The transverse diameter of the heart is moderately enlarged. There is a bulge of the lower half of the left heart border extending down to the apex. This bulge is due to the aneurysm itself. (b) Apical four-chamber view echocardiogram of a left ventricular aneurysm in a different patient.

rest and on exercise. Alternatively, changes in ejection fraction between rest and exercise can be used. A fall of greater than 5% on exercise would indicate ischaemia, provided valvular disease or cardiomyopathy are excluded. A ventricular aneurysm can be readily recognised by viewing the gated blood pool studies. It appears as an area of paradoxical movement which bulges outward when the remainder of the ventricle contracts.

Acute myocardial infarcts can be imaged by nuclear medicine techniques. In practice, however, these tests are rarely performed. Technetium-99m pyrophosphate—the bone scanning agent—may concentrate in necrotic tissue, including myocardial infarcts, producing a 'hot spot'. The main disadvantage is the delay of 12–36 hours before the appearance of detectable uptake. Thallium-201 is sometimes used to image

acute myocardial infarction; it is not taken up by the infarcted tissue and, therefore, gives rise to a 'cold spot', a feature that can be identified after 6 hours.

Magnetic resonance imaging has been used to show areas of myocardial thinning following infarction and even to show altered signal in subacute infarction, but there is little clinical utility for MRI in ischaemic heart disease.

Demonstrating the state of the coronary arteries is

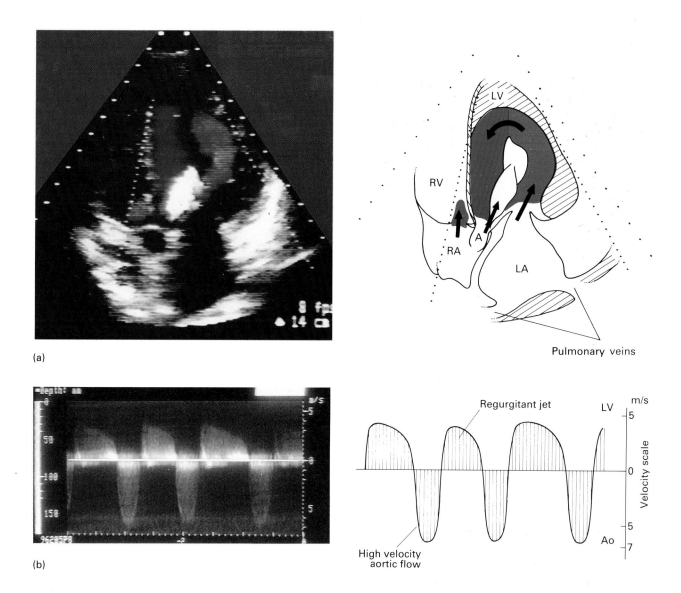

(a)

(b)

Plate 3 Aortic valve disease.

(a) Colour flow Doppler in a patient with aortic regurgitation. Apical four-chamber view showing turbulent jet (white) of regurgitant blood impinging on anterior leaflet of mitral valve to mix with the stream (red) passing from left atrium to left ventricle. Note change in colour to blue as the stream is directed by the ventricular apex towards the aortic valve. A small portion of right atrial to right ventricular flow is depicted in red.

(b) Continuous wave Doppler from the apical position in a patient with aortic stenosis and regurgitation showing a high velocity (7 m/s) jet into the aorta. There is immediate diastolic flow back into the left ventricle representing aortic regurgitation.

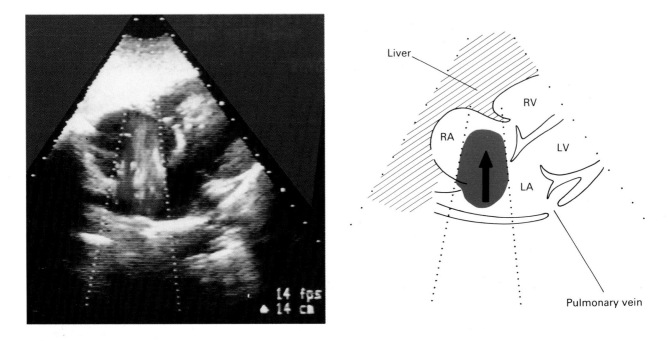

Plate 4 Atrial septal defect. Colour flow Doppler in the subcostal four-chamber view showing substantial flow (red) passing from left to right atrium.

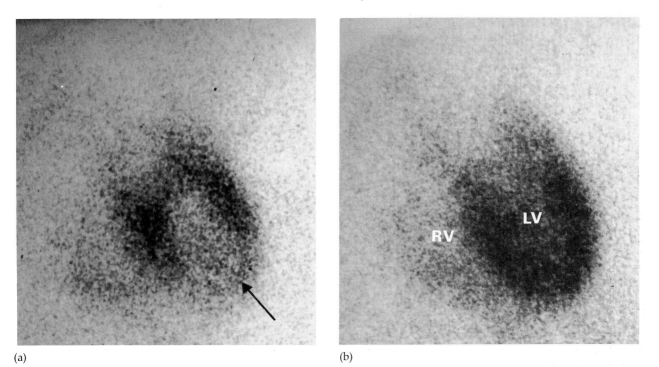

(a) (b)

Fig. 3.31 Thallium-201 myocardial perfusion scans. (a) Exercise scan showing an extensive area of poor perfusion in the apical region of the left ventricle (arrow). (b) The same patient, following surgical revascularisation, showing a normal appearance. LV, left ventricle; RV, right ventricle.

the province of coronary arteriography — a technique that is beyond the scope of this book.

Hypertensive heart disease and other myocardial problems

As discussed previously, ventricular hypertrophy without dilatation does not cause recognisable abnormality on plain chest films. Therefore, in systemic hypertension and various forms of cardiomyopathy the chest x-ray only becomes abnormal once ventricular dilatation has taken place. If there is a rise in left ventricular end-diastolic pressure, moderate left atrial enlargement and the signs of elevation of the pulmonary venous pressure may be seen. The shape of the heart is the same regardless of the cause of the myocardial disorder. The aorta is, however, large only in systemic hypertension.

Echocardiography in systemic hypertension shows a symmetrical increase in the thickness of the left ventricular wall with a normal aortic valve. Once decompensation occurs, the cavity will enlarge. The pattern of hypertrophy is different in idiopathic hypertrophic cardiomyopathy (also known as idiopathic hypertrophic subaortic stenosis or IHSS), in which the hypertrophy is much greater in the ventricular septum than in the free wall. This asymmetrical septal hypertrophy is diagnostic of the condition (Fig. 3.32).

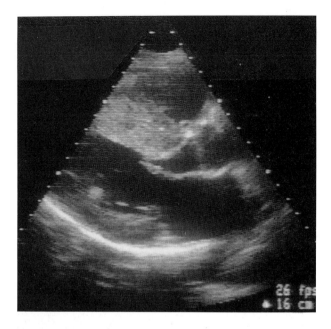

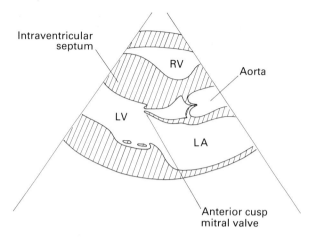

Fig. 3.32 Hypertrophic cardiomyopathy, parasternal long axis view echocardiogram. Note very thickened septum (almost 3 cm) and thickened ventricular walls. The anterior cusp of the mitral valve contacts the septum during diastole—a diagnostic feature of this condition.

Congenital heart disease

There are a large number of congenital malformations of the heart and great vessels. Frequently they are multiple. Echocardiography, MRI or angiocardiography are usually necessary for their elucidation, topics which are beyond the scope of this book. Only the plain film findings in a few selected disorders are discussed here. A major role of the chest radiograph is to assess pulmonary vascularity (Table 3.2)

Atrial septal defect, ventricular septal defect and patent ductus arteriosus

All these conditions give rise to cardiac enlargement and enlargement of the main pulmonary artery, large hilar arteries and pulmonary plethora (Fig. 3.33). These signs are usually only visible when the shunt through the defect is 2 : 1 or more. The value of plain film radiology is that it provides a simple method of estimating the degree of shunting in a patient known to have a left to right shunt. It is, however, of limited value in making a diagnostic distinction between the three major causes of left to right shunt. In cases of clinical diagnostic doubt (notably pulmonary stenosis which can be confused with atrial septal defect, and mitral regurgitation which can be confused with a ventricular septal defect), the presence of plethora indicates that the patient has a left to right shunt.

Echocardiography will show the size of the various cardiac chambers and a defect in the atrial or ventricular septum can be visualised directly. Even if the defect is not seen it may be possible to make the correct diagnosis by knowing which chambers are enlarged, e.g. absence of left ventricular enlargement in the presence of substantially increased pulmonary flow suggests an atrial septal defect. Colour Doppler is particularly useful in demonstrating septal defects (see Plate 4, opposite p. 127).

Pulmonary valve stenosis

Stenosis of the pulmonary valve can give rise to a specific appearance on plain chest radiography

Table 3.2 Commoner congenital heart disease: diagnosis based on blood vessel pattern

Plethora	*Normal vascularity*	*Oligaemia*
Not cyanosed		Severe pulmonary stenosis
ASD ⎫	ASD ⎫	
VSD ⎬ shunt > 2 : 1	VSD ⎬ shunt < 2 : 1	
PDA ⎭	PDA ⎭	
	Pulmonary stenosis	
	Coarctation of aorta	
Cyanosed		
Transposition of great arteries	Fallot's tetralogy	Fallot's tetralogy
Total anomalous pulmonary venous drainage	Pulmonary atresia	Pulmonary atresia
Truncus arteriosus		Tricuspid atresia
Eisenmenger ASD, VSD, PDA		

ASD, atrial septal defect; VSD, ventricular septal defect; PDA, patent ductus arteriosus.

(Fig. 3.34), namely enlargement of the main pulmonary artery and enlargement of the left pulmonary artery, the remainder of the lung vasculature being normal. The dilatation of these vessels is due to the phenomenon of poststenotic dilatation. Usually, the heart is not enlarged.

Coarctation of the aorta (Fig. 3.35)

An abnormal aortic arch is the commonest finding in coarctation of the aorta. The site of narrowing may be seen as an indentation and there is sometimes a bulge above the coarctation due to dilatation of the left subclavian artery, as well as a bulge below, due to poststenotic dilatation of the aorta. The heart is often enlarged, as is the ascending aorta, due to the long-standing hypertension.

Rib notching is a frequent sign in older childhood and in adults. It is due to the enlargement of intercostal arteries which act as collateral vessels, and which produce one or more small corticated indentations on the inferior margins of the posterior halves of the ribs from the third or fourth ribs downwards. Rib notching is not seen until late childhood.

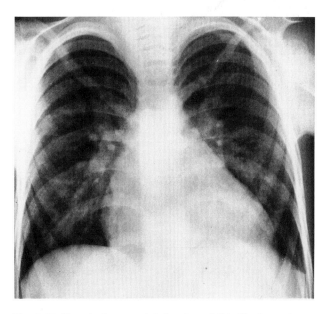

Fig. 3.33 Ventricular septal defect in a child. The heart is enlarged and there is obvious enlargement of the pulmonary vessels. The left-to-right shunt in this case was 3 : 1.

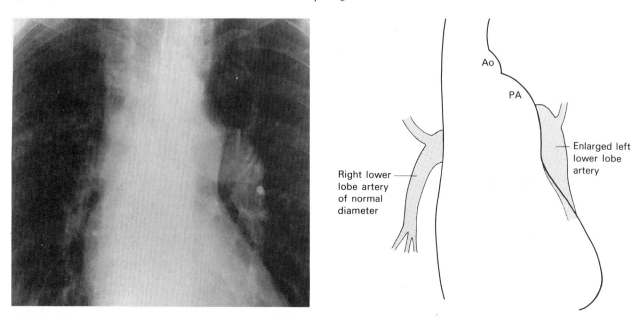

Fig. 3.34 Pulmonary valve stenosis. The heart is normal in size and the main pulmonary artery is enlarged. The left lower lobe artery is enlarged, whereas the right lower lobe artery is of normal diameter. The appearances are otherwise normal. PA, pulmonary artery; Ao, aorta.

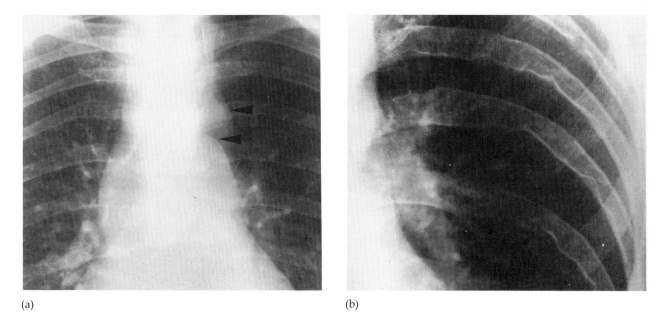

(a)   (b)

Fig. 3.35 Coarctation of the aorta. (a) Abnormal aortic knuckle: the lower arrow points to the poststenotic dilatation of the aorta immediately below the coarctation. The upper arrow indicates the dilated left subclavian artery above the coarctation. (b) Rib notching: portion of the ribs in another patient showing notching on the under surfaces.

Tetralogy of Fallot

Fallot's tetralogy consists essentially of a ventricular septal defect and right ventricular outflow obstruction, usually subvalvar or valvar stenosis. Right ventricular hypertrophy and the aorta overriding the ventricular septal defect are the other features that make up the tetralogy.

Approximately half the cases have a normal chest film. The abnormal radiological signs, when present, are an upturned cardiac apex and a bay in the region of the main pulmonary artery (Fig. 3.36), a shape sometimes referred to as a 'boot-shaped heart'. An important diagnostic feature is oligaemia of the lungs. The aorta is right-sided in 25% of patients.

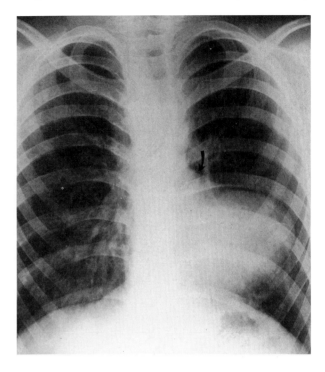

Fig. 3.36 Tetralogy of Fallot. The heart is not increased in overall size but shows a very abnormal outline. The apex is lifted up and there is a bay in the region of the main pulmonary artery (arrow). This combination is known as 'coeur en sabot' (boot-shaped heart). The aorta is right-sided as it is in 25% of cases. The hilar vessels are very small and the vessels in the lungs are also small.

4

Plain Abdomen

The standard plain films of the abdomen are the supine and erect AP views. An alternative to the erect AP view in patients unable to sit or stand is to take a lateral decubitus view (i.e. an AP film with the patient lying on his or her side). This view, like the erect view, utilises a horizontal x-ray beam. The main purpose of horizontal beam films is to detect air—fluid levels and free intraperitoneal air.

How to look at a plain abdominal film (Fig. 4.1)

• Relatively large amounts of gas are usually present in the stomach and colon in a normal patient. The stomach can be readily identified by its location above the transverse colon, by the band-like shadows of the gastric rugae in the supine view, and by the gas—fluid level beneath the left hemidiaphragm in the erect view. The duodenum often contains air and shows a fluid level. There may be some gas in the normal small bowel, but it is rarely sufficient to outline the whole of a loop. Short fluid levels in the small and large bowel are normal. Fluid levels become abnormal when they are seen in dilated loops of bowel or when they are very numerous. If the bowel is dilated it is important to try and decide which portion is involved.

• Look for any gas outside the lumen of the bowel. Its location and pattern often give valuable diagnostic information.

• Look for ascites and any soft tissue masses in the abdomen and pelvis.

• If there is any calcification try to locate exactly where it lies.

• Identify the liver and spleen. The liver is seen as a homogeneous opacity in the right upper quadrant, usually extending into the left upper quadrant. Occasionally, there is a tongue-like extension of the right lobe into the right iliac fossa. This is a normal variant known as a Reidl's lobe and should not be confused with generalised liver enlargement. The lower border of the liver is often difficult to see but its position can be predicted by the position of the gas in the hepatic flexure and transverse colon.

• Identify the borders of the kidneys, bladder and psoas muscles.

Dilatation of the bowel

The distinction between dilatation of the large and small bowel can be difficult. It depends on the appearance of the dilated bowel, the position and number of the bowel loops, and the presence of solid faeces. The presence of solid faeces is a useful and reliable indication of the position of the colon.

The colon can be recognised by its haustra, which usually form incomplete bands across the colonic gas shadows. They are always present in the ascending and transverse colon but may be absent distal to the splenic flexure. When the jejunum is dilated the valvulae conniventes can be identified. They are always closer together than the colonic haustra and cross the width of the bowel, often giving rise to the appearance known as 'a stack of coins' (Fig. 4.2). Problems may be encountered in distinguishing the lower ileum from the sigmoid colon since both may be smooth in outline. The radius of curvature of the loops is sometimes helpful in this respect: the tighter the curve the more likely it is to be a dilated loop of small bowel.

The small bowel usually lies in the centre of the

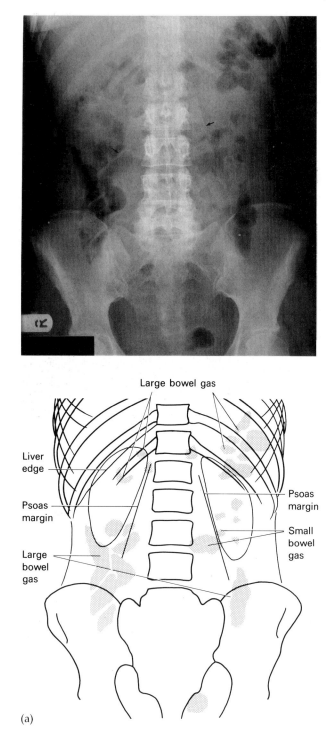

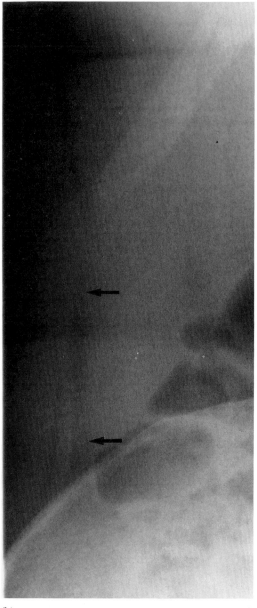

(b)

Fig. 4.1 Normal plain abdominal film. (a) Normal abdomen.
The arrows point to the lateral borders of the psoas muscles.
The renal outlines are obscured by the overlying colon;
(b) Normal extraperitoneal fat stripe. Part of the right flank
showing the layer of extraperitoneal fat (arrows) which
indicates the position of the peritoneum.

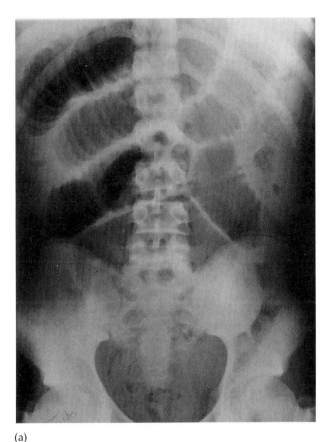 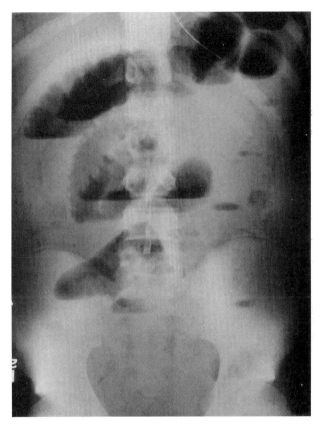

(a)   (b)

Fig. 4.2 Small bowel obstruction due to adhesions. (a) Supine. (b) Erect. The jejunal loops are markedly dilated and show air–fluid levels in the erect film. The jejunum is recognised by the presence of valvulae conniventes. Note the large bowel contains less gas than normal.

abdomen within the 'frame' of the large bowel, but the sigmoid and transverse colon are frequently very redundant and may also lie in the centre of the abdomen, particularly when dilated.

The number of dilated loops is a valuable distinguishing feature between small and large bowel dilatation, because even with a very redundant colon one does not see the numerous layered loops that are so often present with small bowel dilatation.

Dilatation of the bowel occurs in mechanical obstruction, paralytic ileus, acute ischaemia and inflammatory bowel disease. The radiological differential diagnosis of these phenomena depends mainly on the

distribution of the dilated loops. The following patterns can be recognised:

1 *Mechanical obstruction of the small bowel* (Fig. 4.2) causes small bowel dilatation with a normal or reduced calibre to the large bowel.

2 *Obstruction of the large bowel* (Fig. 4.3) causes dilation of the colon down to the point of obstruction, and may be accompanied by small bowel dilatation if the ileocaecal valve becomes incompetent.

3 In *generalised paralytic ileus* (Fig. 4.4) both the large and the small bowel will be dilated. The dilatation often extends down into the sigmoid colon and gas may be present in the rectum. It may be difficult

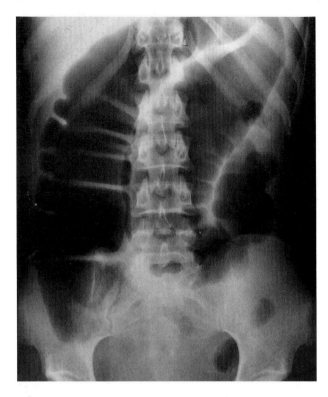

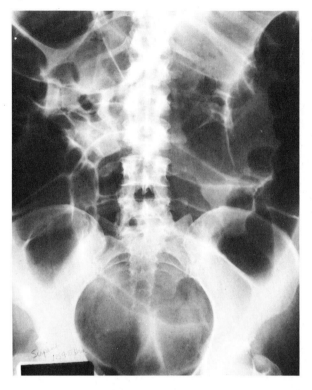

Fig. 4.3 Large bowel obstruction due to carcinoma at the splenic flexure. There is marked dilatation of the large bowel from the caecum to the splenic flexure.

Fig. 4.4 Paralytic ileus. There is considerable dilatation of the whole of the large bowel extending well down into the pelvis. Small bowel dilatation is also seen.

to differentiate such cases from low large bowel obstruction.

4 *Local peritonitis* often results in dilatation of the loops adjacent to the inflammatory process, giving rise to the so-called 'sentinel loops' which may be seen, for example, in appendicitis and pancreatitis.

5 Patients with *gastroenteritis* may show a number of patterns: some patients have a normal film and some show excess fluid levels without dilatation, whereas some mimic paralytic ileus and others small bowel obstruction.

6 *Small bowel infarction* may mimic both obstruction of the small bowel and obstruction of the large bowel.

7 *Closed loop obstruction*. The diagnosis depends on whether the loop in question contains air. If it does, as for example in a caecal or sigmoid volvulus, the dilated loop is seen filled with gas in a characteristic shape (Fig. 4.5). If the closed loop is filled with fluid it may not be visible—the common situation in most obstructed hernias.

8 *Toxic dilatation of the colon*. Should this occur in patients with ulcerative colitis, or more rarely Crohn's disease, the large bowel becomes distended (Fig. 4.6). In most of the patients maximal dilatation occurs in the transverse colon; indeed, the descending colon may be narrower than normal. The haustra are lost or grossly abnormal and the swollen islands of mucosa between the ulcers can be recognised as polypoid shadows. If the transverse colon is more than 6 cm in diameter in a patient with colitis, toxic dilatation should be strongly suspected. One cannot, however, make the diagnosis of 'toxic' dilatation from radio-

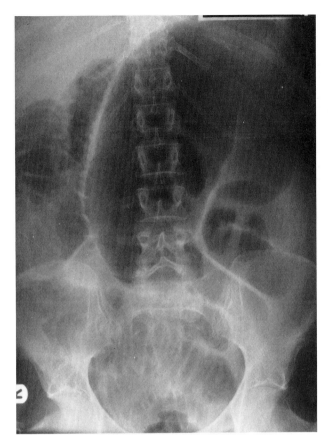

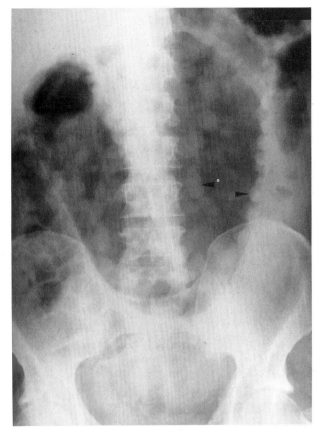

Fig. 4.5 Volvulus of the caecum. The twisted obstructed caecum and ascending colon now lie on the left side of the abdomen and appear as a large gas shadow. There is also extensive small bowel dilatation due to obstruction by the volvulus.

Fig. 4.6 Toxic dilatation of the large bowel due to ulcerative colitis. The dilatation is maximal in the transverse colon. Note the loss of haustra and islands of hypertrophied mucosa. Two of these pseudopolyps are arrowed.

logical findings alone since not all patients with these findings are toxic on clinical examination.

Gas outside the lumen of the bowel

Gas outside the lumen of the bowel is abnormal. Its location can usually be assessed by plain films.

● *Gas in the peritoneal cavity* (Fig. 4.7) is almost always due to perforation of the gastrointestinal tract, or follows surgical intervention in the abdomen. The most common cause of spontaneous pneumoperitoneum is a perforated peptic ulcer and two-thirds of such cases are recognisable radiologically. The largest quantities of free gas are seen after colonic perforation and the smallest amounts with leakage from the small bowel. A pneumoperitoneum is very rare in acute appendicitis even if the appendix is perforated.

Free intraperitoneal air is a normal finding after a laparotomy. In adults, all the air is usually absorbed within 7 days. In children, the air absorbs very much

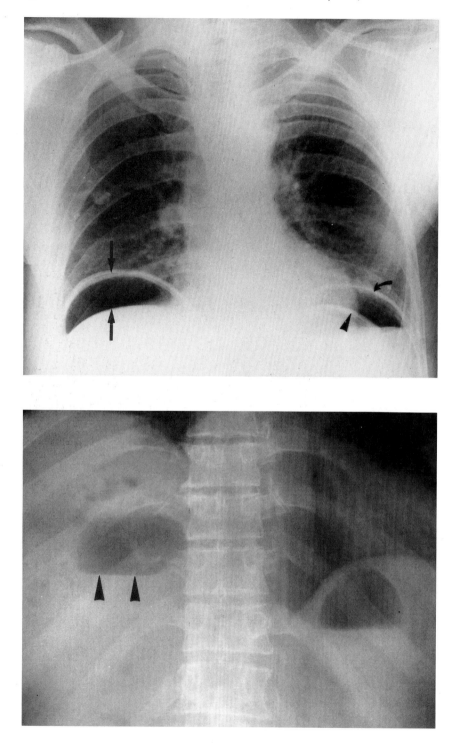

Fig. 4.7 Free gas in the peritoneal cavity. On this chest radiograph air can be seen under the domes of both hemidiaphragms. The curved arrow points to the left hemidiaphragm and the arrow head to the wall of the stomach. The two vertical arrows on the right point to the diaphragm and upper border of the liver.

Fig. 4.8 Gas in a right subphrenic abscess. There are several collections of gas within the abscess. The largest of these contains a fluid level (arrows). The air–fluid level under the left hemidiaphragm is normal. It is in the stomach.

faster, usually within 24 hours. An increase in the amount of air on successive films indicates continuing leakage of air.

Air under the right hemidiaphragm is usually easy to recognise on an erect abdominal or chest film as a curvilinear collection of gas between the line of the diaphragm and the opacity of the liver. Free gas under the left hemidiaphragm is more difficult to identify because of the overlapping gas shadows of the stomach and splenic flexure of colon. Gas in these organs may mimic free intraperitoneal air when none is present. Gas under the diaphragm is much easier to diagnose on an erect chest film than on an upright abdominal film. If there is doubt about the presence of a pneumo-peritoneum, a lateral decubitus film will show the air collected beneath the flank. It is important to realise that when the patient is lying flat the free gas collects centrally beneath the abdominal wall and is very difficult to identify on the conventional supine film.

• *Gas in an abscess* (Fig. 4.8) produces a very variable pattern on plain films. It may form either small bubbles or larger collections of air, both of which could be confused with gas within the bowel. Fluid levels in abscesses may be seen on a horizontal ray film. Since abscesses are mass lesions they displace the adjacent structures, e.g. the diaphragm is elevated with a sub-phrenic abscess, and the bowel is displaced by pericolic and pancreatic abscesses. Pleural or pulmonary shadows are very common in association with sub-phrenic abscess. Ultrasound, radionuclide examin-ations and computed tomography are extensively used to evaluate abdominal abscesses (see p. 285).

• *Gas in the wall of the bowel.* Numerous spherical or oval bubbles of gas are seen in the wall of the large bowel in adults in the benign condition known as *pneumatosis coli.* Linear streaks of intramural gas have a more sinister significance as they usually indicate infarction of the bowel wall. Gas in the wall of the bowel in the neonatal period, whatever its shape, is diagnostic of necrotising enterocolitis (Fig. 4.9), a dis-

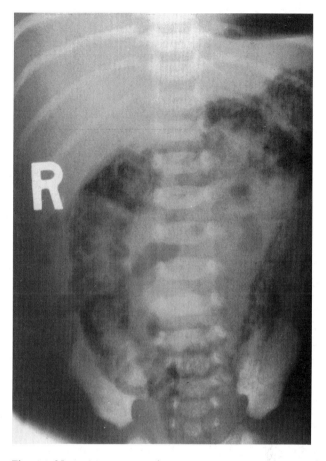

Fig. 4.9 Necrotising enterocolitis in a neonate. There is intramural gas throughout the colon.

ease that is fairly common in premature babies with respiratory problems.

• *Gas in the biliary system* is seen on plain films follow-ing sphincterotomy or anastomosis of the common bile duct to the bowel (Fig. 4.10). It is also seen with a fistula due to erosion of a gallstone into the duodenum or colon, or following penetration of a duodenal ulcer into the common bile duct.

Gas may be seen, very occasionally, in the wall or lumen of the gall bladder in acute cholecystitis due to gas-forming organisms.

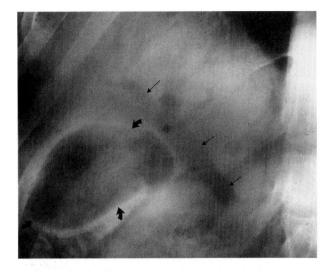

Fig. 4.10 Gas in the biliary tree. The gall bladder (curved arrows) and the duct system (straight arrows) have been outlined with air. The patient had an anastomosis of the common bile duct to the bowel.

Ascites

Small amounts of ascites cannot be detected on plain films. Larger quantities separate the loops of bowel from one another and displace the ascending and descending colon from the fat stripes which indicate the position of the peritoneum along the lateral abdominal walls (see Fig. 4.1, p. 134). The loops of small bowel float to the centre of the abdomen (Fig. 4.11).

In practice, plain films are of very limited value in the diagnosis of ascites, since the signs are so difficult to interpret confidently except when large amounts of ascites are present. Ascites is readily recognised at ultrasound or computed tomography (see p. 285).

Abdominal calcifications

An attempt should always be made to determine the nature of any abdominal calcification. The first essential is to localise the calcification; for this, a lateral or oblique view may be necessary. Once the organ of origin is known, the pattern or shape of the

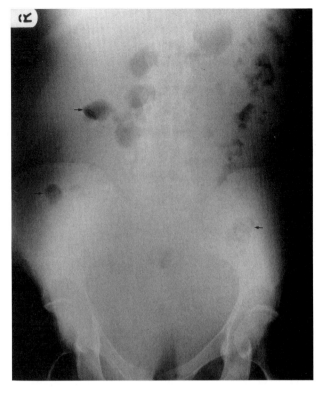

Fig. 4.11 Ascites. Note how the gas in the ascending and descending colon (arrows) is displaced by the fluid away from the side walls of the abdomen.

calcification will usually limit the diagnosis to just one or two alternatives.

The most common calcifications are of little or no significance to the patient. These include phleboliths, calcified lymph nodes, costal cartilages and arterial calcification. Calcifications in the abdomen are likely to be as follows:

• *Pelvic vein phleboliths* (Fig. 4.12) are very common; the only problem they cause is that they may be difficult to distinguish from urinary calculi and faecaliths. As with phleboliths, calcified *mesenteric lymph nodes*, due to old tuberculosis, are important only in that they may be difficult to differentiate from other more important calcifications. Their pattern is often specific: they are irregular in outline and very dense and since they lie in the mesentery they are often

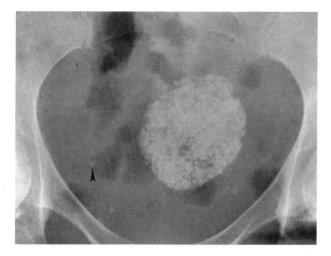

Fig. 4.12 Calcification in a large uterine fibroid. There are also several phleboliths, one of which is arrowed.

mobile. It is usually possible to see that they are composed of a conglomeration of smaller rounded calcifications.

● *Vascular calcification* occurs in association with atheroma, but there is no correlation with the haemodynamic severity of the vascular disease.

Calcification is frequently present in the walls of *abdominal aortic aneurysms*. It is usually easier to assess the size of such aneurysms on the lateral projection (Fig. 4.13).

● *Uterine fibroids* (Fig. 4.12) may contain numerous irregularly shaped well-defined calcifications conforming to the spherical outline of fibroids. Again, the calcification is by itself of no significance to the patient.

● *Malignant ovarian masses* occasionally contain visible calcium. The only benign ovarian lesion that is visibly calcified is the *dermoid cyst*, which may contain various calcified components, of which teeth are the commonest.

● *Adrenal calcification* (Fig. 4.14) occurs after adrenal haemorrhage, after tuberculosis and occasionally in adrenal tumours. However, the majority of patients with adrenal calcification are asymptomatic healthy people in whom the cause of the calcification is unclear.

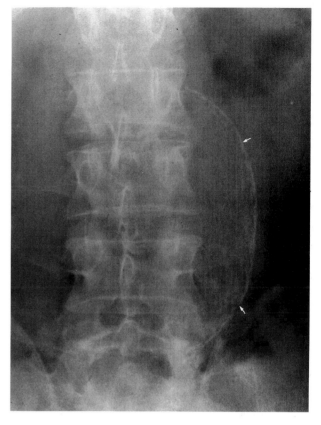

Fig. 4.13 Calcified abdominal aortic aneurysm (arrows). The aneurysm measured 8 cm in diameter on the lateral view.

Only a minority of patients with Addison's disease have adrenal calcification.

● *Liver calcification* occurs in hepatomas and rarely in other tumours. Hydatid cysts, old abscesses and tuberculosis may also calcify. Gallstones, renal stones and costal cartilage are common causes of calcification projected over the liver shadow.

● *Splenic calcification* is rarely of clinical significance. It is seen in cysts, infarcts, old haematomas and following tuberculosis.

● *Pancreatic calcification* occurs in chronic pancreatitis. The calcifications are mainly small calculi within the pancreas. The position of the calcification usually enables the diagnosis to be made without difficulty (Fig. 4.15).

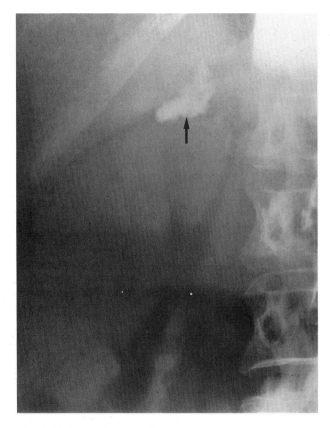

Fig. 4.14 Adrenal calcification.

• *Faecaliths*. Calcified faecaliths may be seen in diverticula of the colon or in the appendix (Fig. 4.16). Appendiceal faecaliths are an important radiological observation since the presence of an appendolith is a strong indication that the patient has acute appendicitis, often with gangrene and perforation. However, only a small proportion of patients with appendicitis have a radiologically visible appendolith.

• *Soft tissue calcification* in the buttocks may be seen following injection of certain medicines. These shadows can at times be confused with intra-abdominal calcifications.

• *Calcification of the urinary tract* is discussed on page 223.

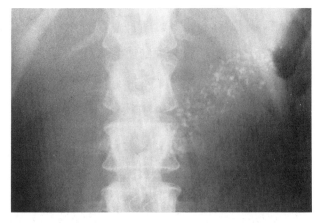

Fig. 4.15 Pancreatic calcification.

Plain films of the liver and spleen

Substantial enlargement of the liver has to occur before it can recognised on a plain abdominal film. As the liver enlarges it extends well below the costal margin displacing the hepatic flexure, transverse colon and right kidney downwards and displacing the stomach to the left. The diaphragm may also be elevated.

As the spleen enlarges the tip becomes visible in the left upper quadrant below the lower ribs. Eventually, it may fill the left side of the abdomen and even extend across the midline into the right lower quadrant. The splenic flexure of the colon and the left kidney are displaced downwards and the stomach is displaced to the right.

Following trauma, rupture of the spleen occurs more frequently than of the liver. As a haematoma forms the plain films may show a mass in the upper abdomen displacing adjacent structures. There may be paralytic ileus and fractures of the lower ribs may also be present. These signs, though helpful if present, are often not seen even with significant lacerations of the liver and spleen. For this reason, ultrasound or computed tomography (CT) is usually carried out in cases of suspected internal abdominal injury (see Chapter 6).

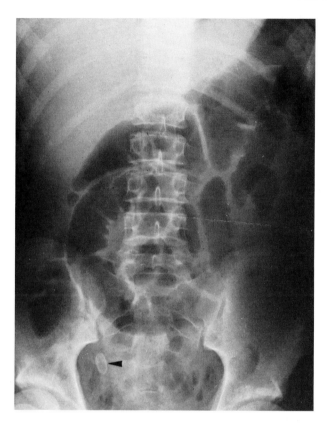

Fig. 4.16 Appendolith. The oval calcified shadow (arrow) is a faecalith in the appendix. The patient had perforated appendicitis. Note the dilated loops of small bowel in the centre of the abdomen due to peritonitis — the so-called 'sentinel loops'.

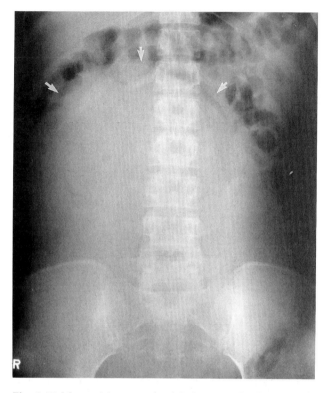

Fig. 4.17 Mass arising out of pelvis (arrows) displacing bowel to the sides of the abdomen. The mass was a large cystadenocarcinoma of the ovary.

Abdominal and pelvic masses

Attempting to diagnose the nature of an abdominal mass on a plain film is notoriously difficult, and resource to ultrasound or CT is invariably necessary. The site of the mass, displacement of adjacent structures and presence of calcification are important diagnostic signs but plain films are unable to distinguish between solid and cystic masses.

An enlarged bladder can be seen as a mass arising from the pelvis displacing loops of bowel. In females, uterine and ovarian enlargement also appear as masses arising from the pelvis. Ovarian cysts can become very large, almost filling the abdomen and displacing the bowel to the sides of the abdomen (Fig. 4.17).

Retroperitoneal tumours and lymph nodes, when large, become visible on plain films. Renal masses, especially cysts and hydronephrosis, can become large and appear as masses in the flank. With retroperitoneal masses the outline of the psoas muscle may become invisible.

5

Gastrointestinal Tract

The previous chapter showed that the plain film can be very informative in patients with an acute abdomen, but for most other intestinal disorders some form of contrast examination is necessary, as the other imaging modalities are only of limited use. Barium sulphate is the best contrast medium for the gastrointestinal tract. It produces excellent opacification, good coating of the mucosa and is completely intert. Its only major disadvantange is that when water is reabsorbed in the colon the barium may solidify and impact proximal to a colonic or rectal stricture. The other available contrast is water-soluble medium, Gastrografin. It has several disadvantages: it is hypertonic and soon becomes diluted; it is irritant should it inadvertently enter the lungs; and it is less radio-opaque than barium. Its major use is for opacifying the bowel prior to computed tomography scanning (CT) of the abdomen.

Gastrointestinal contrast examinations are carried out under fluoroscopic control so that the passage of contrast can be observed on a television monitor. By watching the television screen the radiologist is able to position the patient so that any abnormality is shown clearly. Films are taken to show fine detail and to serve as a permanent record. One of the values of fluoroscopy is to ensure that an abnormality has a constant appearance. Peristaltic waves are transitory and so can be easily distinguished from a true narrowing, which is constant.

The double-contrast examination of the stomach and colon is now widely practised. In the single-contrast method the bowel is filled only with barium. In the double-contrast technique the mucosa is coated with barium and the stomach or colon distended by introducing gas, often in combination with an injection of a short-acting smooth muscle relaxant to paralyse the bowel. The double-contrast method is a little more time consuming but shows the mucosa to advantage and demonstrates small abnormalities which would be obscured by a large volume of barium.

It is important to understand some basic terms applicable to barium examinations of the gastrointestinal tract which are often used in rather a loose way:

The wall of the bowel is never seen as such. What is seen is the outline of the lumen and from this one has to draw conclusions about the state of the wall. Usually, the most reliable information is obtained when the bowel is fully distended.

Mucosal folds are seen when the bowel is in a contracted state so that the mucosa becomes folded (see Fig. 5.5b, p. 148). When the bowel is distended these mucosal folds disappear. The normal mucosal fold pattern may be altered by smoothing out or by abnormal irregularity.

Filling defect is a term used to describe something occupying space within the bowel thereby preventing the normal filling of the lumen with barium. This creates an area of total or relative radiolucency within the barium column. There are three types of filling defects, each having distinct radiological signs:
1 An intraluminal filling defect is entirely within the lumen of the bowel (e.g. food), and has barium all around it (Fig. 5.1a).
2 An intramural filling defect arises from the wall of the bowel (e.g. a carcinoma or leiomyoma). It causes

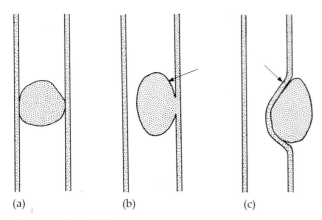

(a)   (b)   (c)

Fig. 5.1 Filling defects shown diagrammatically in the bowel. (a) Intraluminal. (b) Intramural. Note the sharp angle (arrow) made with the wall. (c) Extramural. There is a shallow angle (arrow) with the wall of the bowel.

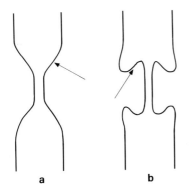

a   b

Fig. 5.2 Stricture. (a) Tapering ends (arrow). (b) Overhanging edges or shouldering (arrow).

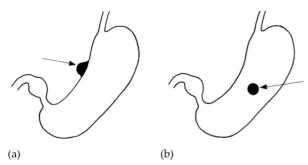

(a)   (b)

Fig. 5.3 Ulceration. (a) In profile the ulcer is seen as an outward projection (arrow); (b) *En face* the ulcer appears rounded (arrow).

an indentation from one side only, making a sharp angle with the wall of the bowel and is not completely surrounded by barium (Fig. 5.1b).

3 An extramural filling defect arises outside the bowel but compresses it, e.g. enlarged pancreas or lymph nodes. It also gives a narrowing from one side only but makes a shallow angle with the wall of the bowel. The mucosa is preserved but stretched over the filling defect (Fig. 5.1c).

A stricture is a circumferential or annular narrowing. A stricture must be differentiated from the transient narrowing which occurs with normal peristalsis. A stricture may have tapering ends (Fig. 5.2a) or it may end abruptly and have overhanging edges giving an appearance known as 'shouldering' (Fig. 5.2b). Shouldering is a feature of malignancy.

Ulceration. An ulcer is a breach of a mucosal surface which becomes visible when the crater contains barium. When viewed in profile it appears as an outward projection from the barium-filled lumen (Fig. 5.3a). When viewed *en face* the ulcer crater appears as a rounded collection of barium (Fig. 5.3b).

The oesophagus

Plain films do not normally show the oesophagus unless it is very dilated (e.g. achalasia), but they are of use in demonstrating an opaque foreign body such as a bone lodged in the oesophagus (Fig. 5.4).

The barium swallow is the contrast examination employed to visualise the oesophagus. The patient drinks some barium and its passage down the oesophagus is observed on a television monitor. Films are taken in an oblique position to project the oesophagus clear of the spine with the oesophagus both full of barium, to show the outline, and empty to show the mucosal pattern.

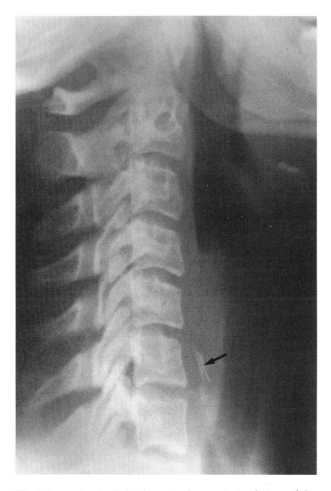

Fig. 5.4 Foreign body in the oesophagus. Lateral view of the neck showing a chicken bone (arrow) lodged in the upper end of the oesophagus.

Normal barium swallow

The oesophagus when full of barium should have a smooth outline. When empty and contracted, barium normally lies in between the folds of mucosa which appear as three or four long, straight parallel lines (Fig. 5.5).

The aortic arch gives a clearly visible impression on the left side of the oesophagus, which is more pronounced in the elderly as the aorta becomes tortuous and elongated. Below the aortic impression there is often a smaller impression due to the left main bronchus. The lower part of the oesophagus sweeps gently forward closely applied to the back of the left atrium and left ventricle.

Peristaltic waves can be observed during fluoroscopy. They move smoothly along the oesophagus to propel the barium rapidly into the stomach even if the patient swallows when lying flat. It is important not to confuse a contraction wave with a true narrowing: a narrowing is constant whereas a contraction wave is transitory. Sometimes the contraction waves do not occur in an oderly fashion but are pronounced and prolonged to give the oesophagus an undulated appearance (Fig. 5.6). These so-called tertiary contractions usually occur in the elderly and in most instances they do not give rise to symptoms. Occasionally, these contractions give rise to dysphagia and the condition is known as diffuse oesophageal spasm.

Abnormal barium swallow

Strictures

Strictures are an important cause of dysphagia. There are four main causes; carcinoma, peptic, achalasia and corrosive. In order to distinguish between these possibilities it is useful to answer the following questions:
• Where is the stricture?
• What is its shape?
• How long is it?
• Is there a soft tissue mass?

Carcinomas rarely arise from only one wall but usually involve the full circumference to form strictures. The stricture, which may occur anywhere in the oesophagus, shows an irregular lumen with shouldered edges and is normally several centimetres in length (Fig. 5.7). A soft tissue mass may be visible.

Computed tomography may be carried out, particularly if surgery is contemplated. Computed tomography shows the tumour causing thickening of the oesophageal wall. In addition it may show invasion of

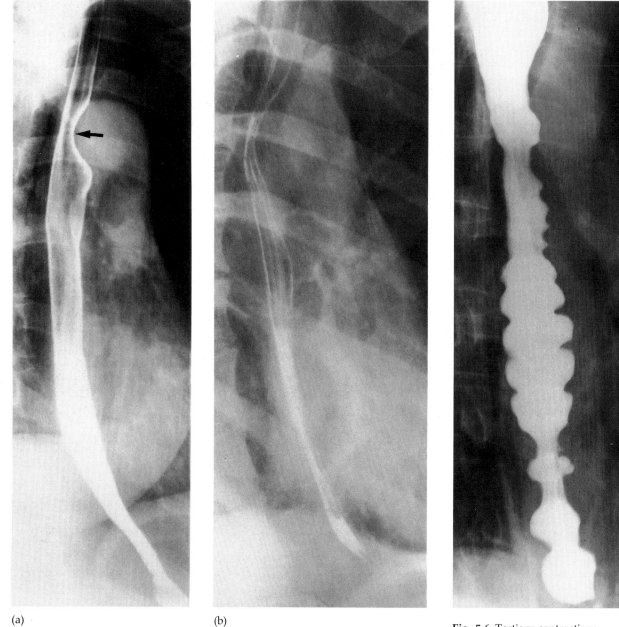

(a)

(b)

Fig. 5.5 Normal oesophagus. (a) Full of barium to show the smooth outline and indentation due to the aortic arch (arrow). (b) Film taken after the main volume of barium has passed, to show the parallel mucosal folds.

Fig. 5.6 Tertiary contractions (corkscrew oesophagus) giving the oesophagus an undulated appearance.

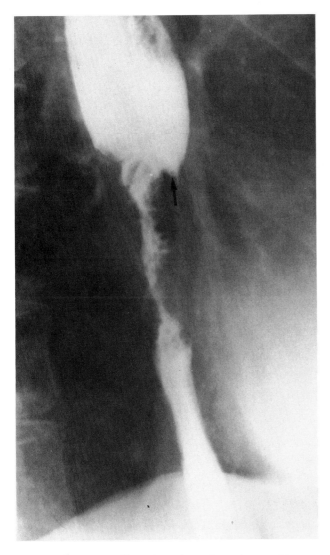

Fig. 5.7 Carcinoma. There is an irregular stricture with shouldering (arrow) at the upper end.

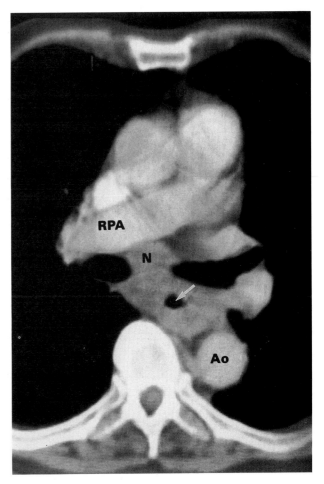

Fig. 5.8 Carcinoma of the oesophagus. The carcinoma is shown as a mass around the lumen of the oesophagus (arrow). Subcarinal nodes (N) are also present. Ao, descending aorta; RPA, right pulmonary artery.

adjacent structures and evidence of spread to draining lymph nodes (Fig. 5.8).

Peptic strictures are found at the lower end of the oesophagus and are almost invariably associated with a hiatus hernia and gastro-oesophageal reflux and, therefore, the stricture may be some distance above the diaphragm. Peptic strictures are characteristically short and have smooth outlines with tapering ends (Fig. 5.9). An ulcer may be seen in close proximity to the stricture.

Achalasia is a neuromuscular abnormality resulting in failure of relaxation at the cardiac sphincter which presents radiologically as a smooth, tapered narrowing which is always at the lower end of the oesophagus

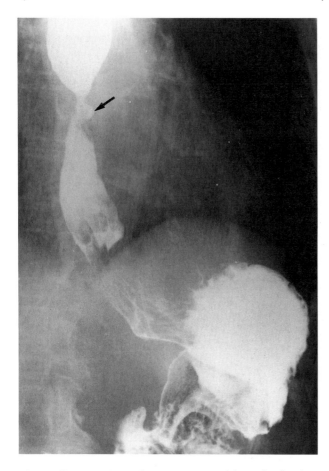

Fig. 5.9 Peptic stricture due to gastro-oesophageal reflux in a patient with a hiatus hernia. There is a short smooth stricture at the oesophagogastric junction with an ulcer crater within the stricture (arrow).

(Fig. 5.10). There is associated dilatation of the oesophagus, which often shows absent peristalsis. The dilated oesophagus usually contains food residues and may be visible on the plain chest radiograph. The lungs may show consolidation and bronchiectasis due to aspiration of the oesophageal contents. The stomach gas bubble is usually absent because the oesophageal contents act as a water seal, but this sign is not diagnostic of achalasia as it is seen in other causes of oesophageal obstruction and can occasionally be observed in healthy people.

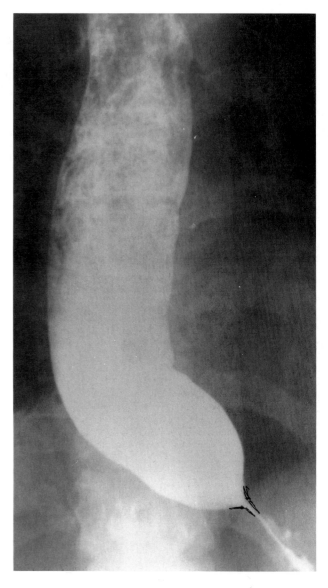

Fig. 5.10 Achalasia. The very dilated oesophagus containing food residues shows a smooth narrowing at its lower end.

Corrosive strictures are the result of swallowing corrosives such as acids or alkalis. They are long strictures which begin at the level of the aortic arch. As with the other benign strictures they are usually smooth with tapered ends, but may be irregular (Fig. 5.11).

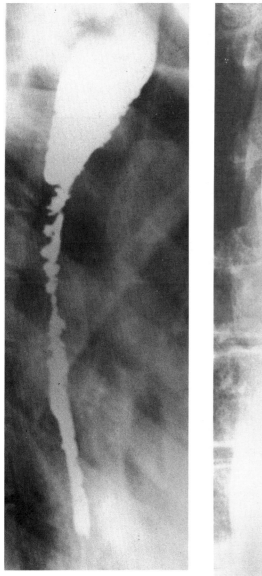

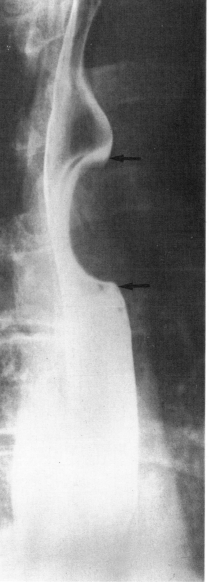

Fig. 5.11 Corrosive stricture.

Fig. 5.12 Leiomyoma. There is an intramural filling defect in the oesophagus below the aortic arch (arrows). The sharp angle this makes with the wall of the oesophagus indicates that the filling defect is due to a mass arising in the wall of the oesophagus.

Filling defects on barium swallow

Filling defects may be caused by a tumour arising in the wall of the oesophagus, by a lesion arising from outside the oesophagus or by objects in the lumen of the oesophagus.

An intramural filling defect is likely to be a leiomyoma (Fig. 5.12). A leiomyoma causes a smooth, rounded indentation into the lumen of the oesophagus. A soft tissue mass may be seen in the mediastinum indicating extraluminal extension.

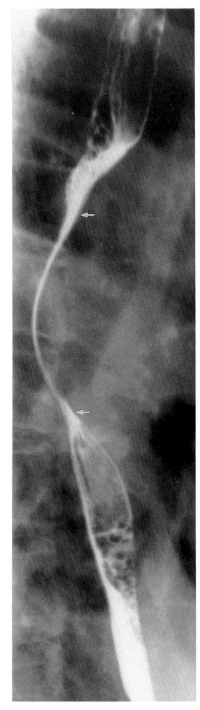

A carcinoma may cause an irregular filling defect, but as mentioned above, carcinomas usually present as strictures.

Extramural lesions compressing the oesophagus include carcinoma of the bronchus (Fig. 5.13), enlarged mediastinal lymph nodes and an aneurysm of the aorta. In all these conditions the chest film or CT will usually show the underlying pathology.

An anomalous right subclavian artery, which instead of coming from the innominate artery, arises as the last major branch from the aortic arch, gives rise to a characteristic short, smooth narrowing as it crosses behind the upper oesophagus (Fig. 5.14).

Intraluminal filling defects. A lump of food may impact in the oesophagus and may cause a complete obstruction (Fig. 5.15). This is usually associated with a stricture.

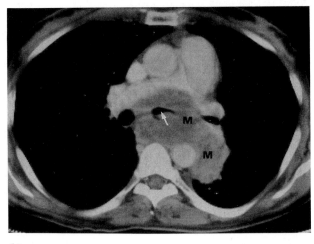

(b)

Fig. 5.13 Extraluminal compression of oesophagus by carcinoma of the bronchus. (a) Barium swallow shows extraluminal compression (arrows) making a shallow angle with the wall of the oesophagus. (b) CT of the same patient shows a very large mass surrounding and indenting the oesophagus (arrow).

(a)

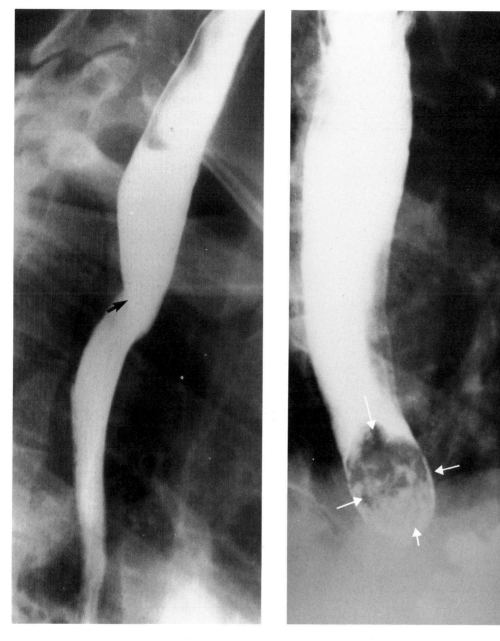

Fig. 5.14 Anomalous right subclavian artery. There is a localised indentation caused by the anomalous artery as it passes behind the oesophagus (arrow).

Fig. 5.15 Impacted food. A piece of meat is lodged at the lower end of the oesophagus and appears as a filling defect (arrows) surrounded by barium.

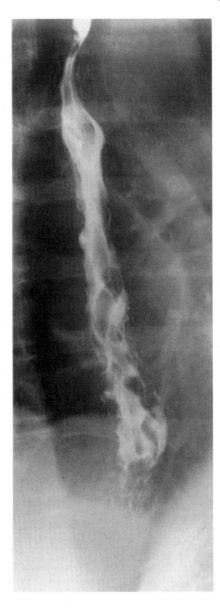

Fig. 5.16 Oesophageal varices. Tortuous, worm-like filling defects are seen in the lower half of the oesophagus.

Dilatation of the oesophagus

There are two main types of oesophageal dilatation — obstructive and non-obstructive.

1 Dilatation due to obstruction is associated with a visible stricture. The patient with a carcinoma usually presents with dysphagia before the oesophagus becomes very dilated. On the other hand, a markedly dilated oesophagus indicates a very long-standing condition, usually achalasia or occasionally a benign stricture.

2 Dilatation without obstruction occurs in scleroderma. The disease involves the oesophageal muscle resulting in dilatation of the oesophagus, which resembles an inert tube wih no peristaltic movement so that barium does not flow from the oesophagus into the stomach unless the patient stands upright.

Varices

Oesophageal varices appear as lucent, tortuous, worm-like filling defects which distort the mucosal pattern so that the folds are no longer parallel (Fig. 5.16). The primary diagnostic test to confirm or exclude varices is endoscopy.

Oesophageal web

A web is a thin, shelf-like projection arising from the anterior wall of the cervical portion of the oesophagus. To demonstrate it, that part of the oesophagus must be full of barium (Fig. 5.17). A web may be an isolated finding but the combination of a web, dysphagia and an iron deficiency anaemia is known as the Plummer Vinson syndrome.

Diverticula

Diverticula are saccular outpouchings, which are often seen as chance findings, in the intrathoracic portion of the oesophagus. One type of diverticulum, the pharyngeal pouch or Zenker's diverticulum (Fig. 5.18), is important as it may give rise to symptoms due to

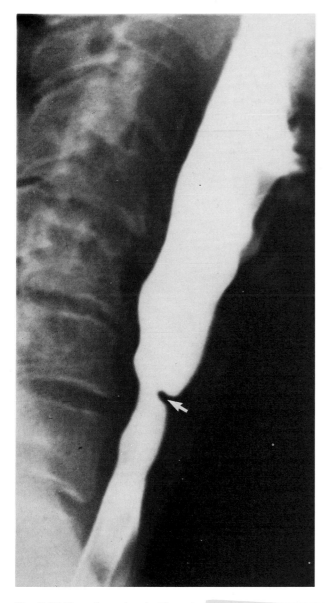

Fig. 5.17 Oesophageal web. There is a shelf-like indentation (arrow) from the anterior wall of the upper oesophagus.

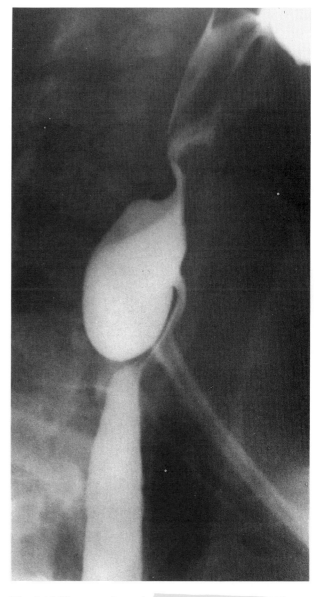

Fig. 5.18 Pharyngeal pouch (Zenker's diverticulum). The pouch is lying behind the oesophagus which is displaced forward.

retention of food and pressure upon the oesophagus. A pharyngeal pouch arises through a congenital weakness in the inferior constrictor muscle of the pharynx and comes to lie behind the oesophagus near the midline. It may reach a very large size and can cause displacement and compression of the oesophagus.

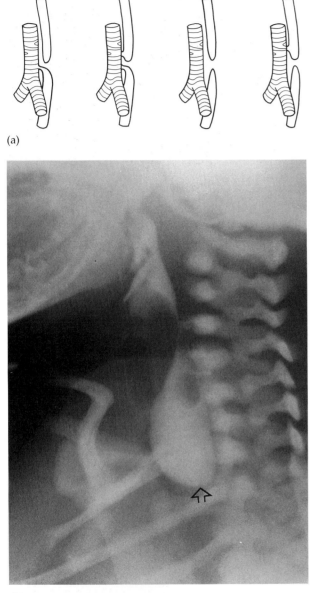

(a)

(b)

Fig. 5.19 Oesophageal atresia. (a) Diagram of the various types. The first two types also have an oesophagotracheal fistula distal to the atretic segment and will show air in the stomach. (b) The dilated oesophagus ends blindly at the thoracic inlet (arrow). There was a fistula from the oesophagus below the atretic segment to the trachea. This is the commonest type of oesophageal atresia.

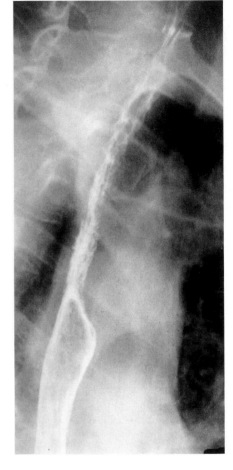

Fig. 5.20 Candidiasis. Mucosal ulceration has caused irregularity of the lumen of the upper oesophagus.

Oesophageal atresia

In oesophageal atresia, the oesophagus ends as a blind pouch in the upper mediastinum. Several different types exist (Fig. 5.19) but the most frequent is for the upper part of the oesophagus to be a blind sac with a fistula between the lower segment of the oesophagus and the tracheobronchial tree. A plain abdominal film will show air in the bowel if a fistula is present between the tracheobronchial tree and the oesophagus distal to the atretic segment.

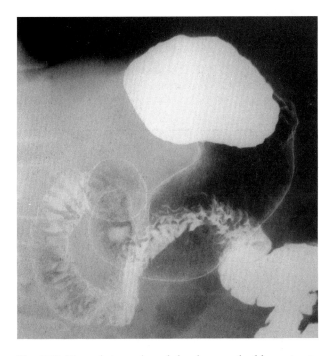

Fig. 5.21 Normal stomach and duodenum: double contrast barium meal. On this supine view barium collects in the fundus of the stomach. The body and the antrum of the stomach together with the duodenal cap and loop are coated with barium and distended with gas. Note how the fourth part of the duodenum and duodenojejunal flexure are superimposed on the body of the stomach.

To confirm the diagnosis of oesophageal atresia it is usually sufficient to pass a soft tube into the oesophagus and show that the tube holds up or coils in the blindly ending pouch. Oily contrast, such as the bronchographic medium Dionosil (0.5–1.0 ml), injected through the tube has been used to outline the oesophagus (Fig. 5.19b), but this is a hazardous procedure because the viscous contrast may cause respiratory obstruction if it spills over into the trachea.

Candidiasis

Involvement of the oesophagus with the fungus Candida (Monilia) occurs in severely ill or immuno-compromised patients. It causes mucosal ulceration

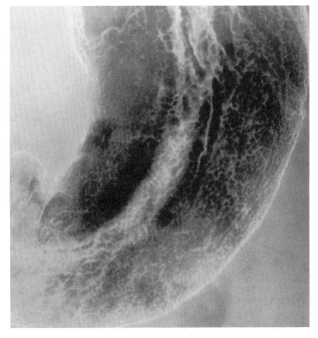

Fig. 5.22 Normal stomach. With a double contrast technique the mucosa is coated with barium and the stomach distended with gas to show the fine mucosal detail, in this case in the body of the stomach.

which is seen as fine irregularities projecting from the lumen of the oesophagus on barium swallow (Fig. 5.20).

The stomach and duodenum

The barium meal is the standard contrast medium to examine the stomach and duodenum. For this the patient drinks about 200 ml of barium. Each radiologist has his own routine but the aim is to take films in various positions with the patient both erect and lying flat, so that each part of the stomach and duodenum is shown distended by barium and also distended with air but coated with barium to show the mucosal pattern (Fig. 5.21). To provide better mucosal detail, the stomach is distended by giving a gas-producing agent and an intravenous injection of a short-acting smooth muscle relaxant is often given (Fig. 5.22).

Food residues in the stomach produce pictures which are very difficult to interpret. For this reason it is most important that the patient fasts for at least 6 hours prior to the examination.

Normal barium meal

Each part of the stomach and duodenum should be checked to ensure that no abnormal narrowing is present. A transient contraction wave must not be confused with a constant pathological narrowing. The outline of the lesser curve of the stomach is smooth with no filling defects or projections visible but the greater curve is nearly always irregular due to prominent mucosal folds. In the stomach the mucosa is thrown up into a number of smooth folds and barium collects in the troughs between the folds. There should be no effacement of the folds or rounded collections of barium.

The duodenal cap or bulb should be approximately triangular in shape. It arises just beyond the short pyloric canal and may be difficult to recognise if deformed due to chronic ulceration.

The duodenum forms a loop around the head of the pancreas to reach the duodenojejunal flexure. Diverticula arising beyond the first part of the duodenum are a common finding (Fig. 5.23) and are usually without significance.

Gastroscopy

Gastroscopy enables the mucosa of the stomach and duodenum to be directly inspected and biopsied. Gastroscopy and barium meal are complementary investigations and nowadays gastroscopy is widely used as the initial investigation in patients with dyspepsia or suspected carcinoma.

Although gastroscopy will not be discussed in detail the main indications for its use are:
- Demonstrating mucosal lesions such as gastritis which cannot be reliably visualised on a barium examination.
- Making a histological diagnosis of an abnormality shown on a barium meal.
- Investigating persistent dyspepsia in a patient with a normal barium meal.
- Assessing healing of an ulcer.
- Examining patients after gastric surgery when the radiological appearances may be difficult to interpret.
- Diagnosing the cause of acute bleeding from the upper gastrointestinal tract.

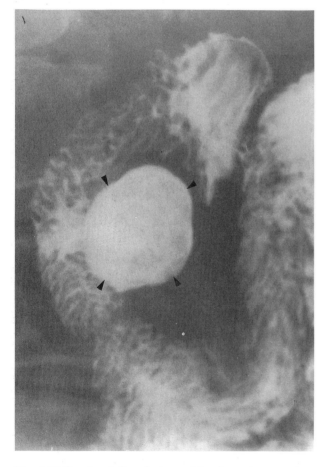

Fig. 5.23 Duodenal diverticulum arising from the second part of the duodenum (arrows).

Abnormal barium meal

Filling defects in the stomach

These may arise from the wall of the stomach or be due to masses that press in from outside the stomach. A few are entirely intraluminal. It should be remembered that carcinoma is by far the commonest cause of a filling defect in an adult.

Carcinoma usually produces an irregular filling defect with alteration of the normal mucosal pattern. The tumour is often larger than is readily appreciated from the barium meal. Overhanging edges or shouldering may be seen at the junction of the tumour and the stomach wall (Fig. 5.24). A carcinoma at the fundus may obstruct the oesophagus while one in the antrum may cause gastric outlet obstruction (see Fig. 5.31, p. 163). Carcinoma diffusely involving the stomach is known as linitis plastica and is discussed below.

Because of the much better prognosis, emphasis has been placed on the diagnosis of early gastric cancer which is confined to the mucosa. It may be flat or appear as a shallow ulcer indistinguishable from a benign ulcer. This stage of cancer is difficult to detect and is usually only diagnosed with a double contrast barium meal.

Leiomyoma. A smooth, round filling defect arising from the wall of the stomach may be caused by a benign tumour such as a leiomyoma (Fig. 5.25). A leiomyoma is a submucosal tumour which, as well as projecting

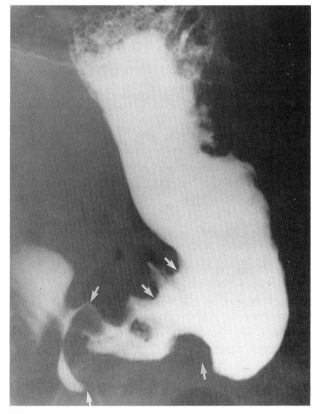

(a)

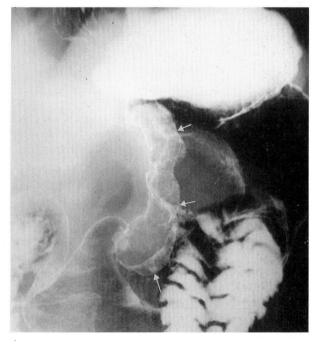

(b)

Fig. 5.24 Carcinoma. (a) There is a large filling defect in the antrum and body of stomach with overhanging edges (arrows). (b) Double contrast examination of different patient showing large carcinoma arising from lesser curve of stomach (arrows).

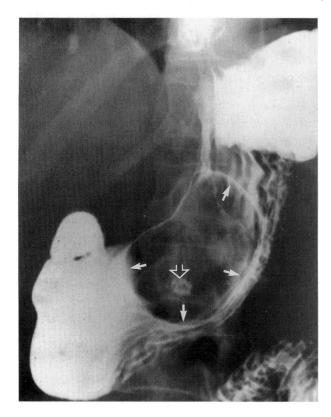

Fig. 5.25 Leiomyoma. There is a large filling defect in the stomach with smooth borders (outer arrows). An ulcer crater (central arrow) is present within the filling defect—a characteristic feature of a leiomyoma.

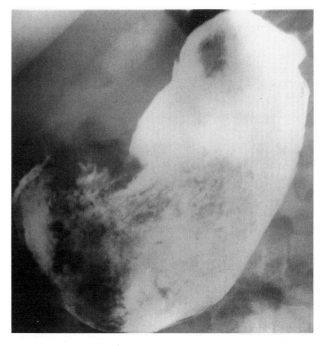

Fig. 5.26 Bezoar. Masses of hair in the stomach have caused irregular filling of the stomach with barium.

into the lumen of the stomach, may show a large extraluminal extension. One of the characteristic features of a leiomyoma is that it may have an ulcer on its surface.

Polyps may be single or multiple. They may be sessile or have a stalk. Even with high quality radiographs it is often impossible to distinguish benign from malignant polyps. For this reason gastroscopy with biopsy or operative removal is invariably carried out on all suspected polyps.

Intraluminal defects are completely surrounded by barium and are often mobile in the stomach. Examples are food or blood following a haematemesis. Sometimes ingested fibrous material such as hair may intertwine forming a ball or bezoar (Fig. 5.26).

Gastric ulcers

Depending on the projection, ulcers may be seen either *en face* as a collection of barium occupying the ulcer crater, or in profile as a projection from the lumen of the stomach.

Gastric ulcers may be benign or malignant. Table 5.1 gives some of the distinguishing features between benign and malignant gastric ulcers though endoscopy and biopsy are usually carried out once a gastric ulcer is diagnosed. Although it may be possible to diagnose an ulcerating carcinoma with confidence it is never possible to be sure that a gastric ulcer is benign until it has healed.

Table 5.1 Distinguishing features between benign and malignant gastric ulcers

Benign (Fig. 5.27 — p.162)	Malignant (Fig. 5.28 — p.162)
1 The ulcer projects beyond the lumen of the stomach	1 The ulcer occurs within an irregular filling defect, which may be difficult to demonstrate, therefore the ulcer appears not to project beyond the original lumen
2 The edge of the ulcer is regular and round when seen *en face*	2 The edge of the ulcer is irregular
3 Usually on lesser curve, rarely on greater curve	3 May occur anywhere but ulcers in the antrum and on greater curve are particularly suspicious
4 Radiating mucosal folds reach the edge or near to the edge of the ulcer crater	4 The mucosal folds are obliterated some distance from the edge of the ulcer

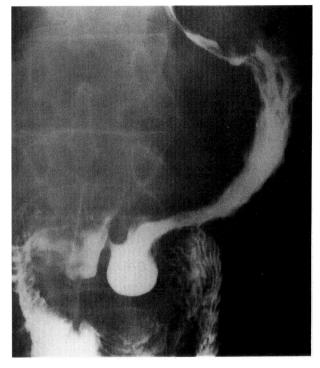

Fig. 5.29 Linitis plastica. The stomach is narrowed by an extensive carcinoma converting it to a rigid tube with obliteration of mucosal folds.

Narrowing of the stomach

If constant, narrowing is an important feature as it may herald malignancy.

When the whole stomach is involved, the narrowing is due to a carcinoma. This is the so-called leather bottle stomach or linitis plastica (Fig. 5.29). The stomach behaves as a thick rigid tube lacking peristalsis with obliteration of the mucosal folds. Rapid gastric emptying takes place because the cardia and pylorus are held open by the rigid stomach wall.

It is when the narrowing is localised that diagnostic difficulties arise as it may be due to either an infiltrating carcinoma, an active ulcer causing spasm or an ulcer which has healed with scarring and fibrosis (Fig. 5.30).

Thick gastric mucosal folds

Enlarged mucosal folds are associated with a high acid secretion. They are seen in patients with duodenal ulcers and also in the Zollinger—Ellison syndrome which comprises a high acid secretion, gastrin secreting tumour in the pancreas and multiple peptic ulcers.

Occasionally, diffuse infiltration of the stomach with malignant lymphoma can produce generalised thickening of the mucosal folds.

Gastric outlet obstruction

Emptying of the stomach can be a difficult feature to assess on a barium meal. In most patients barium rapidly leaves the stomach to enter the duodenum, but in others this only occurs after the patient has been lying on the right side for several minutes. In gastric outlet obstruction less than 50% of the barium leaves the stomach after 4 hours and some may still be present after 24 hours. The stomach will be large and will contain food residues.

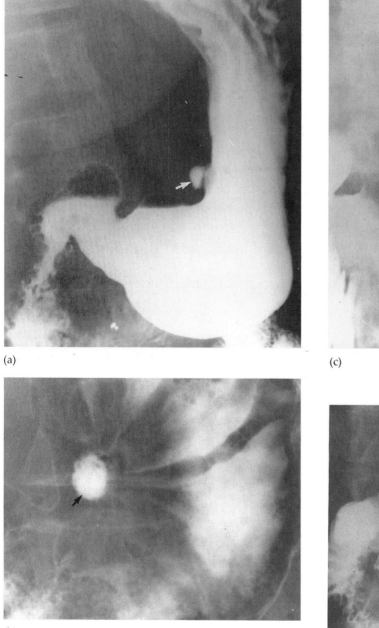

(a)

(b)

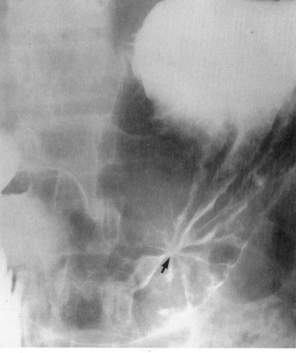

(c)

Fig. 5.27 Benign ulcer. (a) In profile the ulcer (arrow) projects from the lesser curve of the stomach. (b) *En face* the ulcer (arrow) is seen as a rounded collection of barium. (c) Radiating mucosal folds reach the ulcer crater (arrow).

Fig. 5.28 Malignant ulcer. The ulcer (arrow) does not project from the lumen of the stomach. Note how the mucosal folds do not reach the ulcer crater.

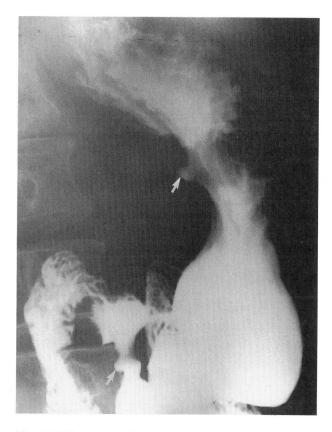

Fig. 5.30 Narrowing of the stomach due to an ulcer. The antrum is narrowed due to spasm resulting from the antral ulcer (arrow). Note the second ulcer on the lesser curve of the stomach (arrow).

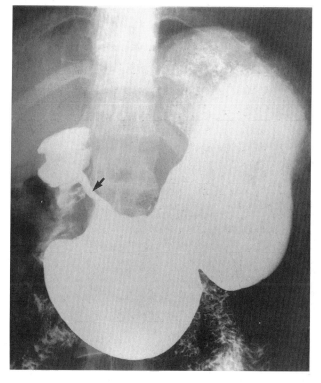

Fig. 5.31 Gastric outlet obstruction. A carcinoma is causing narrowing of the antrum (arrow). The speckled appearance in the fundus of the enlarged stomach is due to food residues.

Gastric emptying can be assessed by giving a radioactive test meal and measuring the disappearance of radioactivity from the stomach, with the patient positioned under a gamma camera. By making corrections for radioactive decay the half-emptying time for the stomach can be calculated.

It is not sufficient merely to diagnose gastric outlet obstruction; an attempt must be made to find the underlying cause, which may be situated in the duodenum, pylorus or antrum. The term 'gastric outlet obstruction' is preferred to the older term 'pyloric stenosis', as the pylorus is often not the site of the obstruction.

In adults the causes of gastric outlet obstruction are:
• *Chronic duodenal ulceration*. The diagnosis depends on demonstrating a very deformed, stenosed duodenal cap. It may or may not be possible to identify an actual ulcer crater.
• *Carcinoma of the antrum* may cause narrowing. The diagnosis is made by recognising an irregular filling defect in the antrum of the stomach (Fig. 5.31).

In infants, pyloric stenosis is by far the commonest cause of gastric outlet obstruction. Often, the diagnosis is made clinically and can be confirmed with ultrasound, which has superseded the barium meal. Ultrasound will show a thickened, elongated pyloric canal (Fig. 5.32).

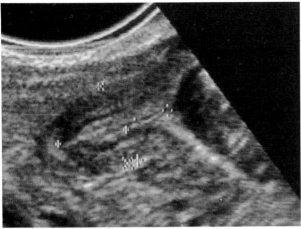

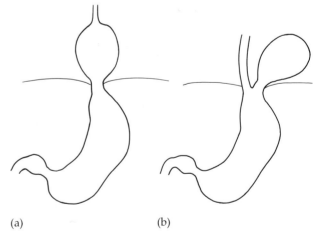

Fig. 5.32 Pyloric stenosis. Ultrasound scan in a neonate showing a thickened elongated pyloric canal.

Gastritis

Often, gastritis may only be diagnosed endoscopically, as the mucosal changes are too slight to be detected on a barium meal. However, erosive gastritis, which is associated with taking alcohol or aspirin, may be seen on a double contrast barium meal. The erosions appear as small, shallow collections of barium surrounded by a radiolucent halo due to oedema (Fig. 5.33).

Hiatus hernia

A hiatus hernia is a herniation of the stomach into the mediastinum through the oesophageal hiatus in the diaphragm. It is a common finding. Two main types of hiatus hernia exist: sliding and rolling. An alternative name for a rolling hernia is 'para-oesophageal' (Fig. 5.34).

The commoner type is the sliding hiatus hernia

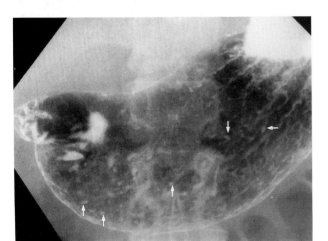

Fig. 5.33 Erosive gastritis. The erosions appear on this double contrast barium meal as many small collections of barium, some of which are arrowed.

Fig. 5.34 Hiatus hernia. (a) Sliding: a portion of the stomach and the gastro-oesophageal junction are situated above the diaphragm. (b) Rolling or para-oesophageal: the gastro-oesophageal junction is below the diaphragm.

where the gastro-oesophageal junction and a portion of the stomach are situated above the diaphragm (Fig. 5.35a). The cardiac sphincter is usually incompetent, so reflux from the stomach to the oesophagus occurs readily and this may cause oesophagitis, ulceration or peptic stricture. A small sliding hernia may be demonstrated in most people during a barium meal examination, provided that enough

manoeuvres have been undertaken to increase intra-abdominal pressure. It is, therefore, difficult to assess the significance of a small hernia with little or no reflux.

In a rolling or para-oesophageal hernia (Fig. 5.35b), the fundus of the stomach herniates through the diaphragm but the oesophagogastric junction often remains competent below the diaphragm.

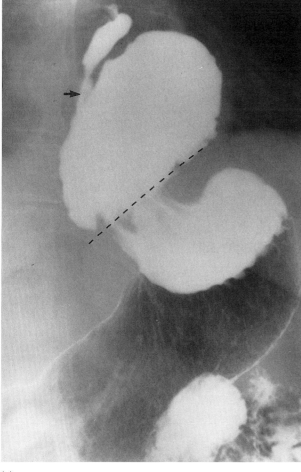
(a)

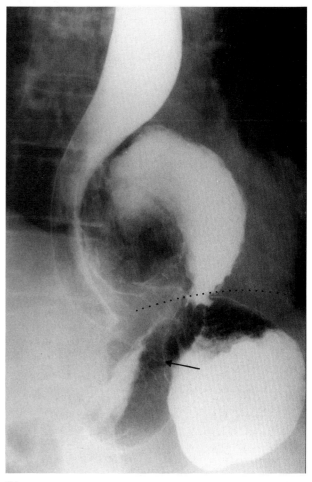
(b)

Fig. 5.35 Hiatus hernia. (a) Sliding: the fundus of the stomach and the gastro-oesophageal junction (arrow) have herniated through the oesophageal hiatus and lie above the diaphragm (dotted line). (b) Rolling. The gastro-oesophageal junction (arrow) is below the diaphragm (dotted line) and the fundus of the stomach has herniated into the chest.

A large hernia, particularly one of the para-oesophageal type, may not be reduced when the patient is in the erect position. In these instances the hiatus hernia will be seen on chest films.

Duodenal ulcer

The great majority of duodenal ulcers occur in the duodenal cap (duodenal bulb) but a few are found just

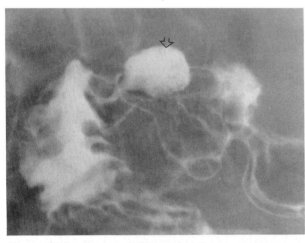

(a)

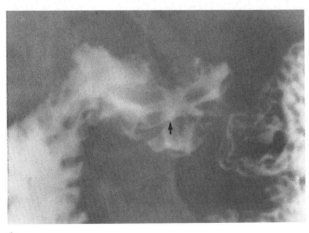

(b)

Fig. 5.36 Duodenal ulcer (two patients). (a) Seen as a large collection of barium in the duodenal cap (arrow). (b) Mucosal folds are radiating to a central ulcer crater (arrow).

beyond the cap and are known as postbulbar ulcers. The ulcer crater (Fig. 5.36a) may have a surrounding lucent zone due to oedema and mucosal folds are often seen radiating towards the ulcer (Fig. 5.36b). With chronic ulceration the cap becomes deformed due to scarring. In a grossly scarred cap it is often impossible to be certain of the presence of an ulcer.

It is not worthwhile carrying out repeat barium meal examinations to assess healing of duodenal ulcers for the following reasons:
• It is often not possible to comment on the presence or absence of an ulcer in a deformed cap.
• Follow-up for malignant change is unnecessary as duodenal ulcers are almost invariably benign and do not undergo malignant degeneration.

Radiology in acute upper gastrointestinal bleeding

The patient presenting with haematemasis and melaena is a common medical emergency. The main causes of bleeding are:
• peptic ulcer
• gastric erosions
• varices
• carcinoma.

Gastroscopy is the key investigation and only rarely is a barium meal performed. Gastroscopy has the advantages of actually demonstrating the site of bleeding and it can show gastric erosions which may be too shallow to be seen on a barium meal.

The small intestine

The standard contrast examination for the small intestine is the barium small bowel follow-through. The patient drinks about 200–300 ml of barium and its passage through the small intestine is observed by taking films at regular intervals until the barium reaches the colon. This can be a time-consuming procedure and usually takes 2–3 hours, but the transit time is very variable.

The normal barium follow-through

The normal small intestine (Fig. 5.37) occupies the central and lower abdomen, usually framed by the colon. The terminal portion of the ileum enters the medial aspect of the caecum through the ileocaecal valve. As the terminal ileum may be the first site of disease this region is often fluoroscoped and observed on a television monitor so that peristalsis can be seen and films can be taken with the terminal ileum unobscured by other loops of small intestine.

The barium forms a continuous column defining the diameter of the small bowel which is normally not more than 25 mm. Transverse folds of mucous membrane project into the lumen of the bowel and barium lies between these folds which appear as lucent filling defects of about 2−3 mm in width. The appearance of the mucosal folds depends upon the diameter of the

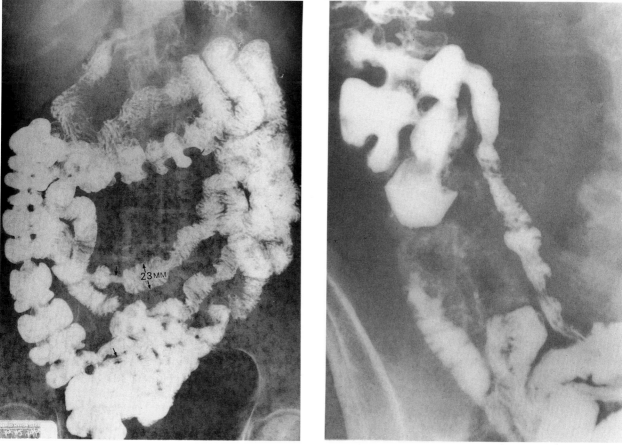

(a) (b)

Fig. 5.37 (a) Normal barium follow-through. The small intestine, ascending and transverse colon are filled with barium. The jejunum in the left side of the abdomen has a much more marked mucosal fold pattern than the ileum which is lying in the pelvis. When a peristaltic wave contracts the bowel the mucosal folds lie longitudinally (arrows). Note the way of measuring the diameter of the bowel. In the pelvis the loops overlap and details of the bowel become hidden. (b) Normal terminal ileum.

bowel. When distended, the folds are seen as lines traversing the barium column known as valvulae conniventes. When the small bowel is contracted, the folds lie longitudinally and when it is relaxed the folds assume an appearance described as feathery. The mucosal folds are largest and most numerous in the jejunum and tend to disappear in the lower part of the ileum.

An alternative method of examining the small bowel is the so-called small bowel enema (enteroclysis) which distends the bowel and gives excellent mucosal detail (Fig. 5.38). The disadvantage is that it requires intubation with a nasoduodenal tube, which is passed to the duodenojejunal flexure. Barium is injected through the tube followed by water or methyl cellulose to propel the barium through the small bowel.

This technique is appropriate for structural de-

formities, e.g. Crohn's disease or tumours, but is not used in cases with the malabsorption syndrome.

The abnormal barium follow-through

The following signs should be looked for:
• *Dilatation* usually indicates either malabsorption, paralytic ileus or small bowel obstruction (Fig. 5.39). If necessary, measure the diameter of the bowel; a value over 30 mm is definitely abnormal but make sure that two overlapping loops are not being measured. As the

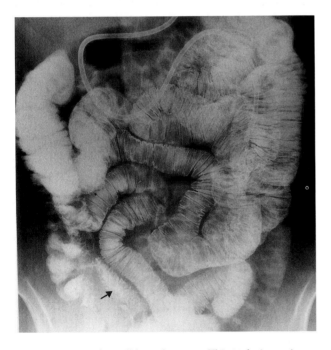

Fig. 5.38 Normal small bowel enema. This technique gives good mucosal detail. The arrow points to the terminal ileum. Note that a tube has been passed through the stomach into the jejunum.

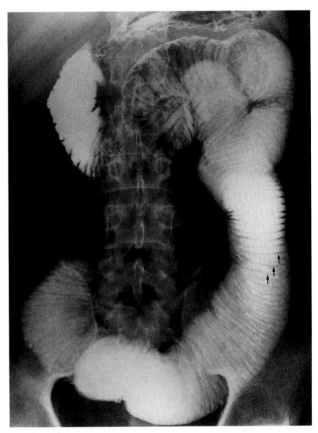

Fig. 5.39 Dilatation due to small bowel obstruction. The diameter of the bowel is greatly increased. The feathery mucosal pattern is lost and the folds appear as thin lines traversing the bowel known as valvulae conniventes (arrows).

bowel dilates the normal mucosal pattern becomes largely effaced and the valvulae conniventes become clearly visible.

• *Mucosal abnormality.* The folds become thickened in many conditions, e.g. malabsorption states, with oedema or haemorrhage into the bowel wall, and when inflamed or infiltrated (Fig. 5.40). Since mucosal fold thickening occurs in many diseases it is not possible to make a particular diagnosis unless other more specific features are present.

• *Narrowing.* The only normal narrowings are those caused by peristaltic waves. They are smooth, concentric and transient with normal mucosal folds traversing them and normal bowel proximally. The common causes of strictures are Crohn's disease (Fig. 5.41), tuberculosis and lymphoma. Strictures do not contain normal mucosal folds and usually result in dilatation of the bowel proximally.

• *Ulceration.* The outline of the small bowel should be smooth apart from the indentation caused by normal mucosal folds. Ulcers appear as spikes projecting outwards which may be shallow or deep (Fig. 5.42). Ulceration is seen in Crohn's disease, tuberculosis and lymphoma. When there is a combination of fine ulceration and mucosal oedema, a cobblestone appearance may be seen.

• *Alteration in position*

(a) Congenital malrotation. During intrauterine life the bowel undergoes a series of rotations. Failure of the normal rotation may result in the small bowel being situated in the right side of the abdomen and the colon on the left side (Fig. 5.43). However, this state of affairs only occasionally gives rise to problems, mainly volvulus associated with abnormal mesenteric attachments.

(b) Displacement by a mass. Because of its mesentery the small intestine is freely mobile and will be displaced by an abdominal or pelvic mass (Fig. 5.44). The bowel will appear stretched around the mass but the mucosal pattern is usually preserved.

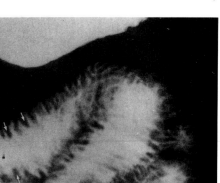

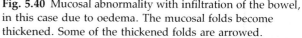

Fig. 5.40 Mucosal abnormality with infiltration of the bowel, in this case due to oedema. The mucosal folds become thickened. Some of the thickened folds are arrowed.

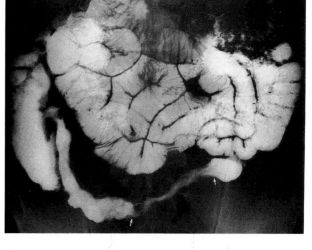

Fig. 5.41 Narrowing. There is a long irregular stricture (arrows) in the terminal ileum due to Crohn's disease. There is an abnormal mucosal pattern in the remainder of the terminal ileum. Note the contracted caecum — another feature of the disease.

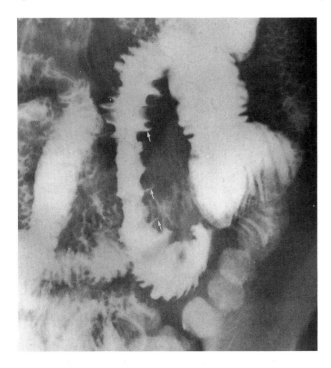

Fig. 5.42 Ulceration. Abnormal loops of bowel in Crohn's disease showing the ulcers as outward projections (arrows).

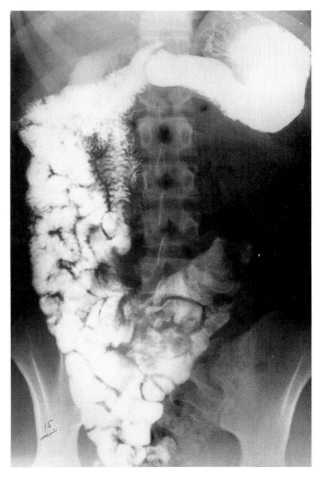

Fig. 5.43 Malrotation. The small bowel is situated in the right side of the abdomen. Later films showed the colon on the left side.

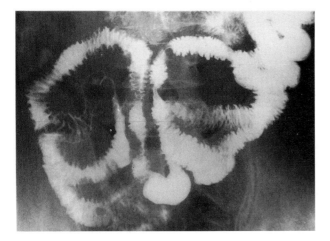

Fig. 5.44 Displacement. The small bowel is displaced around enlarged abdominal lymph nodes due to metastases from a teratoma of the testis.

Crohn's disease

Crohn's disease is a disease of unknown aetiology characterised by localised areas of non-specific chronic granulomatous inflammation, which nearly always affects the terminal ileum. In addition, it may cause disease in several different parts of the small and large intestine, often leaving normal intervening bowel, the affected parts being known as skip lesions. The major signs on the barium follow-through are strictures and mucosal abnormality (Fig. 5.45).

The strictures are extremely variable in length. Sometimes a loop of bowel is so narrow, either due to spasm in an extensively ulcerated loop of bowel or to oedema and fibrosis in the bowel wall, that its appearance has been called 'the string sign'. The bowel proximal to a stricture is often dilated. When there is obvious disease in the terminal ileum the caecum may be contracted.

Ulcers are seen which are sometimes quite deep. Fine ulceration combined with mucosal oedema gives rise to the so-called 'cobblestone' appearance.

Owing to thickening of the bowel wall the mucosal folds may become thickened, distorted or even disappear. When this thickening of the bowel wall is severe then the loops of bowel become separated; the presence of an inflammatory mass will cause even greater displacement of the loops.

Fistulae may occur to other small bowel loops, colon, bladder or vagina. When the fistula is between adjacent loops of small intestine it can be difficult to detect on the barium follow-through.

Crohn's disease may cause malabsorption so the radiological features of this condition may be present as well.

Tuberculosis

Tuberculosis is indistinguishable from Crohn's disease on barium examination. It commonly affects the ileocaecal region and also causes contraction of the caecum.

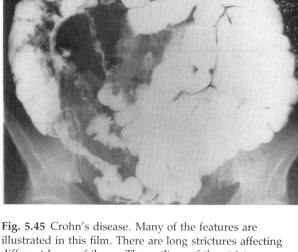

Fig. 5.45 Crohn's disease. Many of the features are illustrated in this film. There are long strictures affecting different loops of ileum. The outlines of the strictures are irregular due to ulceration. Note how the affected loops lie separately, displaced from other loops because of the presence of inflammatory masses.

Lymphoma

The infiltration in the wall of the bowel with lymphoma gives an appearance that is often extremely difficult to distinguish from Crohn's disease. Additional features to look for that may help differentiate the two conditions are small mucosal filling defects due to tumour nodules (Fig. 5.46), and displacement of loops caused by enlarged lymph nodes. Enlargement of the liver and spleen may also be present.

Malabsorption

A number of disorders result in defective absorption of foodstuffs, minerals or vitamins. The definitive test for malabsorption is the jejunal biopsy. Radiology is no substitute for a jejunal biopsy but along with biochemical tests is an important complementary in-

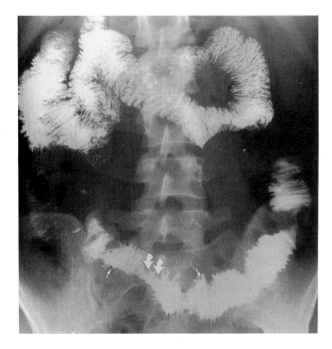

Fig. 5.46 Lymphoma. Lymphomatous infiltration has occurred in the lower loops of bowel causing thickening of the mucosal folds (small arrows) and discrete filling defects due to tumour nodules (curved arrows).

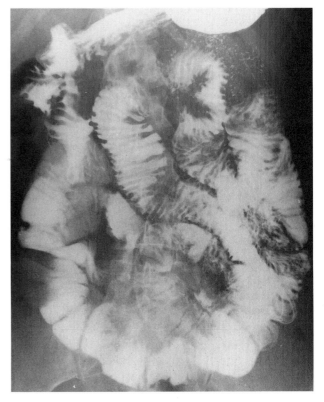

Fig. 5.47 Malabsorption. The bowel is dilated and the mucosal folds thickened. In the lower loops the barium appears less dense due to it becoming diluted. No specific cause for the malabsorption can be detected, which in this case was due to gluten enteropathy.

vestigation. The use of the barium follow-through in malabsorption is twofold:

1 It may show a structural abnormality causing the malabsorption.

2 It may help to make the diagnosis in doubtful cases where the biochemical tests are equivocal or normal.

The signs of malabsorption in the small bowel follow-through are (Fig. 5.47):

• Small bowel dilatation, the jejunum being affected more than the ileum.

• Thickening of mucosal folds.

• Flocculation and dilution of the barium in advanced disease. Instead of the barium forming a continuous column there may be clumping or flocculation so that the barium column is broken up into a number of segments. The barium may become diluted by the excessive fluid in the small bowel and so appears less dense.

The above signs occur with any of the causes of malabsorption.

In the following conditions no clue to the cause can be obtained from a study of the barium follow-through:

1 Diffuse mucosal lesions
  • gluten enteropathy (coeliac disease and idiopathic steatorrhoea)
  • tropical sprue.

2 Deficiency of absorptive factors, e.g. bile or pancreatic enzymes.

3 Postgastrectomy, due to rapid emptying of gastric remnant and insufficient mixing with bile and pancreatic juice.

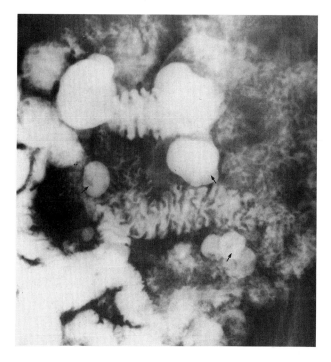

Fig. 5.48 Diverticulosis. A number of diverticula of varying size are arising from the small bowel. Some of these are arrowed.

Those conditions where the cause of malabsorption may be seen include:
1 Crohn's disease (see p. 171).
2 Lymphoma (see p. 171).
3 Anatomical abnormalities
  • Decreased length of small bowel available for absorption, e.g. surgical resection or a fistula short-circuiting a length of small bowel.
  • Stagnation of bowel contents, allowing bacterial overgrowth, which utilises nutrients from the bowel lumen, caused by:
  (a) multiple small bowel diverticula (Fig. 5.48)
  (b) a dilated loop cut off from the main stream of the bowel in which there is delayed filling and emptying (blind loop)
  (c) a dilated loop proximal to a stricture (stagnant loop).

Disaccharidase deficiency

Patients suffering from milk intolerance due to a deficiency of the enzyme lactase in the small bowel mucosa have an abnormal appearance on a barium follow-through if lactose is added to the barium. The small bowel becomes dilated, the barium diluted and the barium rapidly reaches the colon.

Acute small bowel obstruction

A barium examination is not carried out in most cases of obstruction as the diagnosis is usually made on clinical examination with the help of plain abdominal films (p. 135). When barium is given by mouth it shows that the small bowel proximal to an obstruction is dilated, often markedly and the barium becomes diluted by the excess fluid in the bowel (Fig. 5.39, p. 168).

Although a barium follow-through must be avoided in a colonic obstruction owing to the barium becoming solid and impacting proximal to the obstruction, this danger is not present in a small bowel obstruction because the fluid in the bowel prevents the barium solidifying. However, because of the dilution of the barium in the fluid-filled bowel it is often difficult to predict the nature or site of the obstruction.

Worm infestation

Roundworms (Ascaris) are the commonly encountered worms that are large enough to be seen as filling defects in the lumen of the bowel (they may grow up to 35 cm long) (Fig. 5.49). The worms themselves may ingest the barium to have their own barium meal and barium may be seen in their digestive tracts.

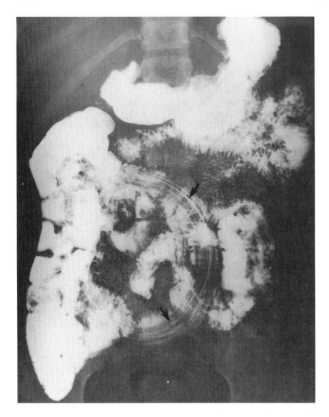

Fig. 5.49 Worm infestation. Several long tubular filling defects (arrows) due to roundworms (Ascaris) in the small bowel.

The large intestine

The standard examination of the large intestine is the barium enema. Barium is run into the colon under gravity through a tube inserted into the rectum. Films are taken in various projections so that all the loops of colon are unravelled. In the 'single contrast method' the whole colon is distended with barium. When a 'double contrast technique' is used only part of the colon is filled with barium and air is then blown in to push the barium around the colon with the result that the colon is distended with air and the mucosa coated with barium.

Prior bowel preparation by means of aperients or washout is most important to rid the colon of faecal material, which might otherwise mask small lesions and cause confusion by simulating polyps.

Endoscopy

Sigmoidoscopy should be performed in every patient in whom a barium enema is requested because lesions in the rectum, especially mucosal abnormalities, may be missed by barium examinations.

Colonoscopy is becoming more widely practised with the advent of flexible endoscopes. Colonoscopy is complementary to a barium enema examination and requires specific indications:

• Inspecting and biopsing abnormalities demonstrated on barium enema.
• Investigating patients with persistent symptoms with a normal barium enema — this applies particularly to rectal bleeding when an undiagnosed polyp may be discovered.
• Performing polypectomy.
• Assessing the extent of ulcerative colitis and Crohn's disease.

The normal barium enema

The radiological anatomy of the normal colon is shown in Fig. 5.50. Certain features are worth emphasising.

The length of the colon is very variable and sometimes there are redundant loops, particularly in the sigmoid and transverse colon. The calibre decreases from the caecum to the sigmoid colon.

The caecum is usually situated in the right iliac fossa but it may be seen under the right lobe of the liver or even in the centre of the abdomen if it possesses a long mesentery. The lips of the ileocaecal valve may project into the caecum and cause a filling defect which must not be mistaken for a tumour. Filling of the terminal ileum and appendix may occur but if they do not fill no significance can be attached to this.

Haustra can usually be recognised in the whole of the colon although they may be absent in the descending and sigmoid regions. The outline of the

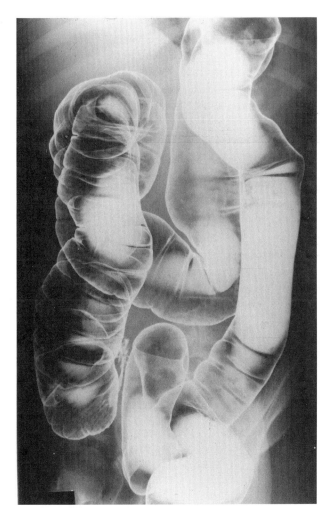

Fig. 5.50 Normal double contrast barium enema.

distended colon, apart from the haustra, is smooth but when the colon is contracted, as in an after evacuation film, the mucosa appears as smooth, regular folds.

The abnormal barium enema

1 *Narrowing of the lumen*

Narrowing of the colon may be due to spasm, stricture formation or compression by an extrinsic mass.

Spasm is often seen in normal patients and providing it is an isolated finding it can be ignored. Spasm is also seen in conjunction with diverticular disease and various inflammatory disorders.

Spasm gives rise to a smooth concentric narrowing which usually varies in severity during the period under observation. It can often be abolished by the intravenous administration of a smooth muscle relaxant, e.g. Buscopan or glucagon.

Strictures. The main causes of stricture formation are:
- carcinoma
- diverticular disease
- Crohn's disease
- ischaemic colitis.

Rarer causes include tuberculosis, lymphogranuloma venereum, amoebiasis and radiation fibrosis.

When attempting to diagnose the nature of a stricture in the colon the following points should be borne in mind:
- *Neoplastic strictures* have shouldered edges, an irregular lumen and are rarely more than 6 cm in length (Fig. 5.51), whereas benign strictures classically have tapered ends, a relatively smooth outline and may be of any length.
- *Ulceration* may be seen in strictures due to Crohn's disease and sacculation of the colon is a feature of ischaemic strictures.
- *Narrowing due to diverticular disease* is usually accompanied by other signs of diverticular disease. It is sometimes impossible to distinguish a stricture due to a carcinoma in an area of diverticular disease from a stricture due to diverticular disease.
- The *site* of the stricture can help in limiting the differential diagnosis. Strictures due to diverticular disease are almost always confined to the sigmoid colon. Ischaemic strictures are usually centred somewhere between the splenic flexure and the sigmoid colon. Crohn's disease and tuberculosis have a predilection for the caecum.

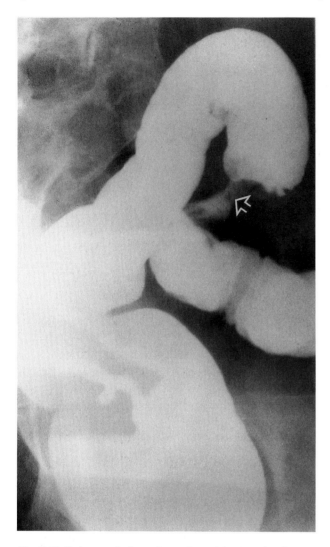

Fig. 5.51 Stricture. A short circumferential narrowing is seen in the sigmoid colon (arrow) due to a carcinoma.

Extrinsic compression by a mass arising outside the wall of the bowel causes a smooth narrowing of the colon frequently from one side only and often displaces the colon, e.g. ovarian and uterine masses (Fig. 5.52). Extrinsic compression causing a smooth indentation on the caecum may be seen with a mucocele of the appendix, appendix abscess (Fig. 5.53) or an inflammatory mass due to Crohn's disease.

2 *Dilatation*

Dilatation of the colon is difficult to assess. The barium enema, particularly the double contrast examination, involves distending the colon, so that its diameter is partly dependent on the amount of barium and air introduced.

The causes of dilatation of the colon are:
- *Obstruction*. Here the important consideration is not the dilatation itself but the nature of the obstructing lesion. In complete obstruction the barium enema may only show one end of the stricture, so some of the valuable signs described above are lost.
- *Paralytic ileus*. This diagnosis is usually made on clinical grounds with the help of plain films of the abdomen (p. 135). In those few cases where it proves difficult to distinguish paralytic ileus from mechanical obstruction to the distal colon, a barium enema can be undertaken. This will show a dilated but otherwise normal colon.
- *Volvulus*.
- *Ulcerative colitis* with toxic dilatation (see Fig. 4.6, p. 137).
- *Hirschsprung's disease and megacolon*.

3 *Filling defects*

Filling defects in the colon, as elsewhere in the gastrointestinal tract, may be intraluminal, arise from the wall or be due to pressure from an extrinsic mass.

In a clean colon, a localised filling defect is likely to be a polyp or a neoplasm. Faeces will cause a filling defect and can be very difficult to distinguish from a polyp or tumour (Fig. 5.54). Faeces have no attachment to the wall of the bowel, are completely surrounded by barium or air, and move freely, varying with the position of the patient. All barium enema examinations should be done with a clean colon in order to avoid misdiagnosing polyps that are in fact faeces.

Intramural haemorrhage, oedema or air in the wall of the colon (pneumatosis coli) all cause multiple smooth filling defects arising from the wall of the bowel.

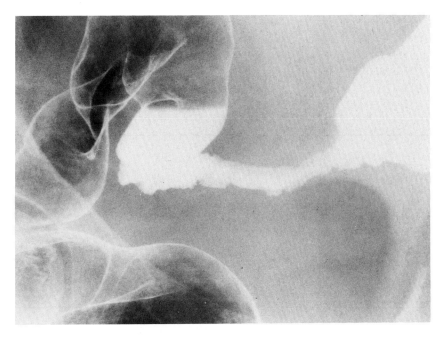

Fig. 5.52 Extrinsic compression. A narrowed length of sigmoid colon is seen due to compression by an adjacent ovarian carcinoma.

A unique type of filling defect is seen in intussusception (p. 187).

4 *Ulceration*

Ulcers of the colonic mucosa can be recognised as small projections from the lumen into the wall of the bowel. This results in the normally smooth outline of the colon having a fuzzy or shaggy appearance (Fig. 5.55). The two major causes of ulceration are ulcerative colitis and Crohn's disease. Rarer causes include tuberculosis, and amoebic and bacillary dysentery.

5 *Diverticula and muscle hypertrophy*

These are seen with diverticular disease (Fig. 5.56) and are discussed on p. 182.

6 *Displacement of the colon*

Displacement of the colon from its normal position may be caused by a variety of abdominal or pelvic masses, e.g. enlargement of the liver and spleen, or ovarian cyst. These masses may also compress the colon. Scrutiny of the plain abdominal films should be made as these may show further details of the mass but ultrasound or CT is usually necessary.

Displacement of the colon is also seen in malrotation.

Ulcerative colitis and Crohn's disease of the colon

Although classical changes are described for both ulcerative colitis and Crohn's disease it is sometimes difficult to distinguish between them. Radiology is important not only to diagnose these conditions but also to assess the extent and severity of the disease and to detect complications.

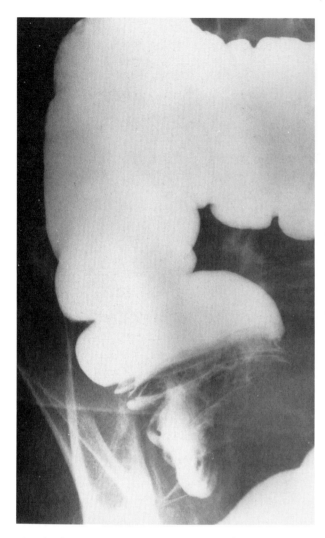

Fig. 5.53 Extrinsic compression. An appendix abscess is compressing and narrowing the caecum.

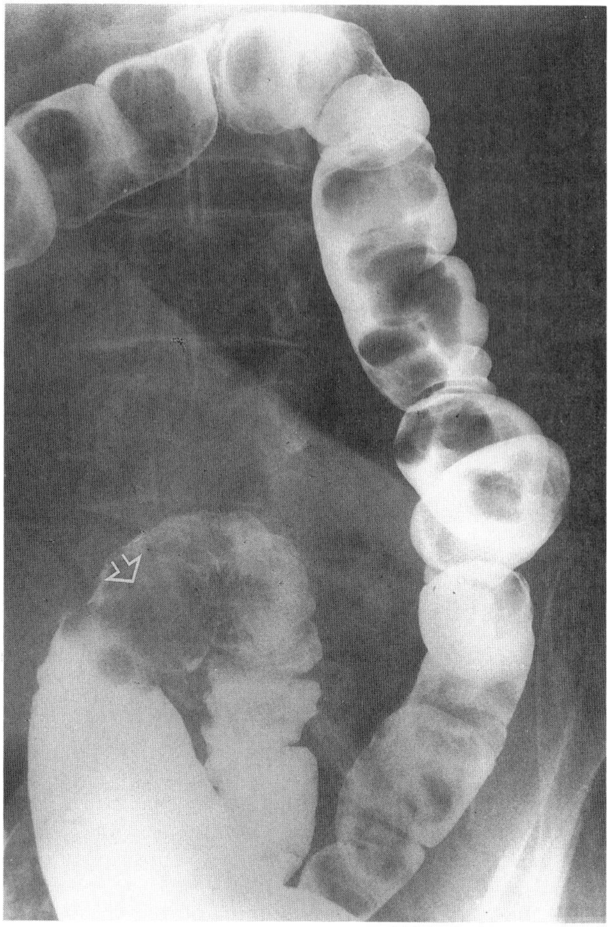

Fig. 5.54 Filling defects. Lumps of faeces have caused smooth filling defects surrounded by barium. However, in the sigmoid colon there is a large filling defect with ill-defined edges (arrow). This is a carcinoma. A clean colon is essential for a satisfactory barium enema.

Ulcerative colitis

Ulcerative colitis is a disease of unknown aetiology characterised by inflammation and ulceration of the colon. The disease always involves the rectum. When more extensive it extends in continuity around the colon, sometimes affecting the whole colon. The cardinal radiological sign is widespread ulceration (Fig.

5.55). The ulcers are usually shallow but in severe cases may be quite deep. In all but the milder cases, there is loss of the normal colonic haustra in the affected portions of the colon. Oedema of the perirectal tissues causes widening of the space between the sacrum and the rectum. Narrowing and shortening of the colon, giving the appearance of a rigid tube (Fig. 5.57), and pseudopolyps are seen in advanced

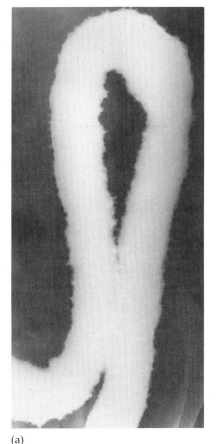

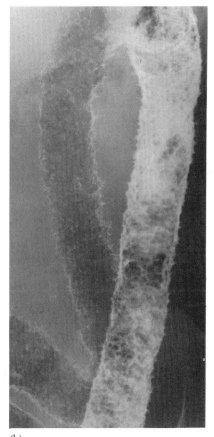

Fig. 5.55 Ulceration. (a) Single contrast. (b) Double contrast. In this case of ulcerative colitis the ulceration causes the normally smooth outline of the colon to be irregular.

(a)

(b)

disease. Pseudopolyps are small filling defects projecting into the lumen of the bowel formed by swollen mucosa in between the areas of ulceration. The swelling of these islands of inflamed mucosa makes it difficult to assess the true depth of the ulceration.

Strictures are rare and when present are likely to be due to carcinoma: the incidence of colonic carcinoma in long-standing ulcerative colitis is significantly increased.

When the whole colon is involved, the terminal ileum may become dilated. Since the ileocaecal valve in this situation is incompetent, the abnormal terminal ileum is usually demonstrated at barium enema.

Toxic dilatation (toxic megacolon) is a serious complication. The diagnosis is made on clinical grounds and on examination of the plain abdominal film. A barium enema should never be performed in the presence of toxic dilatation owing to the risk of perforating the colon.

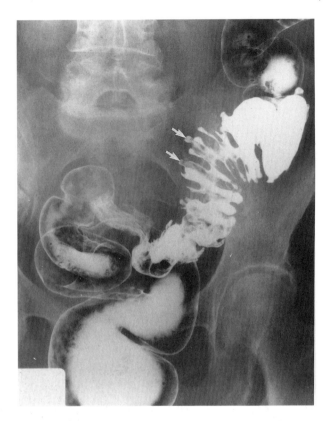

Fig. 5.56 Muscle hypertrophy and diverticula. Muscle hypertrophy gives the sigmoid colon a serrated appearance. Two small diverticula are arrowed.

Crohn's disease of the colon (granulomatous colitis, regional enteritis)

Crohn's disease is a chronic granulomatous condition of unknown aetiology which may affect any part of the gastrointestinal tract, but most frequently involves the lower ileum and the colon. The colon may be the only part of the alimentary tract to be involved, but usually the disease affects the small bowel if the colon is involved.

At an early stage in the disease, the findings at barium enema are: loss of haustration, narrowing of the lumen of the bowel and shallow ulceration. This criss-crossing ulceration combined with mucosal oedema may give rise to a 'cobblestone' appearance of

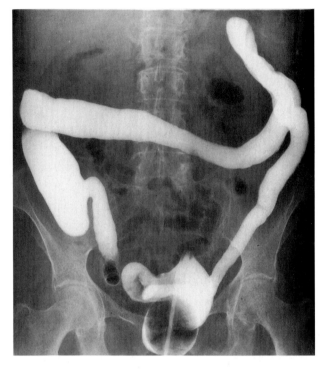

Fig. 5.57 Ulcerative colitis. With long-standing disease the haustra are lost and the colon becomes narrowed and shortened coming to resemble a rigid tube. Reflux into the ileum through an incompetent ileocaecal valve has occurred.

the mucosa (Fig. 5.58). Later, the ulcers become deeper and may track in the submucosa (Fig. 5.59). The ulcers may be very deep, penetrating into the muscle layer, when they are described as rose-thorn ulcers or deep fissures. The deep ulceration in Crohn's disease may lead to the formation of intra- and extramural abscesses. Fistulae are an important complication.

Strictures are a common finding in Crohn's disease (Fig. 5.60). The strictures are smooth and have tapered ends. When the caecum is involved it is usually markedly contracted. Ulcers may or may not be present in the strictured area. The disease is not always circumferential; one of the features that distinguishes it from ulcerative colitis is that it may involve only one portion of the circumference of the bowel.

Another important diagnostic feature is the presence

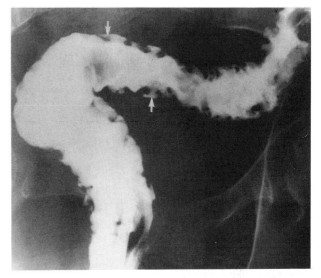

Fig. 5.59 Crohn's disease. Very deep ulcers are present. Two examples of an ulcer tracking in the submucosa are arrowed.

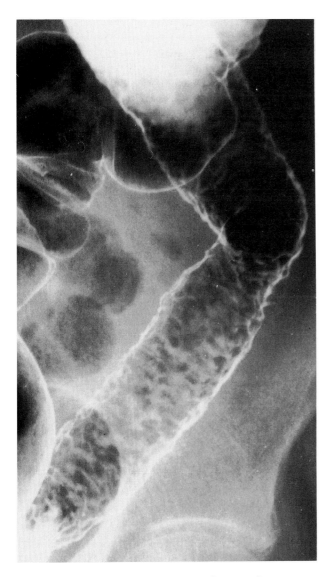

Fig. 5.58 Crohn's disease. The mucosal pattern has a cobblestone appearance due to criss-crossing fine ulceration.

Fig. 5.60 Crohn's disease—strictures. A long stricture is present in the transverse colon (between curved arrows) and a shorter one in the sigmoid colon (between small arrows). In this case the outline of the strictures are irregular, due to ulceration. These two abnormal segments with normal intervening bowel are an example of 'skip lesions'—an important diagnostic feature of Crohn's disease.

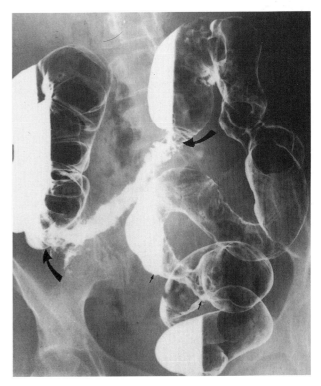

Table 5.2 Differences between Crohn's disease and ulcerative colitis

Crohn's disease	*Ulcerative colitis*
1 Rectum involved in half the cases	1 Rectum involved in all the cases
2 Colon may be affected segmentally	2 Colon always affected continuously
3 Ulcers deep	3 Ulcers shallow
4 Some cases show asymmetrical loss of haustra	4 Symmetrical loss of haustra is the rule
5 Fistulae are a feature	5 Fistulae very rarely occur
6 Anal or perianal lesions frequent	6 Anal or perianal lesions uncommon
7 Small bowel involvement common — particularly of the terminal ileum with narrowing in the region of the ileocaecal valve.	7 Small bowel normal — dilatation of the terminal ileum may be seen

of the so-called 'skip lesion' (Fig. 5.60), namely areas of disease with intervening normal bowel. Skip lesions are virtually diagnostic of Crohn's disease. However, the entire colon may be involved or the disease may be limited to just one segment. There is a predilection for the caecum and terminal ileum. The rectum is often spared — another important differentiating feature from ulcerative colitis. Fistulae may also occur between the colon and the small bowel, bladder or vagina (Fig. 5.61).

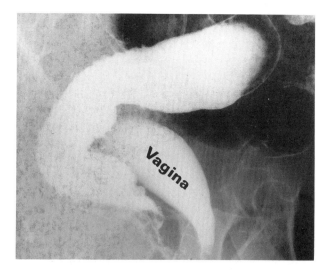

Fig. 5.61 Crohn's disease — rectovaginal fistula. During the barium enema filling of the vagina with barium occurred. Note the ulceration in the rectum.

Differences between ulcerative colitis and Crohn's disease

The only specific features are the presence of skip lesions and a normal rectum providing this is confirmed sigmoidoscopically. If either of these are seen then the diagnosis of Crohn's disease can be confidently made. Other differences are listed in Table 5.2.

Diverticular disease

Diverticula are sac-like out-pouchings of mucosa through the muscular layer of the bowel wall. They are associated with hypertrophy of the muscle layer and are probably due to herniation of mucosa through areas of weakness where blood vessels penetrate the muscle. Diverticula are very common, particularly in the elderly. They are seen in all parts of the colon but are commonest in the sigmoid colon. At one time, the term 'diverticulitis' was applied when infection was thought to be causing symptoms and diverticulosis when the diverticula were considered asymptomatic. As no radiological distinction can be made between these two entities the term 'diverticular disease' is nowadays used to cover both situations.

The diverticula when filled with barium are seen as spherical out-pouchings with a narrow neck (Fig. 5.62). The colon may also show a 'saw tooth' serrated appearance due to hypertrophy of the muscle coats (see Fig. 5.56, p. 180). Sometimes, the signs of muscle hypertrophy are seen in isolation. Some diverticula

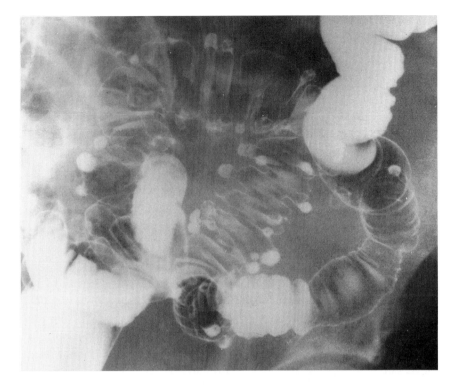

Fig. 5.62 Diverticular disease. Numerous diverticula are seen as out-pouchings from the sigmoid colon.

may not fill; this is particularly true when inflammation occludes the necks of the diverticula.

A diverticulum may perforate, resulting in a pericolic abscess or fistula into the bladder, small bowel or vagina. This is recognised by noting barium outside the colon, either in the pericolic region (Fig. 5.63) or within the structure to which the fistula has occurred. Occasionally, diverticula perforate directly into the peritoneal cavity giving rise to peritonitis, and free intraperitoneal air should be looked for on a plain abdominal film.

A stricture with or without local abscess formation (Fig. 5.64) may occur. Usually, this is clearly within an area of recognisable diverticular disease. It is, however, often impossible to differentiate such a stricture from a carcinoma occurring coincidentally in a patient with diverticular disease.

Ischaemic colitis

Acute infarction of the large bowel is very rare. Ischaemia is usually a more chronic process giving rise, initially, to mucosal oedema and haemorrhage which may resolve. In the later stages a stricture may form. The findings on barium enema depend on the stage at which the examination is performed.

Mucosal haemorrhage and oedema may be recognised by observing multiple smooth indentations into the lumen of the bowel, resembling thumb prints (Fig. 5.65a). If stricture formation occurs, the stricture will be smooth and have tapered ends. The site is usually centred between the splenic flexure and the sigmoid colon since these are the regions of the colon with the most vulnerable blood supply (Fig. 5.65b). Sacculations may be seen arising from one side of the strictured area.

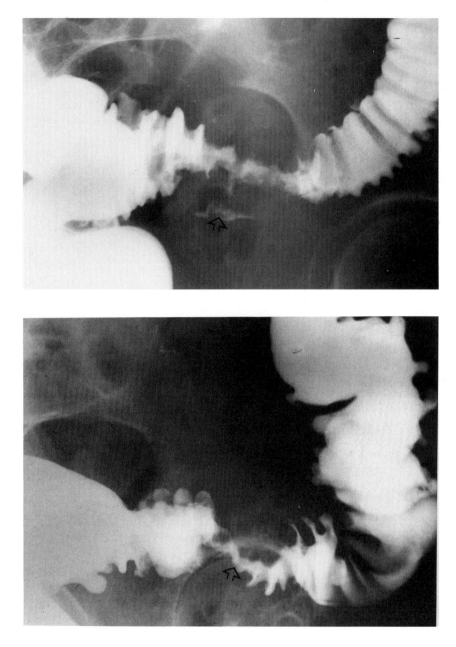

Fig. 5.63 Diverticular disease. Barium is seen outside the lumen of the bowel in a pericolic abscess (arrow). Muscle hypertrophy gives the bowel a serrated appearance.

Fig. 5.64 Diverticular disease. A stricture is present (arrow). Although there is recognisable diverticular disease at both ends of the stricture it is impossible to exclude definitely a carcinoma.

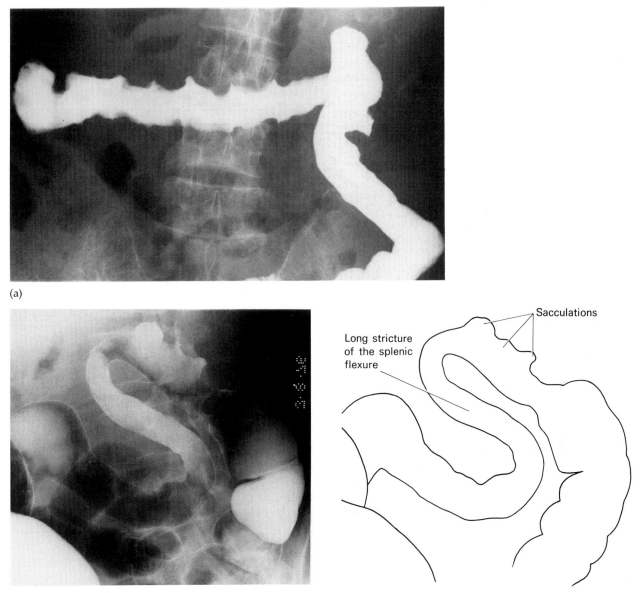

(a)

(b)

Fig. 5.65 Ischaemic colitis. (a) Mucosal haemorrhage and oedema have caused indentations resembling thumb prints in the transverse colon. (b) A long smooth stricture involving the splenic flexure with sacculation arising from one side of the colon in another patient.

Pneumatosis coli

In this unusual condition gas-filled spaces are present in the wall of the bowel. These cyst-like spaces do not communicate with the lumen. They can be identified on a plain film of the abdomen but the diagnosis is much easier with a barium enema where the cysts cause smooth translucent filling defects projecting from the wall of the bowel (Fig. 5.66). The appearance could be confused with intramural haemorrhage and oedema, or with colitis if the presence of air within the cysts is not appreciated.

Volvulus

In a volvulus a loop of bowel twists on its mesentery. This happens most frequently in the sigmoid colon, particularly when it is redundant, and less often in the caecum. The twisted loop becomes greatly distended and the bowel proximal to the volvulus is obstructed by the twist and may, therefore, also be dilated.

The diagnosis is usually made on the plain abdominal films (see p. 136) but a barium enema may be

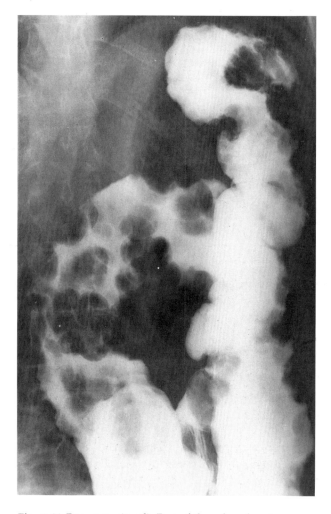

Fig. 5.66 Pneumatosis coli. Part of the colon showing numerous translucencies in the wall of the colon due to many gas-filled cysts.

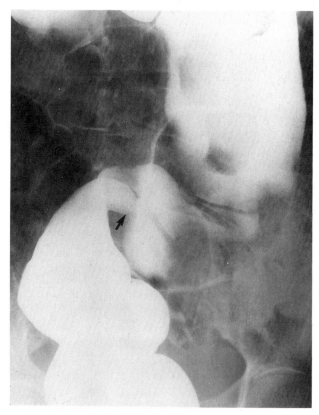

Fig. 5.67 Volvulus. A smooth narrowing is seen in the sigmoid colon where the colon has twisted (arrow). Note the dilated colon proximal to this.

helpful in doubtful cases so that if confirmed, non-operative reduction of the volvulus may be attempted. This will show a smooth, tapered narrowing (Fig. 5.67) due to twisting of the colon, with marked dilatation of the bowel proximal to the twist.

Intussusception

An intussusception is the invagination of one segment of the bowel into another. Infants are much more liable to intussusception than adults.

By far the commonest type is the ileum invaginating into the colon, which is known as an ileo-colic intussusception. Other types are colo-colic, when the colon invaginates into another part of the colon, and ileo-ileal when the ileum invaginates into a more distal segment of ileum.

At barium enema the flow of barium is obstructed by the leading edge of the intussusception, which causes a convex filling defect. This filling defect may show stretched mucosal folds on its surface giving the so-called 'coiled spring' appearance (Fig. 5.68). In infants and young children, an intussusception can sometimes be reduced with a barium enema, so avoiding a laparotomy. If such a reduction utilising hydrostatic pressure is to be safely carried out, the child should have no clinical signs of peritonitis. The longer the symptoms have been present, the greater

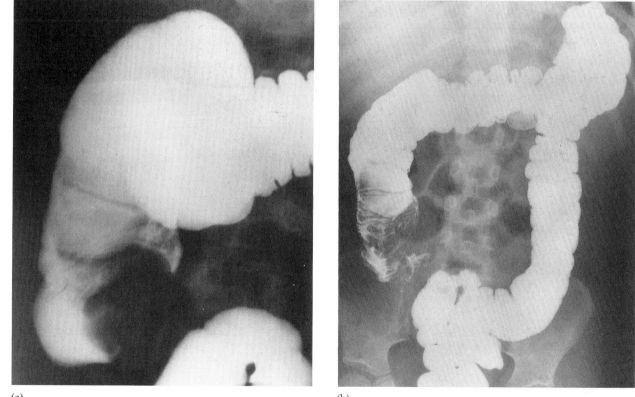

(a)   (b)

Fig. 5.68 Intussusception. A 2-year-old child. (a) Film taken during reduction of the intussusception with a barium enema showing a filling defect in the caecum due to ileum invaginated into the colon. (b) Later film showing a 'coiled spring' appearance in the caecum due to stretched mucosal folds of the invaginated ileum.

the risk of perforating gangrenous bowel. The leading edge of an intussusception may be detected as a mass, using ultrasound. Reduction using a water enema may be monitored with ultrasound, so avoiding the use of ionising radiation.

In adults, surgical treatment is invariable as an intussusception is usually caused by a tumour.

Tumours

Polyps

The word 'polyp' means a small mass of tissue arising from the wall of the bowel projecting into the lumen. Polyps may be sessile or on a stalk, single or multiple. They are best demonstrated with a double contrast barium enema. Polyps may be neoplastic, inflammatory or occasionally developmental in origin.

It is often impossible on radiological grounds to exclude malignancy in a polyp. However, only a tiny minority of polyps less than 1 cm in size and very few less than 2 cm are cancers.

The features that suggest malignancy are: a diameter of more than 2 cm; a short thick stalk; irregular surface; rapid rate of growth as judged by serial barium enema examinations.

The common polyps are:
1 *Adenomatous polyp* (Fig. 5.69). This is a benign neoplasm; there is controversy as to whether such lesions are pre-malignant. They may be single or multiple and are found most frequently in the rectosigmoid region. In familial polyposis they are numerous and one or more will, in time, undergo malignant change (Fig. 5.70). *Villous adenoma* is a benign sessile tumour showing a sponge-like appearance due to barium trapped between the villous strands. They are usually large when first discovered and are frequently mistaken for faeces. The common sites are the rectum and the caecum. There is a high incidence of malignant change.
2 *Polypoid adenocarcinoma.*
3 *Juvenile polyps.* Almost all isolated polyps in children are benign. They are probably developmental in origin.

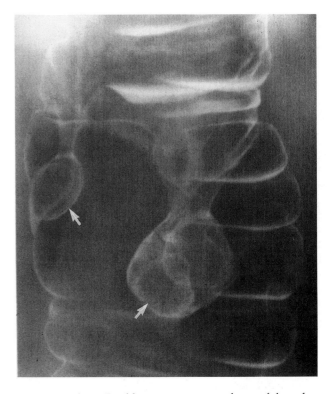

Fig. 5.69 Polyps. Double contrast enema of part of the colon showing two pedunculated adenomatous polyps (arrows).

4 *Inflammatory polyps (pseudopolyps)* are seen in ulcerative colitis.
5 *Hyperplastic or metaplastic polyps.*

Carcinoma

Carcinomas may arise anywhere in the colon but they are commonest in the rectosigmoid region and the caecum. The appearance and behaviour of a carcinoma in these two sites are usually quite different. The patient with a rectosigmoid carcinoma often has an annular stricture and presents with alteration in bowel habit and obstruction, whereas with a caecal carcinoma the tumour can become very large without obstructing the bowel, so anaemia and weight loss are the common presenting features.

A barium enema shows the annular carcinoma as an

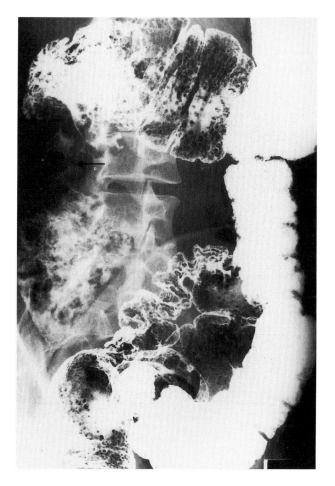

Fig. 5.70 Familial polyposis. Numerous small polyps are present throughout the colon. An annular carcinoma has developed in the ascending colon (arrows).

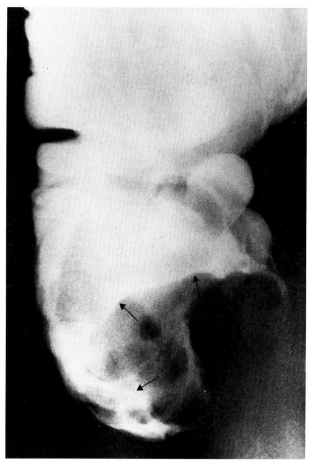

Fig. 5.71 Polypoid carcinoma. A large irregular filling defect is present in the caecum. The extent of the tumour is indicated by the arrows.

irregular stricture with shouldered edges (see Fig. 5.51, p. 176). Such strictures are rarely more than 6 cm in length. The polypoid or fungating carcinoma (Fig. 5.71) causes an irregular filling defect projecting into the lumen of the bowel.

Multiple primary tumours must be excluded, as the patient with one carcinoma of the colon has a higher than normal risk of developing a second colonic cancer. This may be present at the time of the diagnosis or may present after the first tumour has been removed.

CT/MRI of rectal carcinoma (Fig. 5.72)

The main value of CT and MRI is to demonstrate any tumour that has spread through the wall of the rectum and also to diagnose postoperative recurrence. Pelvic fat surrounds the rectum, and tumour infiltrating this fat can be readily recognised. Invasion into adjacent organs, the pelvic side walls, sacrum and lymph node metastases may also be demonstrated. Often, images of the abdomen are also taken in order to detect any para-aortic adenopathy or liver metastases.

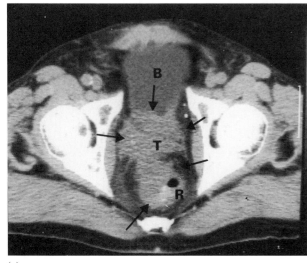

(a)

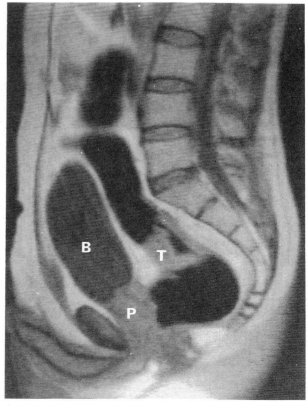

(b)

Fig. 5.72 Carcinoma of the rectum. (a) CT scan showing the tumour (T) invading the peripelvic fat and the bladder (B). The extent of the tumour is indicated by the arrows. (b) Sagittal MRI scan showing a tumour (T) confined within the rectum (R). P, prostate; R, rectum.

Hirschsprung's disease (congenital aganglionosis)

This condition is due to absence of ganglion cells beyond a certain level in the colon, usually in the sigmoid or rectosigmoid region. In time, the colon proximal to the aganglionic segment becomes grossly distended, but in those patients who present soon after birth the dilatation may not be obvious.

The aganglionic segment, usually the rectum, is either normal or small at barium enema and the diagnosis depends on recognising the transition from the normal or reduced calibre colon to the dilated colon (Fig. 5.73). To prevent the danger of water intoxication from the dilated colon, the colon is not washed out before the barium enema. The barium introduced is usually limited to the amount required to show the zone of transition from aganglionic to dilated bowel.

Idiopathic megacolon (functional megacolon)

The cause is believed to be chronic constipation. At barium enema both the rectum and colon are dilated and contain large amount of faeces. The large-sized rectum serves as a differentiating feature from Hirschsprung's disease.

Radiology in acute bleeding from the small and large bowel

A Meckel's diverticulum, if it contains ectopic gastric mucosa, may be responsible for unexplained bleeding, particularly in children. A Meckel's diverticulum is very difficult to demonstrate on a barium follow-through but may be visualised with radionuclide techniques. An intravenous injection of technetium-

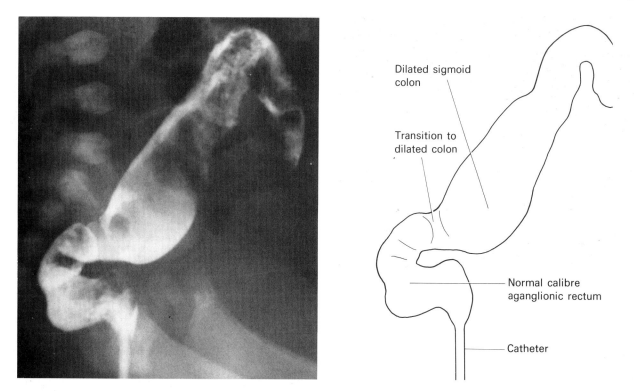

Fig. 5.73 Hirschsprung's disease. Note the transition between the normal calibre aganglionic rectum and the dilated sigmoid colon.

99m (^{99m}Tc-pertechnetate) is given, which localises in gastric mucosa. High uptake will be seen in the stomach and in any gastric mucosa within a Meckel's diverticulum (Fig. 5.74).

Acute bleeding may occur in large and small bowel tumours. The condition angiodysplasia, a disorder comprising dilated vessels in the caecum, is a fairly common cause of bleeding in elderly patients. A barium enema should be avoided as the first examination because the presence of barium in the colon may preclude other investigations. Colonoscopy is usually performed but may be unrewarding as it is sometimes

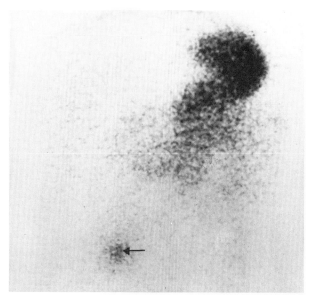

Fig. 5.74 Meckel's diverticulum. ^{99m}Tc-pertechnetate scan showing an isolated area of uptake in ectopic gastric mucosa in a Meckel's diverticulum (arrow). Normal uptake of radionuclide is seen in the stomach.

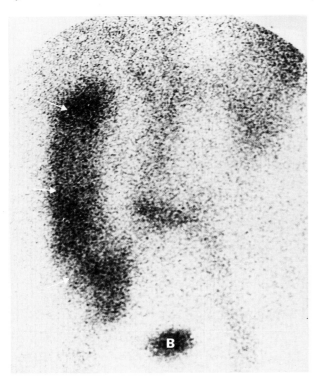

Fig. 5.75 Gastrointestinal bleeding. The patient's red blood cells have been labelled with ^{99m}Tc. Blood has collected in the ascending colon (arrows) from an active bleeding site in the caecum. B, bladder.

not possible to reach the right side of the colon. Even when the caecum is reached, angiodysplasia may not be visible through the colonoscope.

Arteriography may demonstrate the bleeding site, provided the patient is actively bleeding, by showing contrast in the lumen of the bowel. Sometimes arteriography also permits a diagnosis to be made, e.g. angiodysplasia or small bowel tumour. Embolisation of the feeding vessel can be carried out to arrest bleeding at the time of arteriography when appropriate.

If the patient is actively bleeding at a rate of more than 0.5 ml/min then nuclear medicine techniques can be employed to localise the bleeding. Two different methods are available. The patient's red blood cells are labelled with ^{99m}Tc and the patient is then imaged under a gamma camera, so that any blood collecting in the bowel will be visualised (Fig. 5.75). Alternatively, the patient can be given an intravenous injection of ^{99m}Tc labelled colloid, the agent used for liver scanning. This is rapidly cleared from the circulation by the reticuloendothelial system. Any bleeding into the bowel can readily be demonstrated. Nuclear medicine techniques are simpler but almost as accurate as arteriography in localising active haemorrhage and will assist in planning possible surgery or subsequent arteriography.

Hepatobiliary System, Pancreas and Spleen

Many different methods of imaging the hepatobiliary system and pancreas are available, including plain films, contrast examinations of the biliary system, ultrasound, computed tomography (CT), radionuclide imaging, and now magnetic resonance imaging (MRI). Invasive studies such as percutaneous or operative cholangiography and endoscopic retrograde cholangiopancreatography (ERCP) may be indicated, as may selective arteriography. Each of these tests has its own advantages and disadvantages. Ultrasound, for example, is particularly useful for diagnosing gall bladder disease, recognising dilated bile ducts, diagnosing cysts and abscesses, and defining perihepatic fluid collections, whereas CT and MRI are particularly sensitive for detecting mass lesions such as metastases and abscesses. Often the various methods complement each other. Since the roles of the individual procedures are not clear cut, practice will vary from one centre to another.

In order to simplify the presentation, we will discuss the liver parenchyma separately from the biliary tract, though in clinical practice they usually need to be considered together.

Interventional techniques designed to treat or remove gallstones and to drain the biliary system are described on page 434.

LIVER

Ultrasound of the liver

The *normal hepatic parenchyma* (Fig. 6.1) is of uniform echoreflectivity, composed of low and medium amplitude echoes, interspersed with the bright echoes of the portal triads and echo-free areas corresponding to large hepatic veins.

The normal liver displays considerable variation in size and shape. The right hepatic lobe is much larger than the left, which may even be diminutive. The falciform ligament, which contains the ligamentum teres, lies between the medial and lateral segments of the left lobe. The ligamentum teres is often surrounded by fat; the resulting echo pattern should not be confused with a mass (Fig. 6.2).

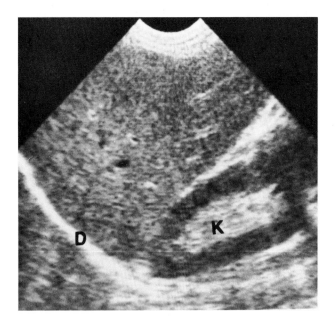

Fig. 6.1 Ultrasound of normal liver. Longitudinal scan showing uniform echo pattern interspersed with bright echoes of portal triads and echo-free areas of hepatic veins. D, diaphragm; K, right kidney.

The portal vein is an important landmark to hepatic anatomy (Fig. 6.3). Within the liver it divides into right and left branches. Running alongside the portal veins are the hepatic arteries and bile ducts, both of which are usually too small to be visualized within the liver. Surrounding these portal triads is an echo-reflective sheath of fibrous and fatty tissue. The hepatic veins run separately, increasing in diameter as they drain towards the inferior vena cava at the level of the diaphragm (Fig. 6.4).

Focal masses are recognised sonographically as alterations of the normal echo pattern. They can be divided into cysts, solid masses, or complex combinations of the two. Cysts which are echo free and have thin or invisible walls can be assumed to be non-neoplastic (Fig. 6.5). Solid and complex masses (Figs 6.6 and 6.7) within the liver may be either benign or malignant in nature. Theoretically, most benign solid masses are encapsulated and should demonstrate a relatively sharp margin with the adjacent hepatic parenchyma, whereas malignant lesions should demonstrate a more irregular border. However, in practice it is often difficult to distinguish benign from malignant lesions unless the mass is clearly a simple cyst.

When multiple solid or complex masses are seen within the liver, metastatic disease is the likely diagnosis, especially in patients with a known primary tumour. The prime differential diagnoses of multiple

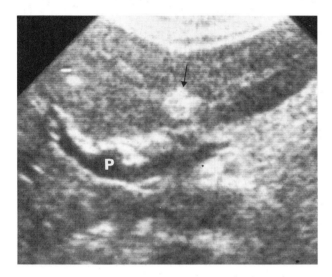

Fig. 6.2 Ultrasound of normal liver. Transverse scan showing ligamentum teres (arrow) which should not be confused with a mass. P, portal vein.

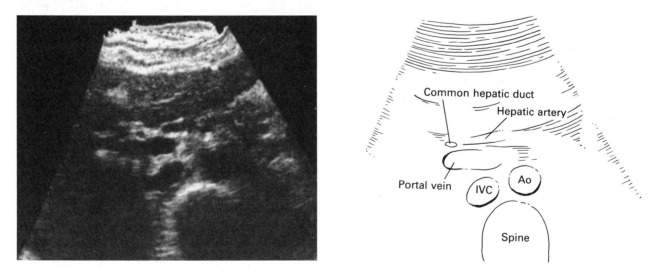

Fig. 6.3 Ultrasound of normal liver. Transverse scan across the porta hepatis. Ao, aorta; IVC, inferior vena cava.

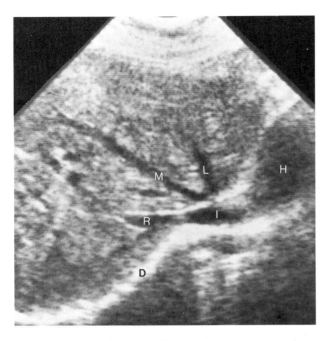

Fig. 6.4 Ultrasound of normal liver. Transverse scan through the superior portion of the liver showing the right (R), middle (M) and left (L) hepatic veins draining into the inferior vena cava (I) as it penetrates the diaphragm (D) to enter the chest. H, heart.

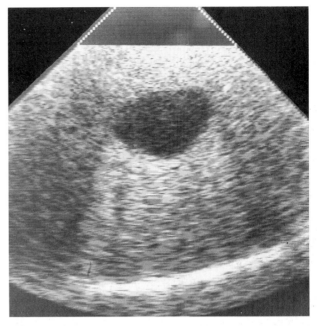

Fig. 6.5 Ultrasound of benign cyst. Note the imperceptible walls and acoustic enhancement behind the cyst. (CT scan of same case is shown in Figure 6.17a.)

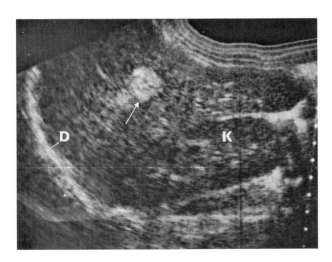

Fig. 6.6 Ultrasound of solid mass. Longitudinal scan. The arrow points to a highly reflective mass which proved to be a metastasis. K, right kidney; D, diaphragm.

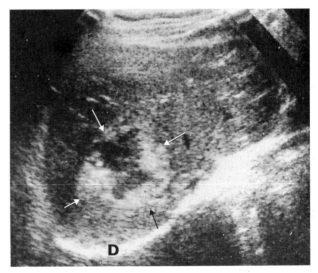

Fig. 6.7 Ultrasound of complex mass. Transverse scan showing spherical mass (arrows) with areas of reflectivity both greater and less than normal liver. D, diaphragm.

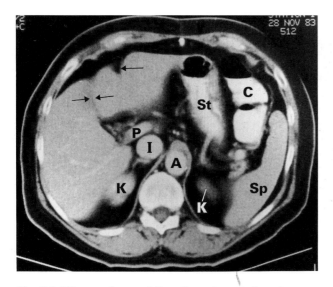

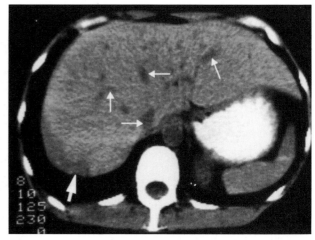

Fig. 6.8 CT scan of normal liver through porta hepatis (enhanced scan). A, aorta; C, colon; I, inferior vena cava; K, kidney; P, portal vein; Sp, spleen; St, Stomach; Single arrow = fissure for falciform ligament, Double arrow = fissure for gall bladder which divides liver into right and left lobes.

Fig. 6.9 CT scan showing unopacified hepatic veins (arrows) which should not be confused with metastases. Comparison with true metastases can be made since a metastasis is present in this case at the periphery of the right lobe (large arrow).

masses are multiple abscesses, regenerating nodules in cirrhosis of the liver, and multiple haemangiomas.

Diffuse parenchymal diseases such as diffuse chronic inflammation, and diffuse neoplastic infiltration can cause a generalised increase in the intensity of echoes from the liver parenchyma, and are difficult to distinguish from one another.

Computed tomography of the liver (Fig. 6.8)

The usual technique is to perform contiguous 10 mm sections through the liver. Intravenous contrast medium is often given in order to increase the density of normal liver parenchyma and to emphasise the density difference between the normal parenchyma and lesions which enhance poorly, such as tumours, abscesses or haematomas. Occasionally, very vascular lesions such as haemangiomas and a few neoplasms show greater enhancement than the surrounding parenchyma.

The lobar anatomy of the liver is defined by the fissure of the gall bladder, which divides the right and left lobes. The fissure for the falciform ligament is also clearly shown dividing the left lobe into medial and lateral segments.

The normal hepatic parenchyma has a relatively high density prior to contrast enhancement; higher than that of muscle and higher or equal in density to the spleen. On images taken without intravenous contrast medium, the hepatic veins are seen as branching, low density structures coursing through the liver. Since CT is a sectional technique, some of these branches may be seen as round or oval low-density areas which should not be confused with metastases (Fig. 6.9). After contrast enhancement, the hepatic veins opacify to become similar or higher in density than the surrounding parenchyma. Because the normal intra-hepatic bile ducts are not visible and hepatic vessels opacify with contrast medium, the normal hepatic parenchyma after contrast shows either uniform density, or shows the hepatic veins clearly opacified against a background of uniform density. The region

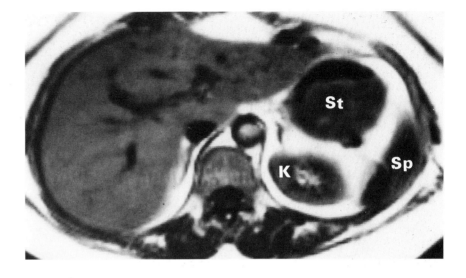

Fig. 6.10 Normal MRI scan of liver (T_1-weighted image). The liver parenchyma shows intermediate signal. The blood vessels within the liver (predominantly the portal and hepatic veins) show no signal. K, kidney; Sp, spleen; St, stomach.

of the porta hepatis is recognisable as the entrance and exit points of the major vessels and bile ducts. The biliary system distal to the right and the left hepatic ducts can be identified on good quality images, but the smaller intrahepatic bile ducts are not visible in the normal patient.

Radionuclide liver imaging

Radionuclide liver scanning (^{99m}Tc labelled sulphur or tin colloid) has been largely replaced by ultrasound, CT and MRI. The hepatobiliary agents which are discussed on page 205 also show the liver parenchyma, but their primary indication is to show disease of the extrahepatic biliary system.

Two further tests are occasionally performed. Technetium-99m may be tagged to the patient's own red blood cells to act as a blood pool agent in order to diagnose haemangiomas in the liver and, secondly, indium-111 can be tagged to the patient's white blood cells in order to demonstrate accumulation of these cells in abscesses.

Magnetic resonance imaging of the liver (Fig. 6.10)

The basic principles of MRI of the liver are similar to CT. MRI appears to be more sensitive than CT for detecting liver masses, notably metastases. It also shows considerable promise for characterising liver masses into cysts, haemangiomas or solid tumours. The major disadvantages of MRI at present are cost, availability and the inability to provide acceptable images of the rest of the abdomen, largely because image quality is degraded due to the motion of breathing, cardiac pulsation and peristalsis.

Liver masses

Ultrasound, CT, MRI and angiography are all good methods of deciding that a mass is present. Occasionally, as for example with cysts and haemangiomas, it is possible to predict the nature of a mass, but more often the definitive diagnosis will depend on the clinical features or biopsy.

Liver neoplasms

Metastases, notably from carcinoma of the stomach, colon, pancreas, lung and breast are much more common than primary carcinoma (hepatoma and malignant lymphoma, both of which can be multifocal).

Metastases are often multiple, situated peripherally

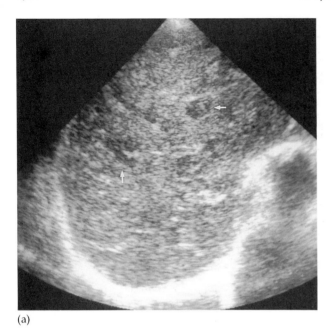

(a)

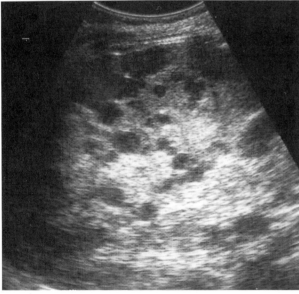

(b)

Fig. 6.11 Ultrasound of liver metastases. (a) Multiple, rounded areas of reduced echogenicity are seen scattered throughout the liver. Arrows point to two of these lesions. (b) Multiple cystic metastases are shown as clearly defined, round, echo-free lesions scattered through the liver.

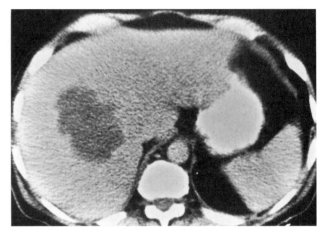

Fig. 6.12 CT scan of metastasis. This large low density mass is situated deeply in the right lobe of the liver.

and of variable size. At ultrasound, they show increased reflectivity (Fig. 6.6) or, more usually, decreased reflectivity compared with the surrounding parenchyma (Fig. 6.11a). At times, they show a complex echo pattern (Fig. 6.7) and when they undergo central necrosis they may even resemble cysts (Fig. 6.11b). Some metastases have an echo pattern virtually identical to that of the surrounding parenchyma which means they cannot be identified at sonography. At CT, metastases are seen as rounded areas, usually lower in density than the contrast enhanced surrounding parenchyma (Fig. 6.12). Most are well demarcated from the adjacent parenchyma. Intense contrast enhancement is sometimes seen within the tumour, or immediately surrounding it—a useful differentiating feature, which is not seen with cysts. MRI is an excellent method of demonstrating metastases (Fig. 6.13). With the increased availability of CT and ultrasound, ^{99m}Tc labelled colloid scans are rarely performed; they show reduced activity in the areas of liver replaced by tumour.

Primary carcinomas of the liver are usually solitary, but may be multifocal. Their CT, ultrasound and MRI features are similar to metastatic neoplasm; they may even be multifocal (Fig. 6.14).

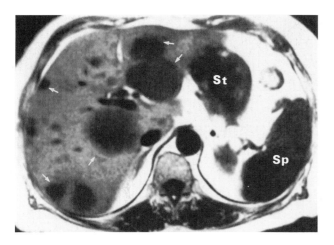

Fig. 6.13 Metastases. MRI scan showing multiple rounded low signal areas in the liver (arrows) on this T_1-weighted image. Compare with the normal image shown in Figure 6.10. Sp, spleen; St, stomach.

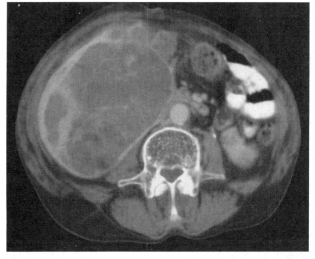

Fig. 6.14 Hepatoma. The CT scan shows a large, well-defined mass of variable density.

Haemangiomas of the liver (Figs 6.15 and 6.16)

One or more haemangiomas of the liver are common incidental findings and rarely require surgical resection. Occasionally they can cause significant haemorrhage, especially following trauma, and therefore percutaneous biopsy should be avoided, if possible. Haemangiomas of the liver resemble neoplasms and other masses at ultrasound. At CT, there is one feature that permits a differentiation to be made. Initially, a haemangioma appears as a rounded, low density lesion but when sections are repeated after contrast, at intervals of a few minutes, the density increases to become similar with that of the surrounding liver. This phenomenon of blood pooling in haemangiomas can also be demonstrated by radionuclide blood pool scans. Magnetic resonance imaging shows uniform very high intensity on T_2 weighted images (Fig. 6.16), a characteristic that is shared with benign cysts, but which is very unusual with malignant neoplastic lesions.

Liver cysts

Simple cysts of the liver, both single and multiple, are usually congenital in origin; some are due to infection. Multiple hepatic cysts occur in adult polycystic disease, which not only affects the kidneys but may also involve the liver and other organs. These cysts are variable in size and are scattered through the liver.

At ultrasound, liver cysts show the typical features of cysts elsewhere in the body, namely: sharp margins; no echoes within the lesion; and intense echoes from the front and back walls with acoustic enhancement deep to the larger cysts (see Fig. 6.5, p. 195).

At CT, cysts show very well defined margins and have attenuation values similar to that of water (Fig. 6.17a). Lesions below 2 cm in diameter may be difficult to distinguish from solid neoplasms because portions of the normal liver may be present on a particular CT section, and partial volume averaging may then result in a CT number close to that of soft tissues. Below 1 cm in diameter it is almost never possible to distinguish cyst from neoplasm.

At MRI, the features will be similar to those found at CT, the signal corresponding to water.

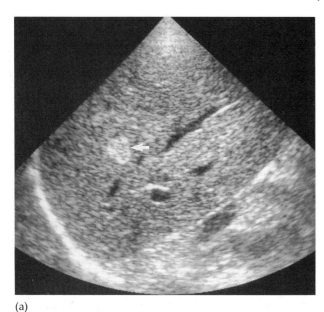

(a)

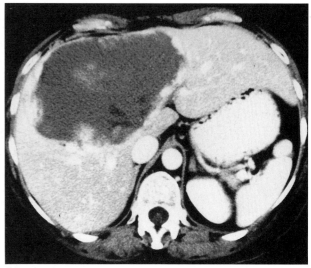

(b)

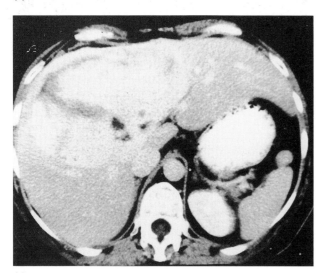

(c)

Fig. 6.15 Haemangioma (incidental finding). (a) Ultrasound scan shows a reflective mass in the right lobe of the liver (arrow). (b) CT scan, in another patient, immediately after intravenous contrast enhancement shows a large, low density lesion in the right lobe of the liver with appearances similar to a tumour. (c) A scan taken 10 minutes later shows that almost the entire lesion enhances to the same or to a greater degree than the normal liver.

Cysts due to echinococcus (hydatid) disease may be single or multiple; a few show calcified walls. Daughter cysts may be seen within a main cyst at both ultrasound and CT (Fig. 6.17b, c). Unless these features are present, hydatid cysts may prove indistinguishable from simple cysts at both ultrasound and CT.

Liver abscess (Fig. 6.18)

Abscesses appear somewhat similar to cysts but usually they can be distinguished. Hepatic abscesses tend to have fluid centres, with walls that are thicker, more irregular and more obvious than those of simple cysts. Although the CT attenuation values in the centre

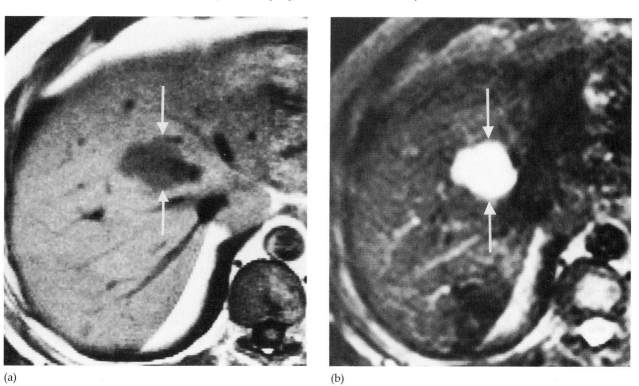

(a) (b)

Fig. 6.16 MRI scan of a haemangioma. (a) Low intensity area (arrows) on a T_1-weighted image. (b) High intensity area (arrows) on a T_2-weighted image. This haemangioma was an incidental finding.

of an abscess may be the same as water, usually they are higher. At ultrasound, a layer of necrotic debris may be seen within the abscess. (It should be noted that even simple cysts may demonstrate some fine low level echoes within them, believed to be due to cholesterol crystals which are the remnants of old haemorrhages into the cysts.) Occasionally, chronic abscesses calcify.

Scanning with radiolabelled white blood cells will reveal substantially increased uptake in an abscess.

Abscesses cannot usually be distinguished from necrotic tumours at either ultrasound, CT or MRI, but the clinical situation should aid in making the distinction.

Liver trauma

Trauma to the liver is the commonest abdominal injury that leads to death. Parenchymal lacerations are the most frequent injury and they are often accompanied by subcapsular haematomas (Fig. 6.19). Both are recognised as low density areas on CT; occasionally iso-dense or high density blood clots are seen. The major differential diagnoses are artefacts from surrounding structures, and pre-existing mass lesions. Although ultrasound, MRI and radionuclide scans can demonstrate liver injuries, CT is the best technique because it also surveys other injured organs (e.g. kidneys, and spleen) and can identify small quantities of fluid in the peritoneal cavity.

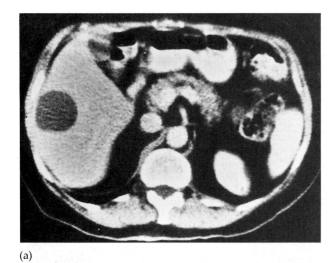

(a)

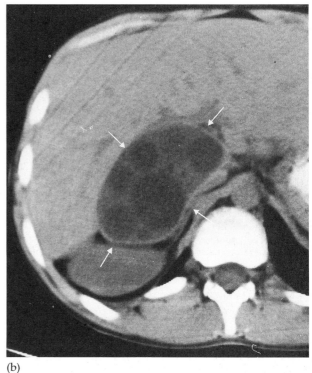

(b)

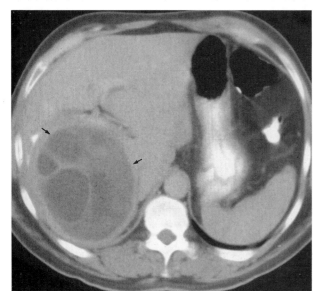

(c)

Fig. 6.17 Liver cysts. (a) Simple cyst of liver. CT scan shows a well-defined lesion of water density. (The ultrasound scan of this patient is shown in Figure 6.5.) (b) CT scan showing a well-defined multilocular hydatid cyst in the right lobe of the liver (arrows). (c) CT scan showing a multilocular hydatid cyst in the right lobe of the liver (arrows) in another patient.

Cirrhosis of the liver and portal hypertension

In portal hypertension the pressure in the portal venous system is elevated due to obstruction to the flow of blood in the portal or hepatic venous systems. Cirrhosis of the liver is by far the most frequent cause.

Other causes include occlusion of the hepatic veins (Budd–Chiari syndrome) and thrombosis of the portal vein, particularly following infection of the umbilical vein in the neonatal period.

Because the portal venous pressure is raised, blood flows through anastomotic channels, known as porto-

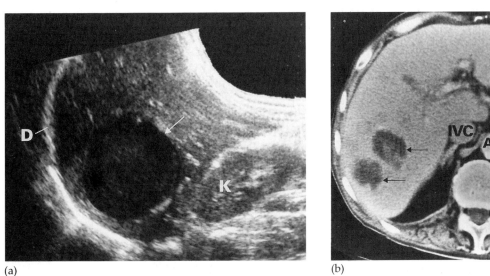

(a)

(b)

Fig. 6.18 Liver abscess. (a) Ultrasound showing a large transonic area (arrow) with echoes arising within it. D, diaphragm; K, kidney. (b) CT scan in another patient showing bilocular area of low attenuation in the right lobe of the liver (arrows). Ao, aorta; IVC, inferior vena cava; S, spleen; St, stomach.

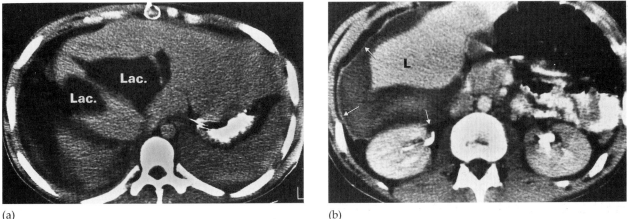

(a)

(b)

Fig. 6.19 Liver trauma. CT scan. (a) Two large lacerations (Lac) are shown in the right lobe of the liver. These contained a mixture of bile and blood. (b) A lower section. Between the liver capsule (arrows) and the liver (L) is an area of soft tissue density representing haematoma.

systemic anastomoses, to enter the vena cavae by-passing the liver. These collateral channels may be found in various sites, but the most important are varices at the lower end of the oesophagus (see Fig. 5.16, p. 154). The collateral channels can sometimes be shown with colour-flow Doppler ultrasound.

The signs of cirrhosis of the liver at CT and ultrasound are reduction in size of the right lobe of the liver together with splenomegaly. The texture of the liver at ultrasound may be diffusely abnormal; at CT, the parenchyma appears normal until late in the disease.

Portal venography may be undertaken to assess the patency of the portal vein but only when surgical portosystemic bypass operations, such as porto-caval shunt, are under consideration. Contrast is injected into the coeliac axis, splenic artery or superior mesenteric artery; films are then taken during the venous phase to show the portal venous system.

Fatty degeneration of the liver

Fatty degeneration of the liver, whilst not normal, is a relatively frequent finding, particularly in those who take alcohol to excess and those who are malnourished or debilitated for any reason. Fatty degeneration may involve the whole liver, or it may just involve individual subsections.

Fatty degeneration leads to a reduction in the attenuation of the affected parenchyma causing low density on CT scans (Fig. 6.20). The vessels are then

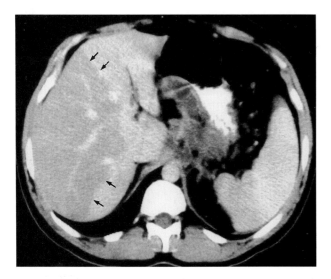

Fig. 6.20 Fatty degeneration of the liver shown by CT as a large focal area of reduced attenuation in the right lobe of the liver (arrows). Note that on this CT scan, taken after intravenous contrast enhancement, the blood vessels within the area of fatty degeneration are seen as relatively high attenuation structures against the background of the low-density parenchyma.

seen as relatively high attenuation structures against a background of low density parenchyma, even on images taken without intravenous contrast medium. On ultrasound, the liver parenchyma shows increased echogenicity, the so-called 'bright liver', in which the echogenicity of the liver is similar to that of the central echo-complex of the kidney. MRI can be very helpful in problem cases because fat gives a characteristic set of signals.

BILIARY SYSTEM

The gall bladder and bile duct system can be demonstrated by a variety of imaging techniques. Ultrasound is the best all-purpose method of investigation, because it is the simplest and best test for showing gallstones and diseases of the gall bladder and is also an excellent test for confirming or excluding bile duct dilatation. Oral cholecystography has a very limited role nowadays and has been largely abandoned as a diagnostic test. Radionuclide examination using hepatobiliary agents has an important role in excluding obstruction to the cystic duct.

Gallstones, gall bladder wall thickening and dilatation of the common bile duct are all recognisable at CT, but since ultrasound provides better information at less cost, CT is not used as the primary method of examination for these problems.

Ultrasound of the gall bladder and bile ducts

As the gall bladder is a fluid-filled structure, it is particularly amenable to sonographic examination. Because it is important that the gall bladder should be full of bile, the patient is asked to fast in order to prevent gall bladder contraction, but no other preparation is necessary. The normal gall bladder wall is so thin that it is sometimes barely perceptible (Fig. 6.21a). *Gall bladder wall thickening* suggests either acute or chronic cholecystitis (Fig. 6.21b). *Gallstones* greater than 1 or 2 mm in size can usually be identified at ultrasound examination. It is usually impossible to diagnose cystic duct obstruction with ultrasound; the

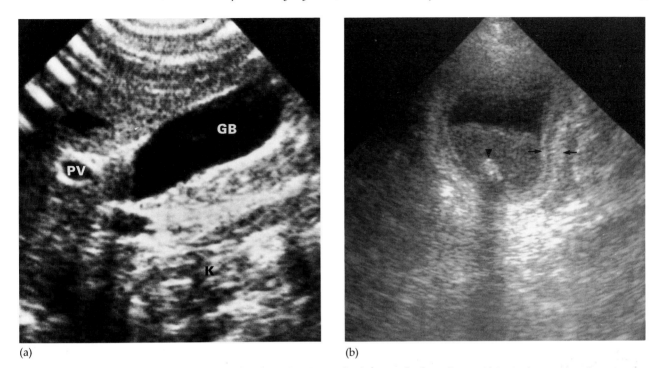

(a)   (b)

Fig. 6.21 (a) Ultrasound of normal gall bladder. Note the thin wall, absence of echoes from within, and acoustic enhancement behind the gall bladder. GB, gall bladder; K, right kidney; PV, portal vein. (b) Thick oedematous gall bladder wall in acute cholecystitis. The arrows indicate the thickness of the gall bladder wall. The gall bladder contains a gallstone (arrowhead) and inflammatory debris.

cystic duct is too small to identify and the stones that impact in it are often too small to see.

Ultrasonography is also the best test for demonstrating the *bile ducts*. The common hepatic or common bile duct can be visualised in almost all patients; it is seen as a small tubular structure lying anterior to the portal vein in the porta hepatis and should not measure more than 7 mm in diameter (Fig. 6.22). The lower end of the common bile duct is often obscured by gas in the duodenum, which lies just anterior to it.

The normal intraphepatic biliary tree is of such small calibre that only small portions a few millimetres long may be seen at ultrasound.

Hepatobiliary radionuclide scanning

Iminodiacetic acid (IDA) pharmaceuticals labelled with

^{99m}Tc are excreted by the liver following intravenous injection and may be used for imaging the bile duct system. Their main use is in patients with suspected acute cholecystitis. Hepatic excretion occurs despite relatively high serum bilirubin levels and, therefore, these agents can be used when the patient is jaundiced, even with serum bilirubin levels of up to 250 μmol/l (15 mg%). All that is required is that the patient fasts for 4 hours prior to the injection of the radionuclide. Normally, the gall bladder, common bile duct, duodenum and small bowel are all seen within the first hour, confirming the patency of both the cystic duct and the common bile duct (Fig. 6.23a). If the common bile duct and duodenum or small bowel are seen within the first hour, but the gall bladder is not visualised, the cystic duct is considered to be obstructed (Fig. 6.23b).

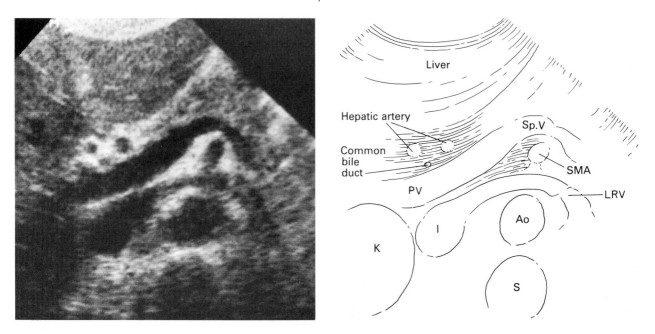

Fig. 6.22 Normal common bile duct. Transverse scan through the porta hepatis. Ao, aorta; I, inferior vena cava; K, kidney; LRV, left renal vein; PV, portal vein; SMA, superior mesenteric artery; S, spine; Sp.V, splenic vein.

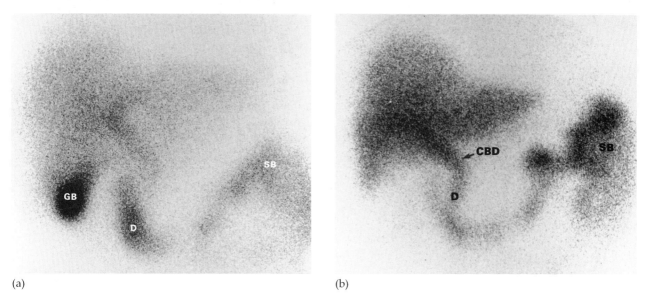

(a)   (b)

Fig. 6.23 Hepatobiliary scan. (a) Normal IDA scan. There is obvious filling of the gall bladder. Activity is also present in the duodenum and small bowel. (b) Cystic duct obstruction. The IDA scan in this patient with acute right upper quadrant pain shows the duct system but no filling of the gall bladder. CBD, common bile duct; D, duodenum; GB, gall bladder; SB, small bowel.

Endoscopic retrograde cholangiopancreatography

Endoscopic retrograde cholangiopancreatography (ERCP) consists of injecting contrast material directly into the common bile duct through a catheter inserted into the papilla of Vater via an endoscope positioned in the duodenum (Fig. 6.24).

The indications are:

• To determine the cause of jaundice, notably in patients with large duct obstruction (Figs 6.24b and c), and to undertake endoscopic treatment (see p. 434).

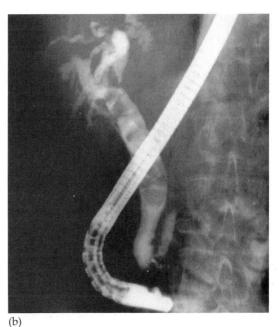

(b)

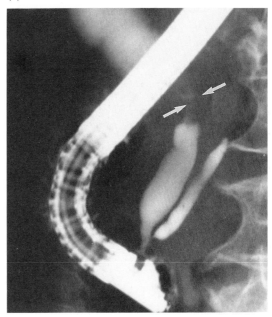

(c)

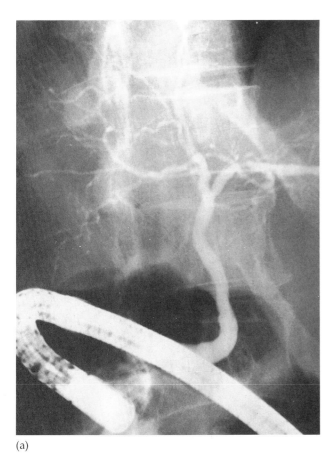

(a)

Fig. 6.24 Endoscopic retrograde cholangiography (ERCP). (a) A normal biliary system has been shown by injecting contrast through a catheter passed from the endoscope into the common bile duct. (b) A dilated ductal system with numerous large calculi in the hepatic and common bile ducts. (c) A localised stricture in the common bile duct due to cholangiocarcinoma (arrow).

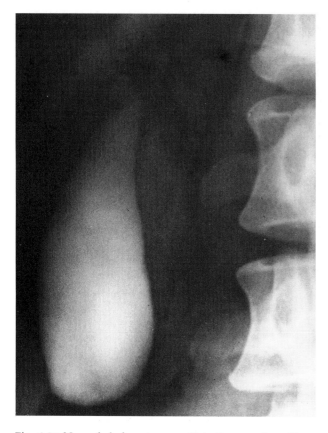

Fig. 6.25 Normal cholecystogram. Note the smooth outline and homogeneous filling of the gall bladder.

• The investigation of unexplained abdominal pain thought to be biliary in origin, when other investigations have been equivocal. An added advantage is that the pancreatic duct system often fills as well.

Oral cholecystography

Oral cholecystography, which used to be the main method of diagnosing gallstones and chronic cholecystitis, has been almost entirely replaced by ultrasound examination and is nowadays used only for very specialised purposes such as equivocal cases on ultrasound and localising the gall bladder for certain types of lithotripsy. On the first day a plain film of the right upper quadrant is taken. The patient takes an iodine-containing contrast medium by mouth at night and films of the gall bladder area are taken the following morning with the patient fasting.

An oral cholecystogram is of no value if the serum bilirubin is above 35 μmol/l (2 mg%).

The outline of the normal gall bladder is always smooth (Fig. 6.25) and its opacification reasonably uniform. Since the colon overlies the gall bladder, superimposed shadowing due to gas and faeces may simulate gallstones.

Other diagnostic procedures

Operative cholangiogram

Operative cholangiography is performed during a surgical operation, usually cholecystectomy. Contrast medium is injected directly into the gall bladder, cystic or common bile duct to show whether there are any stones in the hepatic or common bile ducts and to ensure free passage of contrast into the duodenum. An operative cholangiogram is much better than palpation or surgical exploration for detecting stones within the ducts.

Postoperative T-tube cholangiogram

If the common bile duct is explored at surgery, a T-tube is placed in the duct system to provide biliary drainage. Contrast can be injected through the T-tube about 10 days postoperatively to ensure that no stones are present in the biliary system, and that the contrast flows freely into the duodenum before the T-tube is pulled out (Fig. 6.26).

Percutaneous transhepatic cholangiogram

Percutaneous transhepatic cholangiogram (PTC) is an alternative to ERCP for demonstrating the bile duct system in order to show the site and cause of obstruction. The procedure is carried out under local anaesthesia and because it is far easier and safer to perform

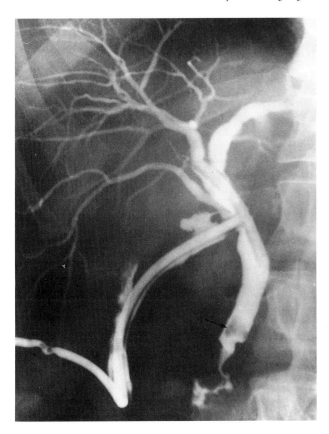

Fig. 6.26 T-tube cholangiogram. There is a stone (arrow) at the lower end of the common bile duct. The intrahepatic ducts are of normal calibre.

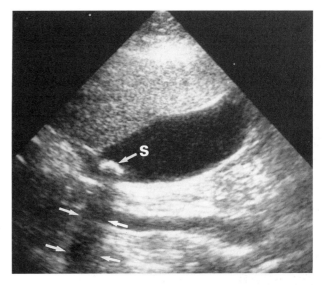

Fig. 6.27 Gallstone. Ultrasound shows a stone (S) in the gall bladder. The arrows point to the acoustic shadow behind the stone.

if the intrahepatic bile ducts are dilated, the patient is usually jaundiced at the time of examination. The examination consists of passing a fine needle (usually 22 or 23 gauge) through the abdominal wall into the liver and injecting contrast directly into an intrahepatic bile duct. Haemorrhage is an occasional problem, as are septicaemia and biliary peritonitis.

Gallstones and chronic cholecystitis

Gallstones are a frequent finding in adults, particularly middle-aged females. Together with accompanying chronic cholecystitis they are a major cause of recurrent upper abdominal pain. The presence of stones within the gall bladder does not necessarily mean the patient's pain in due to gallstones. In the appropriate clinical setting, however, identification of gallstones may be sufficient for many surgeons to take action.

At ultrasound, gallstones are seen as strongly echogenic foci within the dependent portion of the gall bladder. Acoustic shadows are usually seen behind stones, because most of the ultrasound beam is reflected by the stones and only a little passes on through the patient (Fig. 6.27). The presence of an acoustic shadow is an important diagnostic feature. The principles of diagnosing stones in the common bile duct or elsewhere in the biliary tract are similar.

At oral cholecystography, gallstones are usually seen as round or faceted filling defects within the opacified gall bladder (Fig. 6.28). Stones are by far the most frequent cause of filling defects at oral cholecystography, though they may occasionally be mimicked by polyps. Some 20–30% of gallstones contain sufficient calcium to be visible on plain film (Fig. 6.28a). They vary greatly in size and shape and, typically, have a dense outer rim with a more lucent centre. Calcified

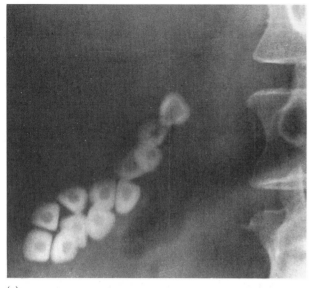

(a)

(b)

Fig. 6.28 Gallstones. (a) Multiple faceted stones showing lucent centres. (b) After oral contrast, the cholecystogram (in a different patient) shows stones which appear as lucent filling defects completely surrounded by contrast.

sludge within the gall bladder is known as 'milk of calcium' bile.

Non-opacification of the gall bladder after administration of oral contrast medium is fairly common in patients with gallstones. When the contrast has definitely been taken, non-opacification in a patient who does not have jaundice is suggestive of chronic cholecystitis.

In *adenomyomatosis* the bladder wall is thickened and may show altered echogenicity due to small projections of the lumen into the wall, known as Rokitansky–Aschoff sinuses. There is dispute as to whether this condition causes symptoms.

Acute choleystitis

In acute cholecystitis, sonography will usually detect gallstones, inflammatory debris and gall bladder wall thickening (see Fig. 6.21b), but unless there is visible oedema adjacent to the wall of the gall bladder, ultrasound cannot distinguish acute from chronic cholecystitis. In patients with abdominal pain and tenderness, ultrasound is sometimes used primarily to locate the gall bladder to determine whether it is truly the gall bladder that is tender.

A hepatobiliary radionuclide scan actually answers the question 'is the cystic duct patent'? No available test is very good at diagnosing the gall bladder inflammation itself, but since the cystic duct is always obstructed in acute cholecystitis, a normal hepatobiliary scan excludes the diagnosis. Conversely, a diagnosis of cystic duct obstruction in the correct clinical setting strongly indicates acute cholecystitis (see Fig. 6.23b).

Jaundice

Clinical examination and biochemical tests often permit the cause of jaundice to be diagnosed. Imaging tests may, however, be required when there is doubt as to the nature of the jaundice. The basis of this distinction is that dilated biliary ducts are a feature of jaundice due to biliary obstruction. More often, imaging is used to determine the site, and if possible, the cause of obstruction in those patients with known large duct obstruction, the common causes of which are:

• impacted stone in the common bile duct
• carcinoma of the head of the pancreas
• carcinoma of the ampulla of Vater.

Dilatation of the intra- and extrahepatic biliary system can be identified at both ultrasound and CT (Fig. 6.29). Ultrasound is the more sensitive test and is usually the first test to be done.

Dilated intrahepatic biliary ducts are seen at ultrasound as serpentine structures paralleling the portal veins, a finding known as 'the double channel sign'.

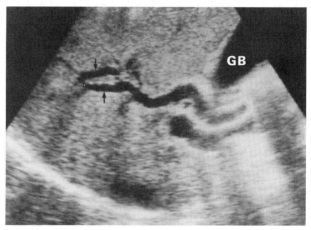

(a)

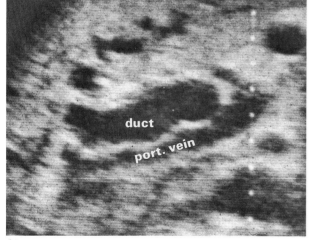

(b)

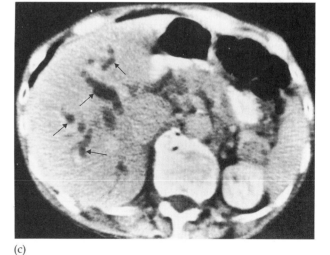

(c)

Fig. 6.29 Dilated intrahepatic ducts. (a) Longitudinal scan through the liver showing dilatation of the biliary system. Dilated intrahepatic ducts are arrowed. GB, gall bladder. (b) Double channel sign. A dilated biliary duct lies in front of a portal vein. Normally the duct is much smaller than the accompanying portal vein. (c) CT scan showing dilated intrahepatic ducts (arrows).

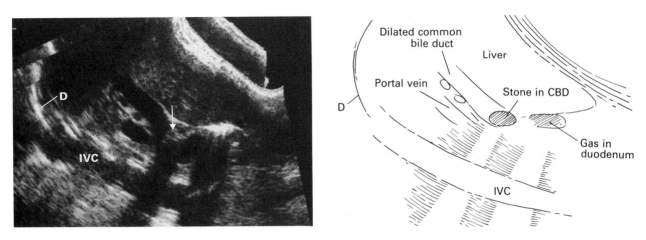

Fig. 6.30 Stone in the common bile duct. The common hepatic and common bile ducts are very dilated and a stone casting an acoustic shadow is seen in its lower portion (arrow). D, diaphragm; IVC, inferior vena cava. The percutaneous cholangiogram in this patient is shown in Figure 6.31a.

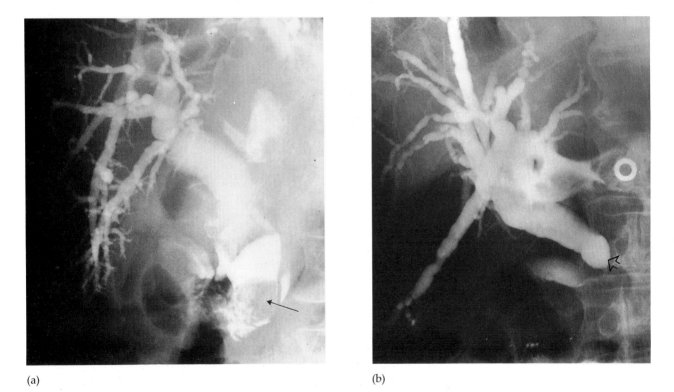

(a)   (b)

Fig. 6.31 Percutaneous cholangiogram. (a) Dilated biliary system. A stone (arrow) is seen in the lower end of the common bile duct. (The ultrasound scan of this patient is shown in Figure 6.30.) (b) Carcinoma of the pancreas. There is complete obstruction of the common bile duct (arrow). Note the dilated intrahepatic ducts.

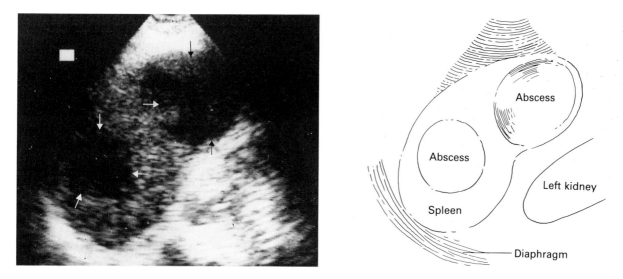

Fig. 6.32 Splenic abscess. Ultrasound scan showing spherical areas of reduced reflectivity in the spleen (arrows).

The common bile duct lies just in front of the portal vein and is dilated when more than 7 mm in diameter.

If there is large duct obstruction, the biliary tree will be dilated down to the level of obstruction. Ultrasound is good for demonstrating the level of obstruction and sometimes the specific cause for biliary obstruction can be seen, e.g. a stone impacted within the common bile duct (Fig. 6.30) or a mass in the pancreatic head. More often, the cause cannot be seen, mainly because associated inflammation causes localised ileus of the duodenum and bowel gas then obscures the common bile duct. Computed tomography may provide useful information about the cause of obstruction. Two points should be appreciated: substantial dilatation of the common hepatic and common bile ducts may be present with only minimal dilatation of the intra-hepatic ducts; and secondly, the intrahepatic biliary tree may not dilate at all within the first 48 hours following obstruction. An ERCP or percutaneous cholangiogram may be needed both to differentiate jaundice due to large duct obstruction from other causes of jaundice and to establish the site and determine the cause of any obstruction that may be present (Figs 6.24 and 6.31) and, if possible, to treat the condition.

Some centres use a radionuclide hepatobiliary agent to confirm or exclude biliary obstruction. The problem with this approach is that with severe jaundice there may be insufficient excretion of the radionuclide to distinguish bile duct obstruction from hepatocellular disease.

SPLEEN

Imaging the spleen is in many respects similar to imaging the liver. At ultrasound, the spleen has a homogeneous appearance with the same echo density as the liver. Computed tomography is an excellent way to examine the spleen; normal CT images are shown in the appendix. Because the spleen contains reticuloendothelial cells it is well demonstrated on a ^{99m}Tc sulphur or tin colloid scan, but the technique has been largely superseded by ultrasound and CT.

The commonly encountered splenic masses are cysts, including hydatid cysts, abscesses (Fig. 6.32) and tumours; lymphoma is much commoner than metastases, which are rare in the spleen.

Many conditions cause enlargement of the spleen but show no change in texture on ultrasound, or any

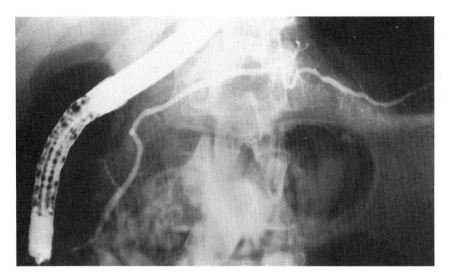

Fig. 6.33 Endoscopic retrograde pancreatography. The pancreatic duct has been cannulated from the endoscope in the duodenum. Contrast has been injected to demonstrate a normal duct system.

change in density on computed tomography. These conditions include lymphoma, portal hypertension, chronic infection and various blood disorders, e.g. haemolytic anaemias and leukaemia. As the appearance of the enlarged spleen in all these conditions is similar, imaging does little except confirm the presence of splenomegaly.

The spleen is the most commonly injured organ in blunt abdominal trauma and lacerations, contusions or haematomas may result. *Splenic injury* may be detected by ultrasound, but CT is a superior method of investigation, since it can show intraperitoneal blood and can visualise injuries to other abdominal organs, particularly the adjacent liver and left kidney.

PANCREAS

Computed tomography and ultrasound have now become the mainstays for imaging the pancreas. A major advantage of CT over ultrasound is that it can image the pancreas regardless of the amount of bowel adjacent to it, whereas the ultrasound beam is absorbed by gas in the gastrointestinal tract. Arteriography and endoscopic retrograde cholangiopancreatography (Fig. 6.33) are used in highly selected cases.

The normal pancreas is an elongated retroperitoneal organ surrounded by a variable amount of fat (Fig. 6.34). The head nestles in the duodenal loop (for CT scanning the duodenum is opacified by an oral contrast agent) and the uncinate process folds behind the superior mesenteric artery and vein; these vessels form a useful landmark to help identify the head of the pancreas. The body of the pancreas lies in front of the superior mesenteric artery and vein, and passes behind the stomach, with the tail situated near the hilum of the spleen. The splenic vein, which can be a surprisingly large structure, is another very useful landmark. Lying behind the pancreas, it joins the superior mesenteric vein posterior to the neck of the pancreas to form the portal vein.

In most people the pancreas runs obliquely across the retroperitoneum, being higher at the splenic end. Because of this oblique orientation, CT shows different portions of the pancreas on the various sections. The normal pancreas shows a feathery texture, corresponding to pancreatic lobules interspersed with fat. At ultrasound, the pancreas gives reasonably uniform echoes of medium to high level compared to the adjacent liver (Fig. 6.35). The pancreatic duct may be seen over short segments as a linear echo in the centre of

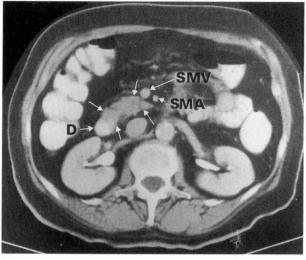

(a)

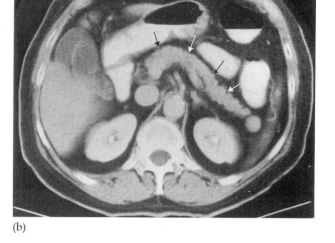

(b)

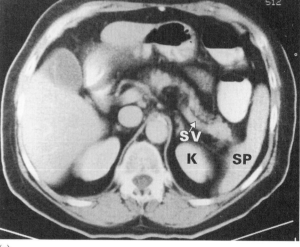

(c)

Fig. 6.34 CT of normal pancreas. Note that several sections are needed to display the pancreas. (a) The head (arrows) nestling between the second part of the opacified duodenum (D) and the superior mesenteric vessels (SMA and SMV). (b) 3 cm higher, showing the body and part of the tail (arrows). Note the feathery texture of the pancreas. (c) 1 cm higher, showing the tail of the pancreas nestling against the spleen. In this patient the splenic vein is particularly well seen and is almost the same diameter as the pancreas. K, kidney; SP, spleen; SV, splenic vein.

the pancreas, the normal lumen being no more than 2 mm in diameter. The normal pancreatic duct is not visible on CT.

The shape and size of the pancreas is so variable that normal measurements have not proved very useful. Atrophy is a common feature with ageing.

Pancreatic masses

The usual causes of masses in, or immediately adjacent to, the pancreas are: carcinoma of the pancreas, neoplasm of the adjacent lymph nodes, focal pancreatitis, pancreatic abscess and pseudocyst formation. Occasionally, congenital cysts may be seen.

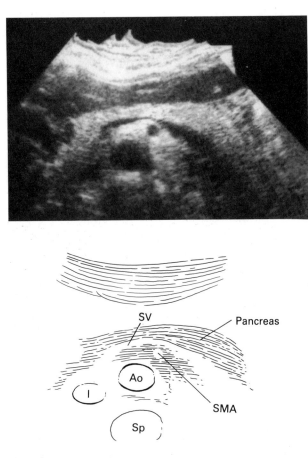

Fig. 6.35 Ultrasound of normal pancreas. Transverse scan. Ao, aorta; I, inferior vena cava; SMA, superior mesenteric artery; Sp, spine; SV, splenic vein.

Most neoplasms of the pancreas are *adenocarcinomas*, two-thirds of which occur in the head of the pancreas. Tumours arising in the head may obstruct the common bile duct giving rise to jaundice and are therefore sometimes diagnosed when relatively small. Tumours arising in the body and tail have to be fairly large to give rise to signs or symptoms, pain being the cardinal symptom. Since the pancreas is so variable, measurements have not proved useful in diagnosing masses. The important sign of carcinoma of the pancreas at both CT and ultrasound is, therefore, a focal mass deforming the outline of the gland (Fig. 6.36). These

neoplasms have frequently already invaded the retroperitoneum at the time of presentation, causing irregular obliteration of the fat around the pancreas, a feature which is readily recognised at CT. Using CT with intravenous contrast enhancement, it is sometimes possible to differentiate the relatively lower density of the tumour from the enhancing normal pancreatic tissue.

Obstructive dilatation of the pancreatic duct can be seen at CT but is more readily apparent at sonography. With obstruction of the common bile duct, it is often possible to recognise dilatation of the duct down to the level of the tumour. The liver, which should always be included in any examination of the pancreas, should routinely be examined carefully for signs of spread of tumour.

Only a few *endocrine secreting tumours* are seen at CT or ultrasound, as they are usually small and do not deform the pancreatic contour. They are best identified at selective angiography where they stand out from the rest of the pancreas by virtue of their hypervascularity.

Acute pancreatitis

Acute pancreatitis causes abdominal pain, fever, vomiting, and leucocytosis together with elevation of the serum amylase. The findings at CT and ultrasound vary with the amount of necrosis, haemorrhage and suppuration. The pancreas is usually enlarged, often diffusely and may show irregularity of its outline, due to extension of the inflammatory process into the surrounding retroperitoneal fat: features that are well seen at CT (Figs 6.37 and 6.38). There may be low density areas at CT and echo-poor areas at sonography, representing oedema and focal necrosis within or adjacent to the pancreas. With very severe disease, large fluid-filled areas representing abscess formation may be seen. Such abscesses occasionally contain gas bubbles.

The diagnosis of pancreatitis is usually made on clinical and biochemical grounds, the purpose of imaging being to demonstrate complications such as abscesses and pseudocysts. Occasionally, CT is used to exclude an underlying carcinoma.

Pseudocysts are a complication of acute pancreatitis in which tissue necrosis leads to a leak of pancreatic secretions, which are then contained in a cyst-like manner within and adjacent to the pancreas. They can be well demonstrated by either CT or ultrasound as thin or thick walled cysts containing fluid, arising

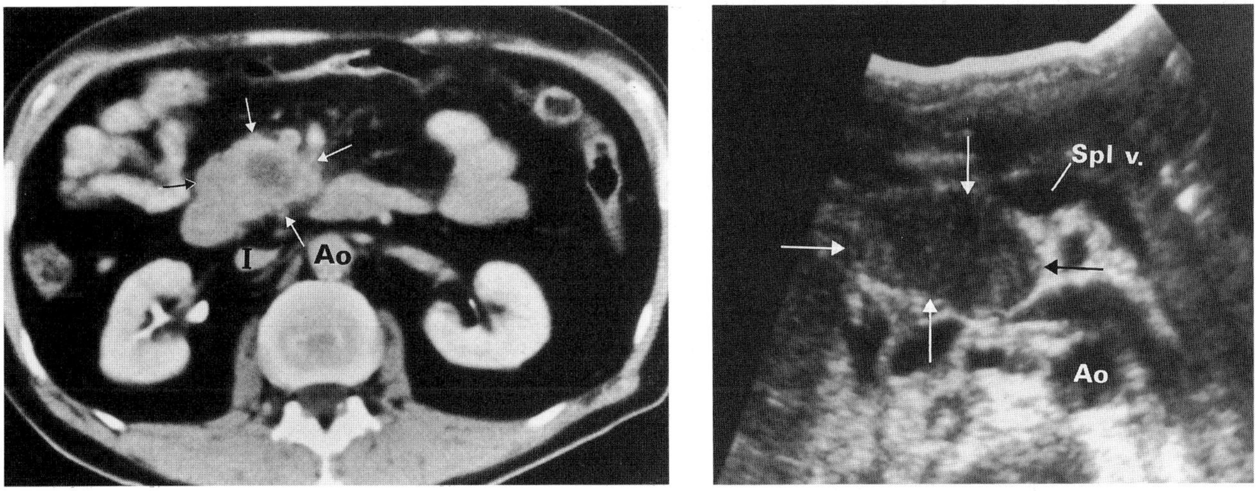

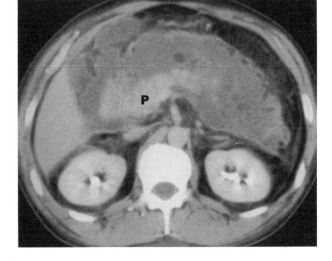

(a)

(b)

Fig. 6.36 Carcinoma of pancreas. (a) CT scan showing focal mass in head of pancreas (arrows). Ao, aorta; I, inferior vena cava. (b) Ultrasound, transverse scan (different patient), showing a similarly situated mass (arrows). Ao, aorta; Spl v., splenic vein.

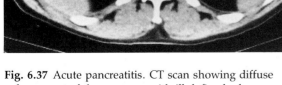

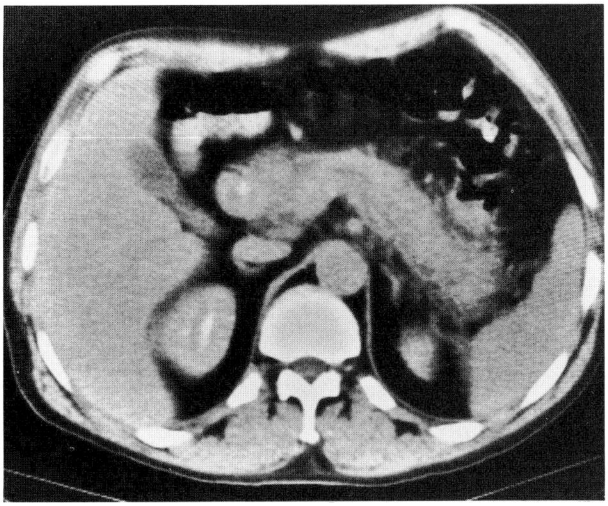

Fig. 6.37 Acute pancreatitis. CT scan showing diffuse enlargement of the pancreas with ill-defined edges.

Fig. 6.38 Acute pancreatitis showing considerable inflammation around the pancreas (P).

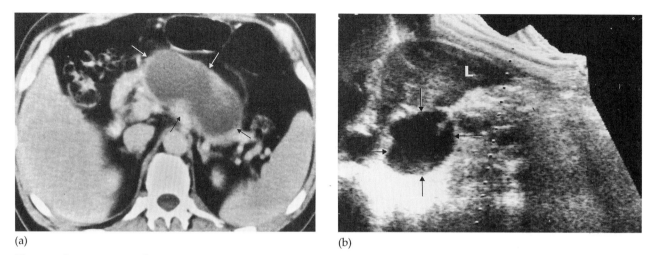

(a)   (b)

Fig. 6.39 Pancreatic pseudocyst. (a) CT scan showing large cyst arising within the pancreas (arrows). (b) Ultrasound. Transverse scan, showing a transonic mass with acoustic enhancement arising from the pancreas (arrows). L, liver.

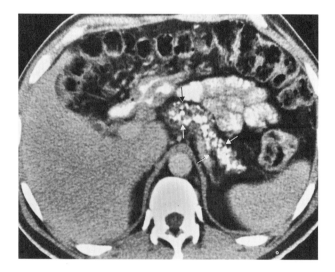

Fig. 6.40 Chronic pancreatitis. CT scan showing numerous small areas of calcification within the pancreas (arrows).

within or adjacent to the pancreas (Fig. 6.39). They vary in size from very small to many centimetres in diameter and may even be seen on a barium meal causing anterior displacement and compression of the stomach and/or duodenum. Many pseudocysts resolve in the weeks following an attack of acute pancreatitis.

Some persist and may need surgical or percutaneous drainage. Both CT and ultrasound are excellent methods of following such cysts and determining the best approach to treatment.

Chronic pancreatitis

Chronic pancreatitis results in fibrosis, calcifications, and ductal stenoses and dilatations. Pseudocysts are seen with chronic pancreatitis (Fig. 6.39), just as they are in the acute form. The calcification in chronic pancreatitis is mainly due to small calculi within the pancreas; they are often recognisable on plain films (see Fig. 4.15, p. 142) and ultrasound, but are particularly obvious at CT (Fig. 6.40). The gland may enlarge generally or focally. Focal enlargement is rare and is then often indistinguishable from carcinoma. Conversely, the pancreas may atrophy focally or generally. Atrophy is a non-specific sign; it is frequently seen in normal elderly people and also occurs distal to a carcinoma. The pancreatic duct may be enlarged and irregular, a feature that is visible at CT, and particularly striking at ultrasound.

Endoscopic retrograde cholangiopancreatography is occasionally used to try and document chronic pancreatitis and exclude carcinoma. The generalised irregular dilatation of the duct system seen with chronic pancreatitis is very well demonstrated with this method.

Pancreatic trauma

Trauma to the pancreas is uncommon but serious. Injuries to other structures are frequent, so CT is the best method of investigation. In addition to lacerations and haematomas, the release of pancreatic enzymes into the surrounding tissues leads to traumatic pancreatitis and tissue necrosis. The features here are similar to other forms of acute pancreatitis (see above), including the subsequent development of pseudocysts.

7

Urinary Tract

The four basic examinations of the urinary tract are the intravenous urography (IVU), computed tomography (CT), ultrasound and radionuclide examinations. Magnetic resonance imaging (MRI), arteriography and studies requiring catheterisation or direct puncture of the collecting systems are limited to highly selected patients.

The IVU used to dominate as the all-purpose examination, but now the newer modalities offer advantages in many areas and often replace the IVU.

Since ultrasound is supreme in showing fluid-filled structures it is used to find or exclude hydronephrosis, particularly in patients with renal failure, and to diagnose cysts and abscesses. It is also able to give valuable information regarding retroperitoneal masses or fluid collections that may be causing urinary symptoms or signs.

Computed tomography is pre-eminent in elucidating focal parenchymal problems such as renal masses. Its other major advantage is the delineation of the adjacent retroperitoneum when searching for tumours, abscesses, and lymphadenopathy.

Both CT and ultrasound are essentially used for anatomical information; the functional information they provide is limited. The converse is true of radionuclide examinations where functional information is paramount.

The IVU provides both functional and anatomical information. It has the advantage that the whole of the urinary tract can be seen on just a few films, and it is the ideal method of investigating calculi.

Intravenous urogram

Contrast medium and its excretion

Urographic media are highly concentrated solutions of organically bound iodine. A large volume, e.g. 50 ml, is injected intravenously and is carried in the blood to the kidneys, where it passes into the glomerular filtrate. Contrast is not absorbed by the tubules, so substantial concentration is achieved in the urine, particularly after fluid restriction. The visualisation of the renal substance (the nephrogram) is dependent on the amount of contrast reaching the kidneys, whereas the visualisation of the collecting systems (the pyelogram) depends mainly on the ability of the kidneys to concentrate the urine.

Adverse reactions to intravenous contrast media are discussed on page 3.

Preparation of the patient

Fluid restriction is an advantage in patients with normal renal function, as this increases the concentration of the urine and produces a dense pyelogram. This does *not* apply to patients in renal failure, since they could be harmed by withholding fluids and there would in any event be no advantage, because many are unable to increase the concentration of their urine.

Routine IVU

One or more plain films are taken to show the whole of the urinary tract. The precise timing of the films following the injection of contrast medium varies in

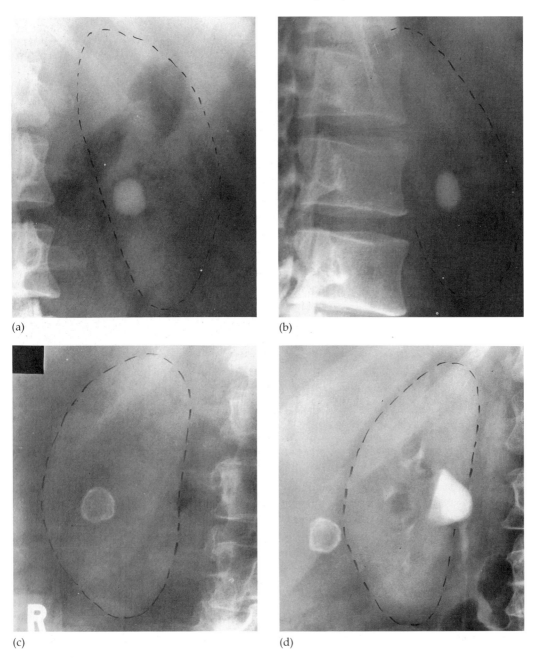

(a)

(b)

(c)

(d)

Fig. 7.1 Oblique views to determine whether calcifications are intra- or extrarenal. (a) A rounded calcification is seen overlying the left kidney in the AP plain film. (b) In the oblique plain film, the calcification is in the same position within the renal shadow and is, therefore, a renal calculus. (c) A rounded calcification is seen over the right renal shadow. (d) An oblique film after contrast shows that the calcification lies outside the kidney. It was later confirmed to be a gallstone.

different hospitals but each film is assessed at the time it is taken, so that appropriate extra views, such as tomography or oblique views (Fig. 7.1), can be obtained. A film taken 1 minute after the injection is designed to show the renal parenchyma, particularly the renal outlines. Further films are then taken to show the kidneys, ureters and bladder (Fig. 7.2).

The following routine is useful when interpreting an IVU.

The plain film

Identify all calcifications. Decide if they are in the urinary tract by relating them to the renal outlines or the expected position of the ureters, bladder, prostate and urethra using oblique plain films where necessary. The major causes of urinary tract calcification are:

- urinary calculi
- nephrocalcinosis
- localised calcification due to conditions such as tuberculosis or tumours
- prostatic calcification

It is important to realise that calcification can be obscured by contrast medium. Stones would often be missed if no plain film were taken (Fig. 7.3).

Look at the other structures on the film, including the bones, just as you would any plain abdominal film. Do not waste time drawing conclusions about the renal outlines on plain films; they are always better seen after contrast has been given.

Films taken after injection of contrast medium

The kidneys

Check that the kidneys are in their normal positions (Fig. 7.2) and that their axes are parallel to the outer margins of the psoas muscles. The left kidney is usually higher than the right.

There are two basic reasons why the position or axis of a kidney might be abnormal: congenital malposition or displacement by a retroperitoneal mass.

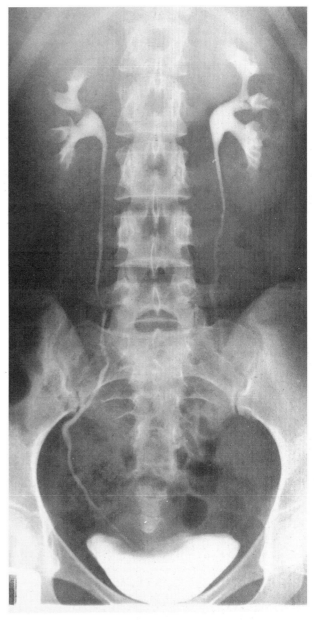

Fig. 7.2 Normal IVU. Full length 15 minute film. Note that the bladder is well opacified. The whole of the right ureter and part of the left ureter are seen. Often, only a portion of the ureter is visualised due to peristalsis emptying certain sections. The bladder outline is reasonably smooth. The roof of the bladder shows a shallow indentation from the uterus.

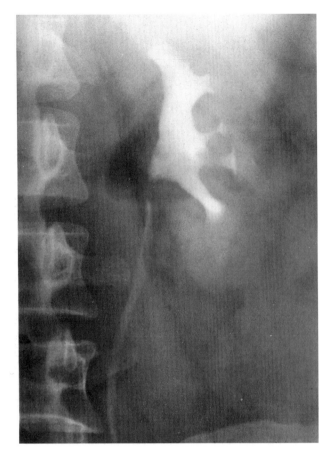

Fig. 7.3 Large calcified calculus in the pelvis of the kidney obscured by contrast medium. This is the same patient as illustrated in Figures 7.1a and b. Since the contrast medium and the calculus have the same radiographic density, the calculus is hidden by the contrast medium.

Fig. 7.4 (a) The distinction between fetal lobulation and renal infarction. With fetal lobulation, indentations in the renal outline are shallow and correspond to the lobules of the kidney, i.e. the indentations are between calices. With renal infarction, the maximal indentation is opposite a calix and there is usually extensive loss of renal parenchyma. (b) Scars in chronic pyelonephritis (drawing of Figure 7.7b) The reductions in renal parenchymal width are opposite calices, and these calices are dilated. The overall kidney size is reduced, as is usual. Scars in tuberculosis have much the same appearance but are usually associated with other signs of tuberculosis.

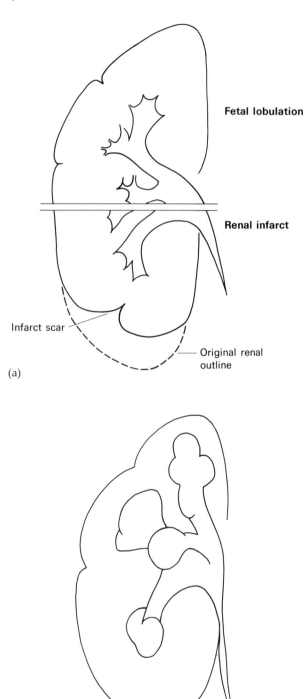

Fetal lobulation

Renal infarct

Infarct scar

Original renal outline

(a)

(b)

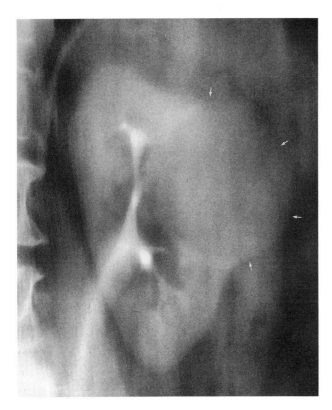

Fig. 7.5 Renal mass. A renal cyst (arrows) has caused a bulge on the lateral aspect of the kidney with splaying of the calices.

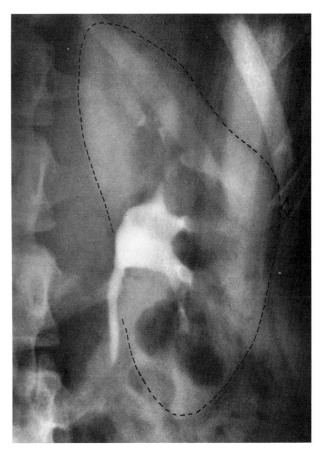

Fig. 7.6 The 'splenic hump'. A bulge is present on the lateral aspect of the left kidney (arrow) but there is no displacement of the calices. This 'splenic hump' is a normal variant.

Identify the whole of both renal outlines. (They are usually better seen on tomography.) If any indentations or bulges are present they must be explained.

• *Local indentations* (Fig. 7.4). The renal parenchymal width should be uniform and symmetrical: between 1.5 and 2 cm, except at the poles where there is an extra centimetre of thickness. Minor indentations between normal calices are due to persistent fetal lobulations. All other local indentations are scars. Visible scars occur with chronic pyelonephritis, tuberculosis and renal infarction.

• *Local bulges of the renal outline.* A bulge of the renal outline usually means a mass. Most masses large enough to deform the renal outline will displace and deform the adjacent calices (Fig. 7.5). An important

normal variant causing a bulge of the outline is the so-called 'splenic hump' (Fig. 7.6).

Measure the renal lengths. The normal adult kidney at IVU is between 10 and 16 cm from top to bottom; the length varies with age, being maximal in the young adult. There may be a difference between the two kidneys, but this is normally less than 1.5 cm. A kidney with a bifid collecting system is usually 1–2 cm larger than expected. Minor changes in size occur in many conditions. Diseases where the increase or decrease in size is sufficient to be recognisable, even without comparison with previous examinations, are listed in Tables 7.1 and 7.2. It will be noted that it is usually possible to diagnose the cause of a unilateral small kidney and bilaterally enlarged kidneys but, except for bilateral chronic pyelonephritis, it is often not possible to distinguish between the various causes of bilaterally small kidneys.

The calices

The calices should be evenly distributed and reasonably symmetrical. The term often used to describe the shape of a normal calix is 'cupped' and that to describe the dilated calix 'clubbed' (Fig. 7.7). The normal 'cup' is due to the indentation of the papilla into the calix.

Caliceal dilatation has two basic causes:
1 Obstruction
2 Destruction of the papilla, the causes of which include:
- chronic pyelonephritis
- tuberculosis
- obstructive atrophy
- papillary necrosis.

The first step, therefore, in sorting out which of these mechanisms is at work is to try and decide whether or not there is obstruction, i.e. dilatation of the collecting system down to a specific point (Fig. 7.7c). If there is no evidence of obstruction, the conditions causing papillary destruction will have to be considered.

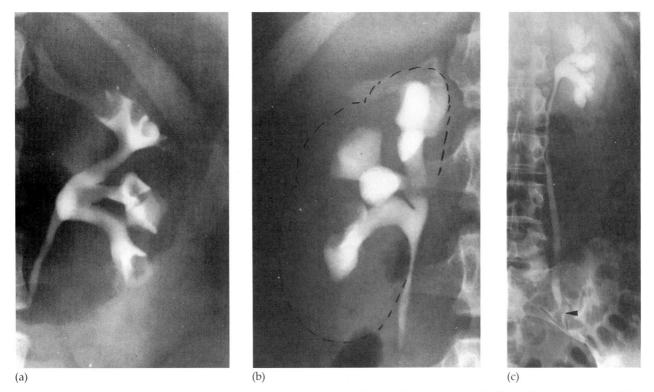

(a)   (b)   (c)

Fig. 7.7 The calices. (a) Normal calices. Each calix is 'cup-shaped'. (b) Many of the calices are clubbed. There is scarring of the parenchyma of the upper half of the kidney indicating that the diagnosis is chronic pyelonephritis. (c) All the calices are dilated, the dilatation of the collecting system extending down to the point of obstruction (arrow), in this case due to a malignant retroperitoneal lymph node.

Table 7.1 Small kidneys

Diagnosis		Comments
Unilateral but may be bilateral	Chronic pyelonephritis	Focal scars and dilated calices
	Tuberculosis	See page 246
	Following acute infection	Very rare
	Obstructive atrophy	Dilatation of all calices with uniform loss of renal parenchyma
	Renal artery stenosis or occlusion	Outline may be smooth or scarred, but the calices appear normal. In severe unilateral cases the density of the pyelogram on the affected side may be increased. If very severe the pyelogram may be delayed by a minute or two.
	Hypoplasia	Very rare; kidneys may be smooth or irregular in outline. Calices may be clubbed.
	Radiation nephritis	
Always bilateral	Chronic glomerulonephritis of many types Hypertensive nephropathy Diabetes mellitus Collagen vascular diseases	Usually no distinguishing features. In all these conditions the kidneys may be small with smooth outlines and normal pelvicaliceal systems
	Analgesic nephropathy	Calices often abnormal (p. 248)

Table 7.2 Enlarged kidneys*

Diagnosis		Intravenous urogram (IVU)
Always unilateral	Compensatory hypertrophy	Opposite kidney small or absent
May be unilateral or bilateral	Bifid collecting system	Diagnosis obvious from abnormalities of collecting systems
	Renal mass	
	Hydronephrosis	
	Lymphomatous infiltration	May show obvious masses; the kidneys may, however, be large but otherwise unremarkable
	Renal vein thrombosis	
Always bilateral	Polycystic disease	Characteristic IVU (Fig. 7.44, p. 257)
	Acute glomerulonephritis	Non-specific enlargement
	Amyloidosis	Non-specific enlargement (rare)
	Diabetic nephropathy	Slight non-specific enlargement (a rare cause of enlarged kidney)

* Minor degrees of enlargement occur in many conditions. Only those conditions that give rise to easily recognised enlargement are listed here.

The pelvis

The renal pelvis is extremely variable in location. It may be almost totally intrarenal or it may be entirely outside the kidney, and yet in both cases be normal. It is also very variable in size and shape. Usually, the inferior border of the pelvis is concave but even normal pelves may show a downward bulge. The pelvi-ureteric junction is usually funnel shaped, but an abrupt change from pelvis to ureter may be normal. True dilatation of the pelvis suggests obstruction.

Filling defects within the pelvis should be looked for. The three common causes of a filling defect in the collecting systems are tumours, calculi and blood clot.

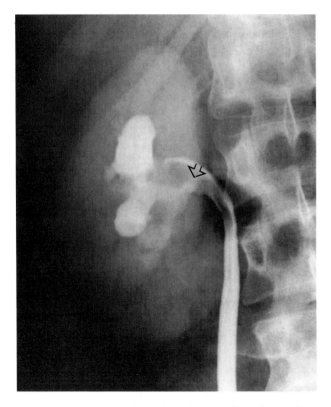

Fig. 7.8 Filling defect due to blood clot in the pelvis and upper ureter (arrow).

Nearly all urinary stones contain visible calcification and virtually all calcified filling defects are stones. Therefore, provided the preliminary film is reviewed, filling defects due to stones very rarely present a diagnostic problem.

The diagnosis of blood clot as the cause of a filling defect rests on knowing that the patient has severe haematuria and noting the smooth outline of the filling defect (Fig. 7.8). Sometimes the distinction between tumour and clot is difficult. A repeat examination after some days will usually show change or clearing if the filling defect is due to blood clot.

The ureters

The ureters are usually seen in only part of their length on any one film owing to obliteration of the lumen by peristalsis. No portion of either ureter should be more than 7 mm in diameter, but the normal effects of pregnancy and the contraceptive pill can cause moderate dilatation. Dilatation is usually due to obstruction. Occasionally, it is due to vesicoureteric reflux without obstruction. Displacement of a ureter may, on rare occasions, be recognisable.

The bladder

The bladder is a centrally located structure which should have a smooth outline. It often shows normal indentations from above due to the uterus or the sigmoid colon, and from below by muscles of the pelvic floor. After micturition the bladder should be empty, apart from a little contrast trapped in the folded mucosa.

Computed tomography of urinary tract

The entire urinary tract can be examined by computed tomography. The technique is virtually the same as for standard abdominal and pelvic CT, except that sections of the kidneys are performed both before and after intravenous contrast medium has been given.

Normal CT (Fig. 7.9)

The basic principles of interpretation are the same as with the IVU. The renal parenchyma should have a smooth outline and opacify uniformly after intravenous contrast administration, although early images may show opacification of the cortex before medullary opacification has had time to occur. The pelvicaliceal system should show cupped calices with uniform width of renal parenchyma from calix to renal edge, and the fat that surrounds the pelvicaliceal system should be clearly visualised. The ureters are seen in cross section as dots lying on the psoas muscles. They lie anterior to the iliac vessels at the pelvic brim and cross the pelvic cavity just prior to entering the bladder. They will not necessarily be seen at all levels because peristalsis obliterates the lumen intermittently. The bladder has a smooth outline contrasted against the pelvic fat; its wall is thin and of reasonably uniform diameter. Contrast opacification of the urine in the bladder is variable depending on how much contrast has reached the bladder. The contrast medium is heavier than urine and therefore, the dependent portion is usually more densely opacified (Fig. 7.9e).

There are many indications for CT. Pre-eminent is the evaluation of mass in or adjacent to the urinary tract. It is also very useful to assess trauma, infarction and neoplastic infiltration of the kidneys.

Ultrasound of urinary tract

Successful ultrasound examination of the kidneys is influenced by the size of the patient and how much fat is present. When examining from the front, the right kidney is often well seen through the liver, but bowel usually masks the left kidney. When examining from the back, the ribs and muscles may interfere with the transmission of sound, and in many patients a lateral approach proves to be the most successful.

Normal ultrasound (Fig. 7.10)

At ultrasound, the kidneys should be smooth in outline. The parenchyma surrounds a central echodense region, known as the central echo complex (also known as the renal sinus), consisting of the pelvicaliceal system, together with surrounding fat and renal blood vessels. In the adult, the renal cortex generates homogeneous echoes which are less intense than those of the adjacent liver or spleen and the renal pyramids are seen as triangular sonolucent areas adjacent to the renal sinus. During the first 2 months of life, cortical echoes are relatively more prominent and the renal pyramids are strikingly sonolucent.

The normal adult renal length, measured by ultrasound, is 9–12 cm. These figures are lower than those for renal size measured by IVU, because there is no swelling due to the action of contrast medium and there is no magnification of the image.

Normal ureters are not usually visualised. The urinary bladder should be examined in the distended state: the walls should be sharply defined and barely perceptible.

The main indications for ultrasound are:
- To demonstrate or exclude hydronephrosis, particularly in patients with renal failure or a non-functioning kidney at IVU.
- Evaluation of renal tumours, cysts and abscesses, including polycystic disease.
- Measurement of renal size. These measurements may be used to follow transplant kidneys and various acute and chronic renal diseases.
- To assess the prostate.
- To guide percutaneous interventional techniques.
- To assess renal blood flow using Doppler techniques.

Radionuclide examination

There are two main radionuclide techniques for studying the kidneys:
1 The renogram which measures renal function.
2 Scans of renal morphology (DMSA scan). The advent

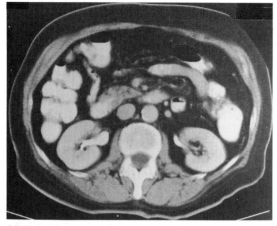

(a)

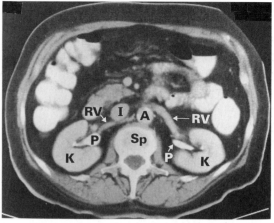

(b)

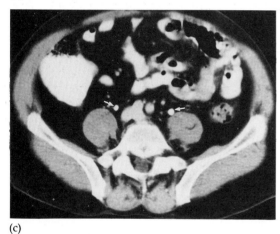

(c)

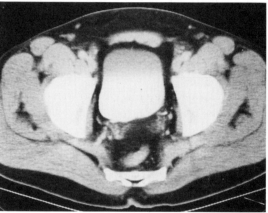

(d)

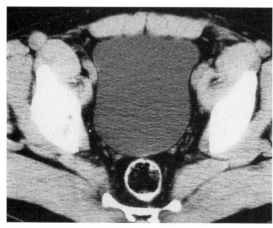

(e)

Fig. 7.9 Normal CT of kidneys and bladder. Adjacent sections, (b) 1 cm higher than (a) showing uniform opacification of parenchyma with well-defined cortical edge. The pelvicaliceal system, which is densely opacified, is surrounded by fat. The renal veins are well shown on the higher section. (c) Section through the level of the ureters (arrows) after contrast has been given. (d) Section through opacified bladder in a male patient shows that the bladder wall is too thin to be seen. Note the layering of contrast medium. (e) Section through bladder without contrast opacification. The bladder wall can be identified as a thin line. A, aorta; I, inferior vena cava; K, kidney; P, pelvis; RV, renal vein; Sp, spine.

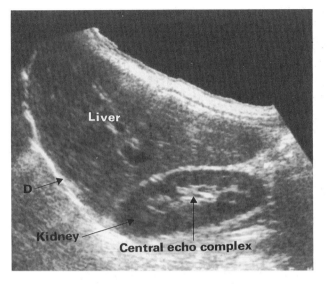

Fig. 7.10 Normal ultrasound of the right kidney. Longitudinal scan. D = diaphragm.

of CT and ultrasound has reduced the need for such scans. They are now used mainly for evaluating renal scarring (see Fig. 7.33c, p. 249).

Renogram (Fig. 7.11)

If substances which pass into the urine are labelled with a radionuclide and injected intravenously, their passage through the kidney can be observed with a gamma camera. The agent of choice for a renogram is technetium-99 m DTPA (diethylenetriaminepentacetic acid). Radio-iodine labelled hippuran is an alternative agent.

The gamma camera is positioned posteriorly over the kidneys and a rapid injection of the radiopharmaceutical is given. Early images show the major blood vessels and both kidneys. Subsequently, activity is seen in the renal parenchyma and by 5 minutes the collecting systems should be visible. Serial images over 20 minutes show progressive excretion and clearance of activity from the kidneys. Quantitative assessment with a computer enables a renogram curve to be produced and the relative function of each kidney calculated.

The indications for a renogram are:
- Measurement of relative renal function in each kidney—this may help the surgeon decide between nephrectomy or more conservative surgery.
- Investigation of urinary tract obstruction.
- Diagnosis of a renovascular cause for hypertension.
- Investigation of renal transplants.

Special techniques

Retrograde and antegrade pyelography

The techniques of retrograde and antegrade pyelography (the term pyelography means demonstrating the pelvicaliceal system and ureters) involve direct injection of contrast material into the pelvicaliceal system or ureters through catheters placed via cystoscopy (retrograde pyelography) or percutaneously into the kidney via the loin (antegrade pyelography). The indications are limited to those situations where the information cannot be achieved by less invasive means, e.g. cases of hydronephrosis where further information about the level and nature of obstruction is required.

Voiding cystourethrogram (micturating cystogram) (see Fig. 7.53, p. 261)

In the technique known as voiding cystourethrography, contrast medium is run into the empty bladder through a catheter. The bladder is filled to capacity and films are taken during voiding. The entire process should be observed fluoroscopically so that any vesicoureteric reflux can be observed and bladder contractility assessed.

The major indications are to:
- Identify and quantify vesicoureteric reflux.
- Investigate the anatomy of the bladder neck and urethra, particularly to show obstructions such as strictures or urethral valves.
- Demonstrate the emptying of the bladder and the control of micturition.

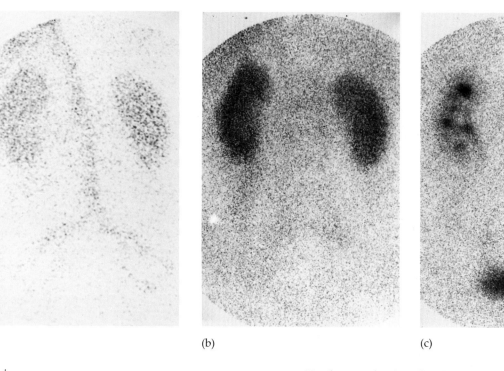

(a)   (b)   (c)

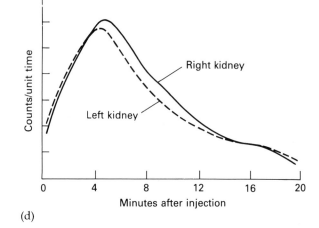

(d)

Fig. 7.11 Renogram, serial images. (a) Vascular phase.
(b) Filtration phase. (c) Excretion phase. (d) The renogram
curve.

Urethrography (see Fig. 7.52, p. 261)

Urethrography can be part of micturating cystography,
or it can be performed by a retrograde injection technique (the retrograde technique is rarely performed in
females). The usual indications for the examination
are the identification of urethral strictures and to
demonstrate extravasion from the urethra or bladder
neck following trauma.

Renal arteriography

Renal arteriography is performed via a catheter introduced into the femoral artery by the Seldinger technique (see p. 427). The usual technique involves
injecting contrast medium into the aorta just above the
origin of the renal arteries, as well as selective injections into one or both renal arteries (Fig. 7.12). CT has
largely replaced the need for arteriography to diagnose
the nature and extent of a renal mass. It is mainly used
to demonstrate the details of vascular anatomy prior
to surgery and to assess renal artery stenosis. Renal

arteriography is an integral part of therapeutic embolisation of the renal artery and percutaneous balloon angioplasty (see p. 430).

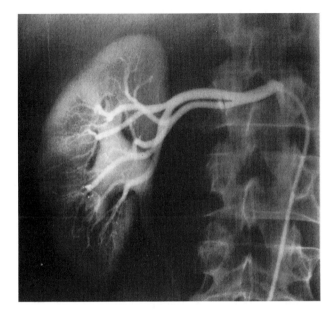

Fig. 7.12 Normal selective right renal arteriogram. Note, that not only are the arteries well shown but there is also an excellent nephrogram. The renal pelvis and ureter are opacified because of a previous injection of contrast.

Urinary calculi

Nearly all urinary calculi are calcified and appear partly or totally opaque on x-ray examinations. Many calculi are uniformly calcified but some, particularly bladder stones, are laminated. Only pure uric acid and xanthine stones are radiolucent.

Small renal calculi are often round or oval; the larger ones frequently assume the shape of the pelvicaliceal system in which they lie and are known as staghorn calculi (Fig. 7.13).

Plain film examination of the urinary tract is the easiest method of identifying calculi. It is essential to examine the preliminary film carefully, because even large calculi can be completely hidden within the opacified collecting system once contrast has been given (see Fig. 7.3, p. 224).

Stones may cause obstruction to the collecting system. Ultrasound and IVU are equally good at assessing the resulting dilatation of the collecting system. The IVU is the best method of showing the precise site of obstruction—information that can be vital if surgical treatment is required—and can also identify any mechanical obstruction or deranged anatomy that may have predisposed to stone formation.

Calculi of more than 5 mm in size are readily seen at

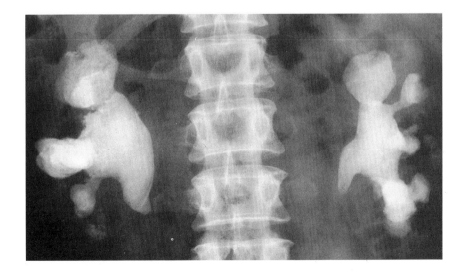

Fig. 7.13 Plain film showing a calcified staghorn calculus in each kidney.

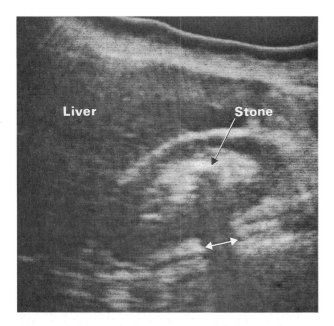

Fig. 7.14 Ultrasound of stone in right kidney. The stone appears as a bright echo partly hidden by the central echo complex. A striking feature is the acoustic shadow of the stone (double headed arrow).

ultrasound but smaller calculi may be missed. They produce intense echoes and cast acoustic shadows. Sometimes the acoustic shadowing is more evident than the echo (Fig. 7.14). Calculi located within the renal sinus may be obscured by echoes from surrounding fat. Staghorn calculi, filling the caliceal system, cast very large acoustic shadows which may even mask an associated hydronephrosis.

Computed tomography, when performed without intravenous contrast, is exquisitely sensitive for the detection of calculi but is not indicated solely for this purpose.

Nephrocalcinosis

Nephrocalcinosis is the term used to describe numerous irregular spots of calcium in the parenchyma of both kidneys (Fig. 7.15). The causes fall into two main categories:
1 Nephrocalcinosis associated with hypercalcaemia

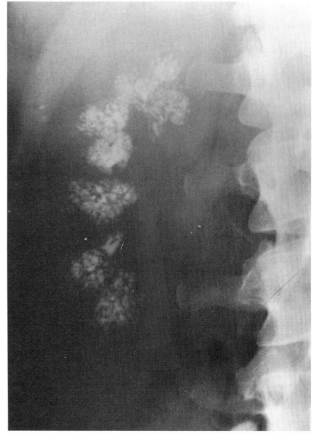

Fig. 7.15 Nephrocalcinosis. There are numerous calcifications in the pyramids of both kidneys (the left kidney is not illustrated).

and/or hypercalcuria: namely hyperparathyroidism, renal tubular acidosis and sarcoidosis.
2 Nephrocalcinosis *not* associated with disordered calcium metabolism: namely widespread papillary necrosis and medullary sponge kidney, a congenital condition with dilated collecting tubules in which small calculi can form.

Urinary tract obstruction

The principal feature of obstruction is dilatation of the collecting system. All the affected calices are dilated to approximately the same degree, the degree depending on the chronicity as well as the severity of the obstruction. The obstructed collecting system is dilated down to the level of the obstructing pathology and demonstrating this level is a prime objective (Fig. 7.16) . The IVU and ultrasound examination play the major roles in evaluating urinary tract obstruction. Computed tomography and radionuclide studies show typical changes, but are rarely the primary imaging procedures.

Intravenous urogram in urinary tract obstruction

Opacification of the urine in an obstructed system usually takes a long time. Delayed films are, therefore, an essential part of any IVU where the level of obstruction is not shown on the routine films. Even if the flow of urine has stopped completely, provided that glomerular filtration is still occurring the collecting system will opacify at IVU, but it may take many hours. In acute obstruction—usually due to a stone in the ureters—contrast accumulates and is concentrated in the tubules producing a very dense nephrogram. The pyelogram phase is greatly delayed, but in time the collecting system and the level of obstruction can be demonstrated (Fig. 7.17). Once the site of obstruction is established, the plain film must be looked at again to confirm or exclude an opaque calculus responsible for the obstruction.

Prolonged obstruction causes atrophy of the kidney substance which is recognised by observing the reduction in renal parenchymal width (Fig. 7.18).

In certain situations obstruction is intermittent. Such patients usually have renal colic and the IVU may be normal between attacks. If, however, the urogram is performed during an attack of colic (the so-called 'emergency urogram') the level of obstruction is nearly always demonstrated.

Ultrasound in urinary tract obstruction

Dilatation of the pelvicaliceal system is demonstrated sonographically as a spreading apart of the central echo complex, due to pooling of urine within the

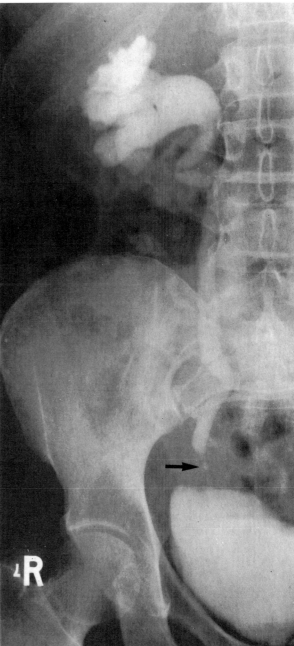

Fig. 7.16 Ureteric obstruction. The pelvicaliceal system and ureter are dilated down to the level of the obstructing pathology (arrow)—in this instance a small calculus.

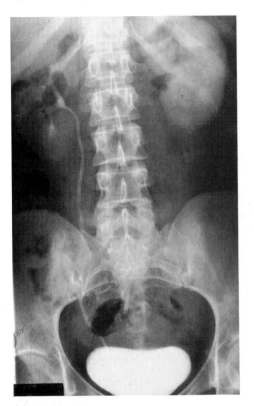
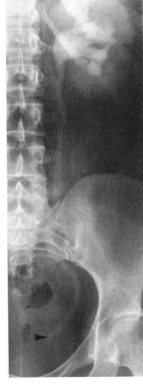

(a)   (b)

Fig. 7.17 Acute ureteric obstruction due to a stone in the lower end of the left ureter. (a) A film taken 30 minutes after the injection of contrast medium. There is obvious delay in the appearance of the pyelogram on the left. The left kidney shows a very dense nephrogram which is characteristic of acute ureteric obstruction. (b) A film taken 23 hours later shows opacification of the obstructed collecting system down to the obstructing calculus (arrow).

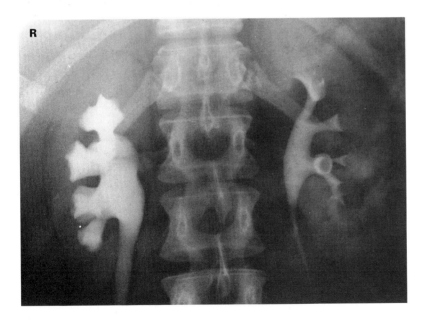

Fig. 7.18 Obstructive atrophy. The right kidney is small with a smooth outline due to reduction in renal parenchyma and shows dilatation of the collecting system. This loss of renal tissue was due to obstruction by a stone in the ureter.

pelvis and calices. Initially, these are seen as fluid collections in the centre of the kidney (Fig. 7.19a). As this distension becomes more severe, the dilated calices can resemble multiple renal cysts, but dilated calices, unlike cysts, show continuity with the renal pelvis (Fig. 7.19b). With prolonged obstruction, thinning of the cortex due to atrophy will be seen.

Proximal ureteric dilatation can frequently be ident-

ified, but dilatation of the distal ureter is often obscured by overlying bowel. It follows, therefore, that while some causes of obstruction are identifiable, e.g. carcinoma of the bladder, it is often not possible to determine the cause of urinary tract obstruction at ultrasound examination. Plain films are useful in this context to demonstrate calculi that may be responsible for the obstruction.

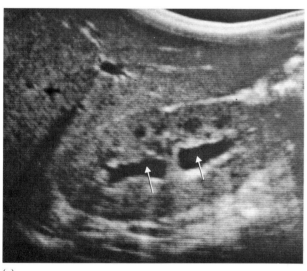

(a)

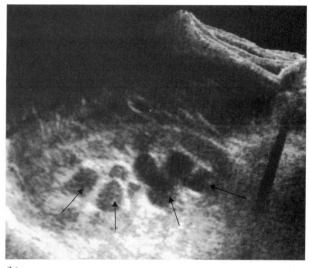

(b)

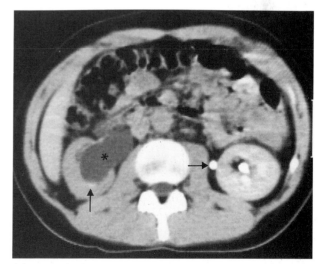

(c)

Fig. 7.19 Dilatation of the pelvicaliceal system.
(a) Longitudinal ultrasound scan of right kidney showing spreading of the central echo complex of the dilated collecting system (arrows). (b) Here the dilation is greater and the calices resemble cysts (arrows). (c) CT scan after contrast showing a dilated renal pelvis (asterisk). The vertical arrow points to a small amount of contrast pooling in a dependent calix. Note the normal left ureter (horizontal arrow).

Computed tomography in urinary tract obstruction

Dilated portions of the collecting systems can be identified on CT both before and after intravenous contrast
administration (Fig. 7.19c). The dilated system can
frequently be traced down to the site of the obstruction. An advantage over the IVU is that tumours
responsible for obstruction may be visualised directly.

Radionuclide examination in urinary tract obstruction

If there is urinary tract obstruction the radionuclide is
filtered by the kidney but not excreted and the retention within the kidney is reflected by the renogram
curve (Fig. 7.20). It is often helpful, particularly in
those cases of possible obstruction at the pelviureteric
junction, to give an intravenous injection of a diuretic,
which washes out the radionuclide from a dilated but
non-obstructed renal pelvis.

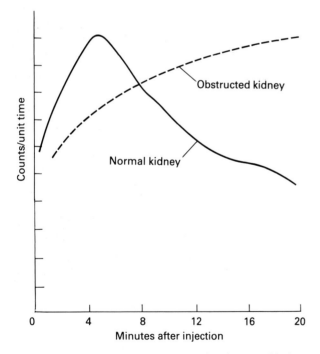

Fig. 7.20 Renogram in obstruction. In the obstructed kidney
there is a slow, continuous accumulation of radionuclide.

A renogram is a very sensitive method of determining the function of an obstructed kidney but,
because of the poor anatomical definition, the renogram cannot reliably predict the site or the cause of the
obstruction.

Causes of obstruction to the ureters and pelvicaliceal systems

There are many causes of obstruction to the ureters
and pelvicaliceal systems. Calculi, tumours or strictures
may be responsible for obstruction at any level. When
obstruction is seen at the pelviureteric junction, an
additional cause to consider is the congenital disorder
'intrinsic pelviureteric junction obstruction'. Aberrant
renal artery, retroperitoneal fibrosis and retroperitoneal tumours are further causes of ureteric obstruction.

Calculi

Calculi are by far the commonest cause of obstruction
of the urinary tract. A calcified opacity will usually be
visible on the plain film, but since parts of the ureter
overlie the transverse processes of the vertebrae
and the wings of the sacrum, the calculus may be
impossible to see on plain film.

Tumours

Transitional cell carcinomas of the calices or pelvis
usually produce a recognisable filling defect at IVU
(see Fig. 7.28, p. 245), but if the tumour is in the ureter
it may not be visible. The best tests to demonstrate the
tumour in such cases are pyelography either retrograde or antegrade. Carcinoma of the bladder causing
ureteric obstruction can usually be easily identified on
IVU, CT or ultrasound, though cystoscopy is the best
method of establishing the diagnosis.

Renal parenchymal masses may narrow and obstruct a
calix or the pelvis but the explanation is usually obvious because of other signs due to the mass (see
p. 240).

Infective strictures

Infective strictures are mostly due to tuberculosis or schistosomiasis. In the case of tuberculosis there is usually other evidence on an IVU to suggest the diagnosis (p. 246).

Congenital intrinsic pelviureteric junction obstruction

In this disorder peristalsis is not transmitted across the pelviureteric junction, i.e. a functional obstruction exists, but there is no naked-eye evidence of the cause. The disease may present at any age but it is usually discovered in children or young adults. The diagnosis depends on identifying dilatation of all the calices and of the pelvis, with an abrupt change in calibre at the pelviureteric junction (Fig. 7.21). Often, the ureter cannot be identified at all. If it is seen, it will be either narrow or normal in size.

Retroperitoneal disease

Tumours. Carcinoma of the cervix and rectosigmoid junction, and malignant lymph node enlargement are frequent causes in this category of ureteric obstruction. The ureters may be visibly deviated by such tumours but frequently the ureteric course is normal. Because some of these tumours originate in the midline or are bilateral, both ureters may be obstructed. Computed tomography, or ultrasound in some cases, is the ideal method of diagnosis because it shows the tumour mass, whereas the IVU only shows the site of obstruction.

Retroperitoneal fibrosis. In most cases, no cause can be found for this benign fibrotic condition which encases the ureters and causes obstruction. When first seen, only one side may be obstructed but eventually the condition becomes bilateral. The affected ureters may be displaced medially. The obstruction is usually at the L.4/5 level. Here again, CT has become the diagnostic method of choice, because it shows the retroperitoneum so well (Fig. 7.22).

Ureteric dilatation in pregnancy

Pronounced unilateral or bilateral ureteric dilatation together with dilatation of the pelvicaliceal systems occurs during the second half of pregnancy, or in

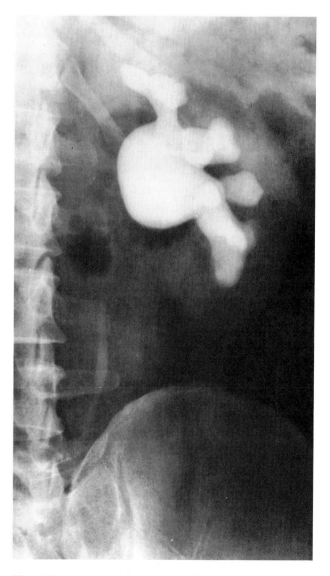

Fig. 7.21 Intrinsic pelviureteric junction obstruction. The pelvicaliceal system is considerably dilated, but the ureter from the pelviureteric junction onward is normal in calibre.

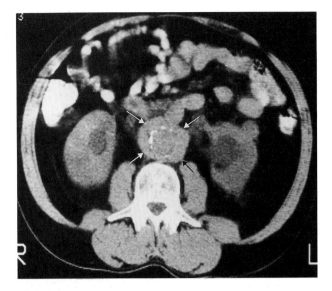

Fig. 7.22 Retroperitoneal fibrosis. CT scan showing bilateral hydronephrosis. The aorta is surrounded by a mass of fibrous tissue (arrows). The position of the aortic wall is shown by its atheromatous calcification. The retroperitoneal fibrosis extended down to the level of aortic bifurcation.

women taking the contraceptive pill. It may take 3 months or more to return to normal. The mechanism is uncertain. It is therefore wise to wait, if possible, for 4 months after pregnancy before evaluating the upper urinary tract.

The unilateral 'non-functioning' kidney at IVU

The phrase unilateral 'non-functioning' kidney implies non-visualisation of the pyelogram of one kidney at IVU, not as the term would suggest a total absence of function by that kidney. Total non-visualisation is rare; a nephrogram is often seen and may show dilated calices as rounded defects in the nephrogram. If this so-called 'negative pyelogram' is seen, the diagnosis of hydronephrosis and, therefore, obstruction is certain. In this situation, delayed films should be taken to show the level of obstruction.

The common cause of a 'non-functioning' kidney,

other than previous nephrectomy, is ureteric obstruction. Other causes are renal agenesis, renal artery occlusion and renal vein thrombosis.

It is worth noting that renal parenchymal tumours (renal cell carcinoma and Wilms' tumour) are very rare causes of 'non-function'. When they do result in absence of a pyelogram, the usual mechanism is obstruction of the ureter by tumour or blood clot. On the other hand, transitional cell carcinomas of the pelvis, ureter and bladder are common causes of 'non-function', since they so readily obstruct the drainage of a kidney.

Most cases of unilateral non-visualisation at IVU require further investigation. It is here that ultrasound is so valuable, since it does not rely on renal function. Ultrasound can demonstrate the renal size, the thickness of the parenchyma and can determine whether there is hydronephrosis.

With *renal artery occlusion* the kidney will be seen on plain film or CT but no nephrogram is seen after contrast is given. Renography will confirm absence of blood flow and function. Ultrasound shows a normal pelvicaliceal pattern.

Acute renal vein thrombosis is a rare cause of non-visualisation. With time, collateral venous channels open up and a visible pyelogram usually returns. The thrombus in the renal veins or inferior vena cava may be detectable with ultrasound or CT.

Renal parenchymal masses

Almost all solitary masses arising within the renal parenchyma are either *malignant tumours* or *simple cysts*. In adults, the malignant tumour is almost certain to be a renal cell carcinoma, whereas in young children the common neoplasm is the Wilms' tumour.

Unusual causes of a renal mass include: renal abscess, hydatid cyst, benign tumours and metastasis.

Occasionally, invagination of normal cortical tissue into the renal medulla (sometimes called a 'renal pseudotumour') may produce the signs of a localised mass at IVU (Fig. 7.23). Here the distinguishing feature

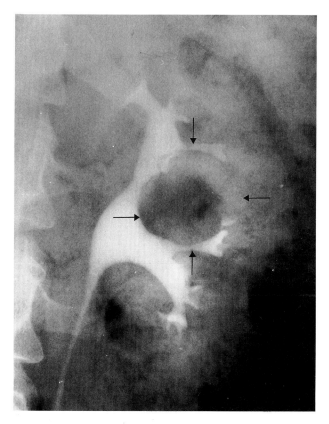

Fig. 7.23 Renal pseudotumour (arrows) which was subsequently shown to be normal renal cortical tissue by DMSA scanning.

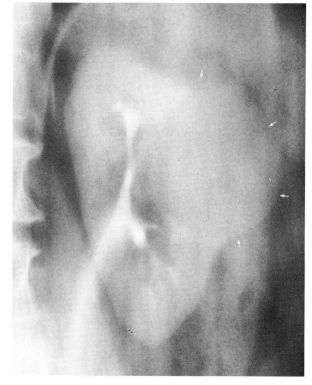

Fig. 7.24 Signs of a renal mass. The renal outline is bulged (arrows) and there is a corresponding displacement of the calices. In this patient the mass is a cyst. Note the lower density of the mass compared with the opacified renal parenchyma and its clear-cut border.

is uniform opacification of the 'mass'. Ultrasound or CT can be used to exclude a true tumour.

Multiple renal masses usually indicate multiple simple cysts, polycystic disease or malignant lymphoma.

Intravenous urogram of renal masses

The basic signs of a renal parenchymal mass on an IVU are (Fig. 7.24):
• Bulging of the renal outline. Sometimes, the outline is so indistinct that the bulge cannot be appreciated.
• Displacement of major and minor calices.
• Increase in renal size, particularly if the mass is at

the upper or lower pole where its bulk adds to the renal length.
• A small proportion of renal carcinomas calcify (Fig. 7.25). When this happens it is always possible to appreciate from the IVU that the calcification is in a renal mass. (Calcification in the wall of a benign cyst is exceedingly uncommon.)

Once a mass is seen or suspected at IVU, the next step is to diagnose its nature using ultrasound or CT. It should be noted that any solitary mass in a young child, or any mass that contains visible calcification, particularly if the calcification is more than just a thin line at the periphery, is likely to be a malignant tumour.

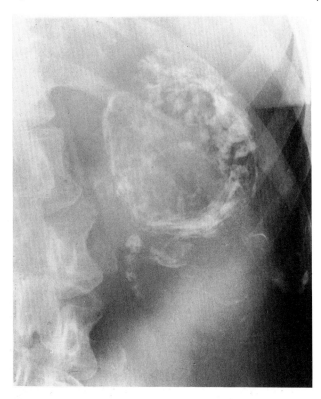

Fig. 7.25 Partially calcified renal cell carcinoma.

Ultrasound of renal masses (Fig. 7.26)

Ultrasound is used to establish whether a mass is a simple cyst, and can therefore be ignored, or whether the lesion is solid and, therefore, is likely to be a carcinoma. A mass with mixed cystic and solid features falls into the indeterminate category and could be a renal tumour, a renal abscess, or possibly a complex benign cyst.

Simple cysts are very common. Being filled with clear fluid, they show obvious echoes from the front and back wall with no intervening echoes. They also show a column of increased echoes behind the cyst; the phenomenon known as 'acoustic enhancement'. Most cysts are spherical in shape. They may be solitary or multiple, unilocular or have septations. Some cysts contain low level echoes in their dependent portions, presumably due to previous haemorrhage. When the

ultrasonographer is sure that the diagnosis is simple cyst, no further investigation is needed.

Solid renal masses have numerous internal echoes of varying intensity. As sound is attenuated during its passage through a solid lesion, the back wall is not as sharp as that seen with a cyst, and there is little or no 'acoustic enhancement' deep to the mass. Solid masses may be irregular in outline.

Computed tomography of renal masses (Fig. 7.27)

Computed tomography has proved very useful in the assessment of renal masses. The alteration of the renal outline and the distortion of the renal collecting systems seen at IVU are well demonstrated at CT. Additionally, it is possible to differentiate cysts from tumours by the differing density of the lesions, particularly after intravenous contrast administration.

At CT, a typical simple renal cyst is a spherical mass with an imperceptible wall. The interior of the cyst is homogeneous with attenuation values similar to those of water. The margins between the cysts and the normal renal parenchyma are sharp. When all of these criteria are met the diagnosis of simple cyst is certain and there is no need to proceed further.

Renal cell carcinomas are approximately spherical, usually lobulated and frequently have poorly defined margins. The attenuation value of renal tumours on scans without intravenous contrast enhancement is often fairly close to that of normal parenchyma, but focal necrotic areas may result in areas of low density and stippled calcification may be present in the interior of the mass. Following intravenous contrast administration, renal cell carcinomas do not enhance to the same degree as the normal parenchyma and they are inhomogeneous in their enhancement pattern.

Tumour extension through the capsule, to adjacent lymph nodes and into the renal vein can be easily evaluated at CT scanning (Fig. 7.27a).

Renal arteriography in renal masses

Renal arteriography used to play a major part in the

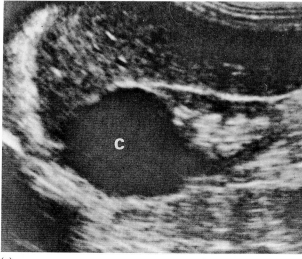

(a)

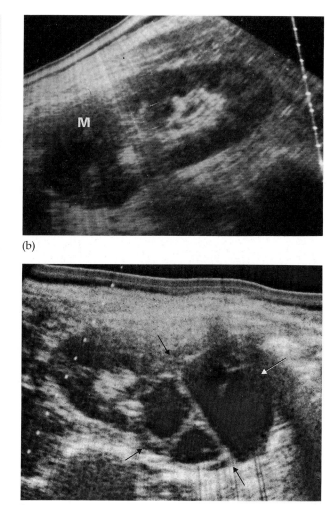

(b)

(c)

Fig. 7.26 Ultrasound in renal masses. (a) Cyst (C) showing sharp walls and no echoes arising within it. Note the acoustic enhancement behind the cyst. (b) Tumour showing echoes arising from within the mass (M). (c) Complex mass due to cystic renal cell carcinoma. The arrows point to the edge of the mass. Note the thick septa within the mass.

diagnosis of renal masses by demonstrating pathological circulation in malignant neoplasm (Fig. 7.27c). Its only diagnostic use nowadays is to demonstrate renal artery anatomy prior to surgery and to perform transcatheter embolisation.

Percutaneous cyst puncture

In those very few cases where the nature of a renal cyst is in doubt after IVU, ultrasound or CT, a percutaneous puncture can be performed and cyst fluid can be obtained for cytology. The procedure is often done under ultrasound guidance.

Urothelial tumours

Almost all the tumours that grow within the collecting systems of the kidneys are *transitional cell carcinomas*. The tumours sometimes occur in multiple sites. In the pelvicaliceal system they are seen as lobulated or, very occasionally, as fronded filling defects either projecting into the lumen or completely surrounded by contrast

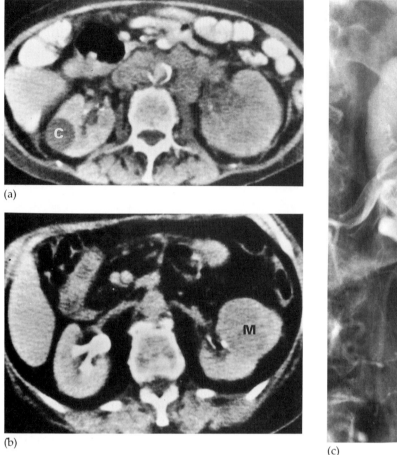

(a)

(b)

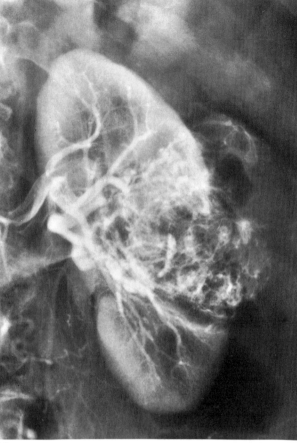

(c)

Fig. 7.27 Computed tomography scans in renal masses. (a) Cyst in right kidney (C) showing a well-defined edge, imperceptible wall and uniform water density. The cyst was an incidental finding. The scan was performed because of the large carcinoma in the left kidney. Metastatic retroperitoneal lymphadenopathy is also present. (b) Renal cell carcinoma. The mass (M) has a thick wall, is not clearly demarcated from the adjacent kidney and is of irregular density. The retroperitoneum is normal. (c) Arteriogram in same patient showing innumerable abnormal vessels within the mass with the remainder of the kidney being normal.

(Fig. 7.28). It is easy to confuse such tumours with overlying gas shadows on an IVU and tomography may be required during an IVU to solve the problem.

At ultrasound, transitional cell carcinomas are difficult to see because they blend with the renal sinus fat.

Urothelial tumours may obstruct the ureter in which they are growing, in which case it is usually only possible to determine the site of obstruction from the IVU or ultrasound. The tumour itself may be visible on antegrade or retrograde pyelography or at CT.

Acute infections of the upper urinary tracts

Acute pyelonephritis

Acute pyelonephritis is usually due to bacterial infection from organisms which enter the urinary system

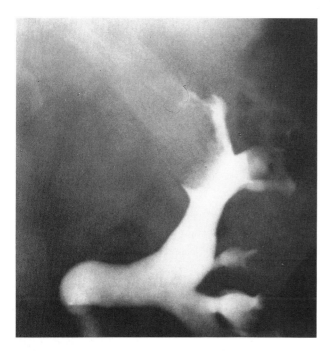

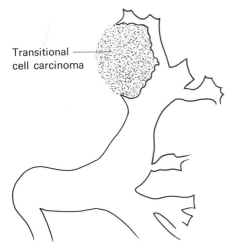

Transitional cell carcinoma

Fig. 7.28 Filling defect in an upper calix due to transitional cell carcinoma.

via the urethra. Anatomical abnormalities such as stones, duplex systems, obstructive lesions and conditions such as diabetes mellitus all predispose to infection.

In most cases, the IVU is normal even during the acute attack. In very severe cases with suppuration of the kidney, the caliceal system is compressed by the swelling of the renal substance and the concentration of contrast on the affected side is reduced or not visible. At ultrasound, one or both kidneys may appear significantly enlarged and show diminished echoes due to cortical oedema. At CT, the pre-contrast scans are usually normal, but may reveal patchy diminished density. Following contrast enhancement, affected portions of the renal cortex show patchy, striated areas of diminished density representing non-functional nephrons.

Renal and perinephric abscesses

Renal and perinephric abscesses are usually difficult to see on IVU, since in many cases there is poor visualisation of the kidneys due to pre-existing hydronephrosis or calculous disease. They are diagnosed by recognising a mass, the clinical setting suggesting the infective nature of the mass. Ultrasound and CT are the best methods of diagnosis.

Most *intrarenal abscesses* (Fig. 7.29) have thick walls and show both cystic and solid components recognisable at both ultrasound and CT. With CT, it is possible to see enhancement of the wall of the abscess following intravenous contrast injection.

Simple cysts may become secondarily infected, in which case the ultrasound and computed tomography features resemble those of a simple cyst, but the wall may be a little thicker and there will frequently be a layer of echogenic debris in the dependent portion of the cyst.

Perinephric abscesses (Fig. 7.30) frequently conform to the shape of the underlying kidney. The CT and sonographic characteristics are variable, usually showing both solid and cystic elements. The cystic portions frequently contain internal echoes at ultrasound due to debris. Since most perinephric abscesses are secondary to an infective focus within the kidney, an underlying renal abnormality is often demonstrable.

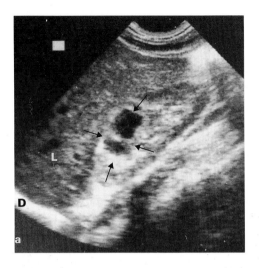

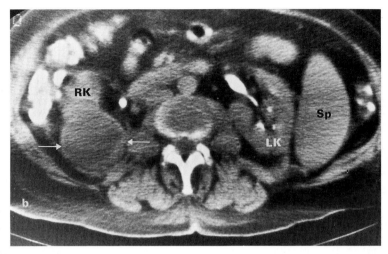

Fig. 7.29 Renal abscess. (a) Ultrasound scan showing a complex mass (arrows) in the right kidney. D, diaphragm; L, liver. (b) CT scan in a different patient showing encapsulated fluid collection in the lower pole of the right kidney (arrows). LK, left kidney; RK, right kidney; Sp, spleen.

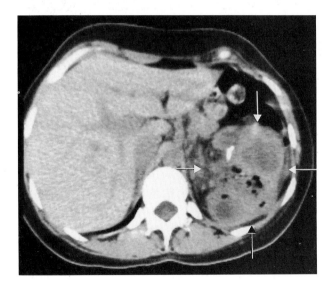

Fig. 7.30 Perinephric abscess. CT scan showing a rounded loculation of fluid and gas in the left perinephric space (arrows).

Pyonephrosis

Pyonephrosis only occurs in collecting systems that are obstructed. At IVU, it may occasionally be possible to identify hydronephrosis, but usually no opacification of the affected side can be seen. It is not possible to differentiate infected urine from sterile urine at IVU. Ultrasound is the most sensitive imaging modality for pyonephrosis. In addition to showing the hydronephrosis it may demonstrate multiple echoes within the urine due to infected debris. At CT, pus is only detectable if it is inspissated.

Tuberculosis

Urinary tuberculosis follows blood-borne spread of *Mycobacterium tuberculosis*, usually from a focus of infection in the lung. A normal chest film, however, does not exclude the diagnosis, since the tuberculous lesion in the lung may be too small to be identified.

The tubercle bacilli infect the cortex of the kidneys and may cause cortical abscesses which can ulcerate into the renal pelvis. The infection may then spread to involve other portions of the urinary and genital systems.

In the early stages of the disease, even though tubercle bacilli can be recovered from the urine, the

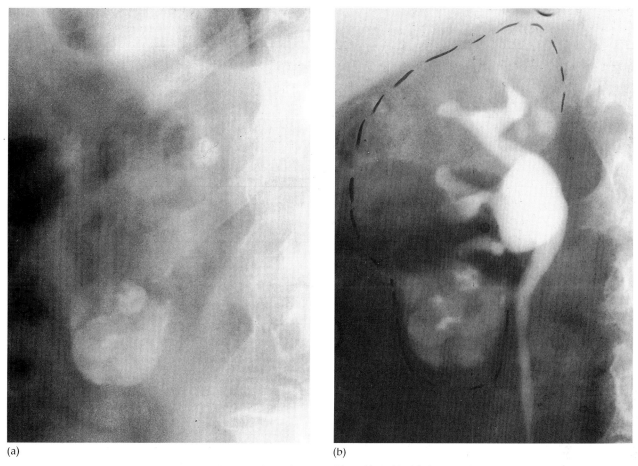

(a)　　　　　　　　　　　　　　　　　　(b)

Fig. 7.31 Renal parenchymal calcification due to tuberculosis. (a) Plain film. (b) After contrast.

IVU may be normal. Signs that develop in the later stages of urinary tuberculosis are:

• Calcification, which is common (Fig. 7.31). Usually, there are one or more patches of irregular calcification, but in advanced cases with long-standing tuberculous pyonephrosis the majority of the kidney and hydronephrotic collecting system may be calcified, leading to a so-called 'autonephrectomy'. Calcification implies healing but does not mean that the disease is inactive. Indeed, the opposite is true; active infection is almost invariably present when untreated calcified tuberculous lesions are first seen in the kidney.

• The earliest change on the post-contrast films is irregularity of a calix. Later, a definite contrast-filled cavity may be seen adjacent to the calix (Fig. 7.32). With progression of the disease the cavities enlarge and the renal substance is destroyed, producing loss of parenchymal width.

• Strictures of any portion of the pelvicaliceal system or ureter may occur, producing dilatation of one or more calices. Multiple sites of stricture are important diagnostic features.

• If the bladder is involved, the wall is irregular due to inflammatory oedema; advanced disease causes fibrosis resulting in a thick-walled small volume bladder. Multiple strictures may be seen in the urethra.

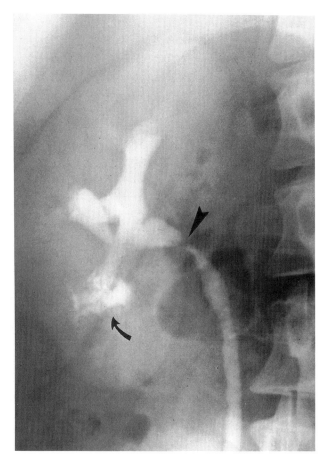

Fig. 7.32 Tuberculosis, showing irregularity of the calices (curved arrow) and stricture formation of the pelvis (arrow head).

Reflux nephropathy (chronic pyelonephritis)

This entity used to be called chronic pyelonephritis but it has now been renamed reflux nephropathy because it is due to reflux of infected urine from the bladder into the kidneys, leading to destruction and scarring of the renal substance. It is believed that scarring only occurs with severe reflux. Most damage occurs in the first year of life. The severity of reflux diminishes as the child gets older and may have ceased by the time the diagnosis of reflux nephropathy is made. The upper and lower calices are the most sus-

ceptible to damage from reflux. The condition is often bilateral.

The usual cause of reflux is a congenital abnormality of the ureterovesical junction, with a shorter than normal intramural section of ureter. A similar arrangement is found in the ureter draining the lower moiety of a kidney with a bifid collecting system. *Vesicoureteric reflux* may be demonstrated at micturating (voiding) cystography.

The signs of reflux nephropathy are (Fig. 7.33):
• *Local reduction in renal parenchymal width (scar formation)*. The distance between the calix and the adjacent renal outline is usually substantially reduced and may be as little as 1 or 2 mm. Since there is no function in these scarred areas, the renal outline is often difficult to see. It may, therefore, be easy to miss the fact that extensive scarring exists. DMSA radionuclide scans and ultrasound are both useful in demonstrating the cortical scars.
• *Dilatation of the calices in the scarred areas*. The dilatation is the result of destruction of the pyramids.
• *Overall reduction in renal size*, which is partly due to loss of renal substance and partly because the scarred areas do not grow.
• *Dilatation of the affected collecting system* due to reflux may be seen.

Papillary necrosis (Fig. 7.34)

In papillary necrosis, part or all of the renal papilla sloughs and may fall into the pelvicaliceal system. These necrotic papillae may remain within the pelvicaliceal system, sometimes causing obstruction, or they may be voided. There are a number of conditions with

Fig. 7.33 (*opposite*) Reflux nephropathy (chronic pyelonephritis). (a) IVU showing reduction in renal parenchymal width due to scarring and dilatation (clubbing) of the adjacent calices. (b) IVU showing a severely shrunken kidney with multiple scars and clubbed calices. (c) DMSA scan (posterior view) showing shrunken left kidney with a focal scar in upper pole (arrow). (d) CT scan (after i.v. contrast enhancement) showing shrunken left pyelonephritic kidney (arrows).

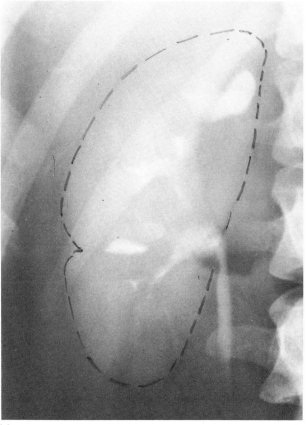

(a)

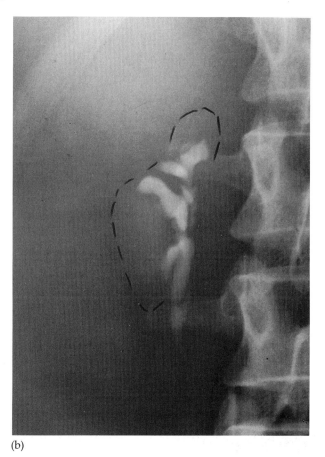

(b)

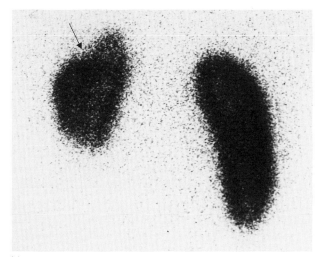

(c)

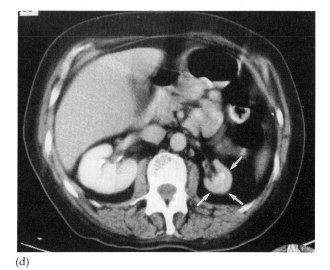

(d)

strong associations with papillary necrosis. The most frequent are:

- high analgesic intake, particularly phenacetin but also aspirin
- diabetes mellitus
- sickle cell disease
- infection, but usually only with very severe infections.

The pattern of destruction of the papilla takes many forms, the disease usually being patchy in distribution and severity. If the papilla is only partially separated, contrast can be seen tracking into it, but if the papilla is totally sloughed the calix appears spherical, having lost its papillary indentation. When sloughed, the papilla may then be seen as a filling defect in a spherical calix or it may have passed down the ureter, often causing obstruction as it does so.

The necrotic papilla can calcify prior to sloughing, so calcification may be seen in the site of the normal papilla, or in the sloughed papilla within the collecting system—in which case it will closely resemble a urinary calculus.

Trauma to the urinary tract

Renal trauma

The kidney, along with the spleen, is the most frequent internal abdominal organ to be injured. Blunt trauma, particularly road traffic accidents and contact sports are the mechanisms of injury in well over three-quarters of patients, the remainder being due to penetrating injury. Loin pain and haematuria are the major presenting features.

The indications for imaging tests depend on the clinical features and surgical approach. The IVU is usually the first test performed, followed by CT if necessary. In general, these tests are used to:

- Demonstrate the presence or absence of perfusion to the injured kidney.
- Ensure that the opposite kidney is normal.
- Show the extent of renal parenchymal damage.
- Demonstrate injuries to other organs, a feature of great importance in penetrating injury, where other organs are frequently lacerated.
- Identify any pre-existing abnormalities of either kidney.

Plain films may show fractures of the vertebrae or ribs. The appearances on IVU or CT depend on the extent of injury. Minor injury (contusion and small capsular haematomas) produces swelling of the paren-chyma which compresses the calices. If the kidney substance is torn, the renal outline is irregular and the calices are separated at the site of rupture. Large sub-capsular and extracapsular blood collections may be present and extravasation of contrast may be seen

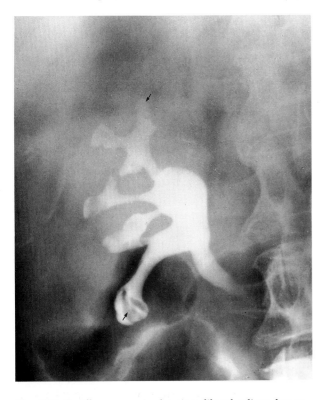

Fig. 7.34 Papillary necrosis showing dilated calices due to loss of the papillae. Some of the papillae have sloughed and appear as filling defects within the calices (lower arrow). The upper arrow points to a contrast-filled cavity within a papilla.

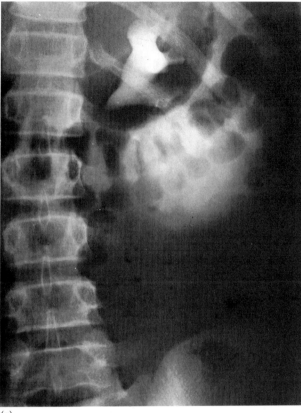

(a)

(b)

Fig. 7.35 Renal trauma. (a) The lower pole of the kidney has been ruptured and a pool of extravasated contrast can be seen. (b) CT scan showing extensive haematoma (arrows) surrounding a fragmented left kidney (K).

(Fig. 7.35). Retroperitoneal haemorrhage may displace the kidney and may cause ureteric obstruction. Fragmentation of the kidney is a serious event, often, though by no means always, requiring nephrectomy or surgical repair. If thrombosis or rupture of the renal artery occurs, there will be no nephrogram. Renal infarction is a very serious condition demanding urgent restoration of blood flow or nephrectomy.

Computed tomography is an excellent method of confirming or excluding significant renal trauma and at the same time will show damage to other abdominal organs. Arteriography is rarely necessary to assess parenchymal damage; its use is confined to detailed evaluation of a renal arterial injury in those cases where reparative surgery is being contemplated.

Trauma to the bladder and urethra

Rupture of the bladder may result from a direct blow to the distended bladder or may be part of extensive injury such as occurs with fractures of the pelvis. If the rupture is intraperitoneal, contrast introduced into the bladder will leak out into the peritoneal cavity.

A common site of rupture is at the bladder base, in which case the bladder shows elevation and compression due to extravasated urine and haematoma.

Rupture of the bladder may be revealed sonographically by the presence of a perivesicular fluid collection but the actual site of a tear will not be seen.

Computed tomography may demonstrate fresh haematomas within the pelvis (which are of high density) or urine collections (which are of low density).

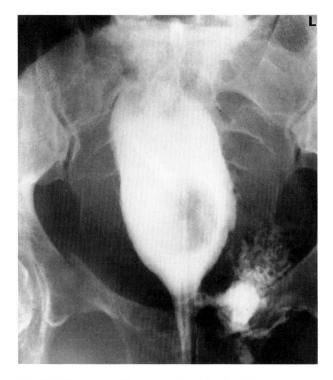

Fig. 7.36 Rupture of the base of the bladder. Cystogram showing extravasation of contrast into the extraperitoneal space on the left, and deformity of the bladder due to surrounding haematoma and urine. There is a fracture of the right pubic bone.

It will also demonstrate the associated fractures, some of which may not be apparent on plain radiographs. Cystography remains the best way of demonstrating the actual site of leakage from the bladder (Fig. 7.36).

Damage to the urethra is a serious complication of pelvic fractures. An ascending urethrogram using a water-soluble contrast medium may show rupture of the urethra with extravasation of contrast into the adjacent tissues.

Hypertension in renal disease

There are a large number of diseases, both renal and non-renal, that are associated with hypertension. The renal conditions include chronic glomerulonephritis, chronic pyelonephritis, renal artery stenosis, polycystic disease, polyarteritis nodosa, Kimmelstiel–Wilson kidney and, occasionally, renal masses. The feature common to all the renal conditions is a reduction in blood supply to all or part of the kidney.

In glomerulonephritis, polyarteritis nodosa and the Kimmelstiel–Wilson kidney, there is usually bilateral uniform reduction in renal size without other specific features. Essential hypertension may cause identical changes at IVU and the decision whether the small kidneys are the cause or the result of hypertension cannot be made radiologically.

Nowadays, because of improved drug therapy, the search for a renal cause is largely limited to children with severe hypertension and those patients whose hypertension is inadequately controlled. Surveys have shown that if a routine IVU is performed in patients with hypertension, 20% will show an abnormality of the urinary tract, but that this leads to a change in management in less than 1% of cases.

Renal artery stenosis

Renal artery stenosis can be a cause of hypertension. It is, however, found fairly frequently at post mortem or angiographically in normotensive patients. The common cause is atheroma.

At IVU, the signs of severe renal artery stenosis are a reduction in size of the affected kidney and delayed visualisation of the pyelogram. Sometimes, the pyelogram on the affected side is denser than normal. These signs are only present in severe renal artery stenosis, and in many cases of hypertension due to renal artery stenosis the diagnosis cannot be made from the IVU.

Renography (Fig. 7.37) is a more sensitive test. It will show delay in peak activity and a relative reduction of function on the affected side if renal artery stenosis is present. Colour-flow Doppler ultrasound is being increasingly used to demonstrate and quantify reduction in blood flow in renal artery stenosis. Arteriography or digital subtraction angiography is the best method of demonstrating the renal artery stenosis

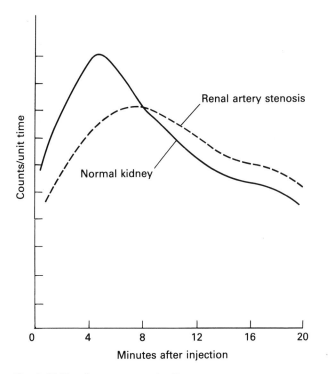

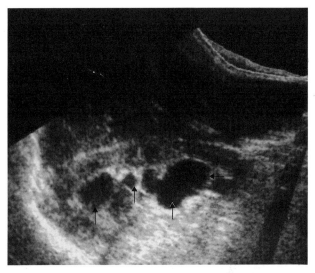

Fig. 7.38 Ultrasound of obstructive renal failure. The dilated collecting system is arrowed. The hydronephrosis was bilateral in this case of retroperitoneal fibrosis.

Fig. 7.37 Renal artery stenosis. Renogram curve. Accumulation and excretion of the radionuclide is delayed and reduced, so the peak of the curve is later and lower than normal.

itself, but it should be realised that it is not always possible to predict the haemodynamic significance of a stenosis from its angiographic appearance.

Renal failure

In patients presenting with renal failure, it is important to confirm or exclude urinary tract obstruction which can sometimes be surgically relieved.

Renal failure due to obstructive uropathy

The cardinal sign of obstructive uropathy is dilatation of the pelvicaliceal system. Ultrasound has now replaced the IVU as the initial investigation to confirm or exclude obstruction (Fig. 7.38). Plain radiographs should be taken to exclude urinary calculi in any patient with renal failure and urinary tract obstruction demonstrated by ultrasound. The demonstration of a normal pelvicaliceal system rules out an obstructive cause for renal failure.

Renal failure due to intrinsic renal disease ('end stage kidney')

Once obstruction and pre-renal conditions have been excluded, intrinsic renal disease is assumed to be responsible for the renal failure.

Chronic pyelonephritis is the only specific diagnosis than can be made with any frequency. Most end-stage kidneys will be small or normal in size with smooth outlines and normal calices. There are many causes for these appearances, notably chronic glomerulonephritis and diabetes (see Table 7.1, p. 227). An alteration of parenchymal texture may be demonstrated by ultrasound, but again the appearances are rarely specific (Fig. 7.39).

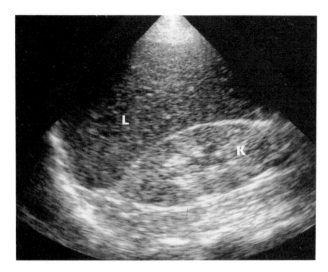

Fig. 7.39 Intrinsic renal disease. Ultrasound of right kidney (longitudinal scan). The kidney is small and the cortical echoes are increased and therefore the central echo is less obvious. Normally, the liver is more echo-reflective than the renal cortex. L, liver; K, kidney.

Acute tubular necrosis

In acute tubular necrosis, from whatever cause, the ultrasound scan shows kidneys that are normal or enlarged with normal pelvicaliceal systems. Early films during an IVU show a definite nephrogram—one which is often denser than normal (Fig. 7.40). The diagnostic feature is that the nephrogram persists for up to 24 hours without visible caliceal filling.

Congenital variations of the urinary tract

Congenital variations in the anatomy of the urinary tract are very common. Only the commoner anomalies are discussed here (congenital pelviureteric junction obstruction is discussed on p. 239).

Bifid collecting systems (Fig. 7.41)

Bifid collecting systems are the most frequent congenital variations. The condition may be unilateral or bilateral. Sometimes just the pelvis is bifid, an

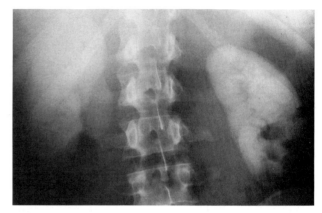

Fig. 7.40 Acute tubular necrosis. This film, taken 9 hours after injection of contrast, shows a dense persistent nephrogram with no opacification of the collecting systems.

anomaly of no importance. At the other extreme, the two ureters may be separate throughout their length and have separate openings into the bladder. The ureter draining the upper moiety may drain outside the bladder, e.g. into the vagina or urethra, producing incontinence if the opening is beyond the urethral sphincter. Such ureters, known as ectopic ureters, are frequently obstructed (Fig. 7.42) and lead to dilatation of the entire moiety; the dilated lower ureter in this condition is known as a ureterocele. The lower end of the dilated ureter often causes a smooth filling defect in the bladder.

Ectopic kidney

During fetal development the kidneys ascend within the abdomen. An ectopic kidney results if this ascent is halted. Such kidneys are usually in the lower abdomen and rotated so that the pelvis of the kidney points forward. The ureter is short and travels directly to the bladder. Chronic pyelonephritis, hydronephrosis and calculi are all more common in ectopic kidneys, but ectopic kidneys are often incidental findings of no consequence to the patient, except as a cause of diagnostic confusion with other causes of lower abdominal masses.

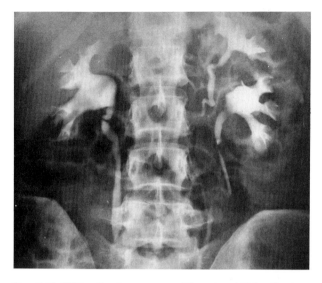

Fig. 7.41 Bifid collecting systems. There is a bifid collecting system on the left with the two ureters joining at the level of the transverse process of L5. Note how the left kidney is larger than the right.

Horseshoe kidney

The kidneys may fail to separate, giving rise to a horseshoe kidney. Almost invariably it is the lower poles that remain fused (Fig. 7.43).

The anomaly may be an incidental finding and of no significance, but obstruction to the collecting systems and calculi formation are both fairly common.

Congenital cystic disease of the kidneys

There are many varieties of cystic renal disease varying from simple cysts (see p. 240), which may be single or multiple, to complex renal dysplasias. The most frequent complex dysplasia encountered in clinical practice is polycystic disease: a familial disorder which, though congenital in origin, usually presents between the ages of 35 to 55 years with features of hypertension, renal failure or haematuria, or by the discovery of bilaterally enlarged kidneys. The reason for the late presentation is that the cysts are initially small and do not cause trouble for a long time.

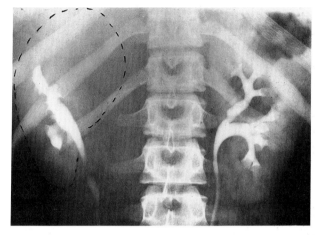

Fig. 7.42 Obstructed ectopic ureterocele. There is a bifid collecting system on the right. The upper moiety is obstructed and dilated causing deformity of the lower moiety. The obstructed moiety does not opacify.

At IVU, both kidneys are enlarged and the calices are stretched and distorted (Fig. 7.44a).

The diagnosis can be readily made at CT or ultrasound examination (Figs 7.44b and c) and is recognisable at an early age, even in childhood. The liver and pancreas may also contain cysts and these organs are routinely examined in such patients.

Renal agenesis

In renal agenesis the opposite kidney, providing it is normal, will show compensatory hypertrophy. Complete absence of blood flow and function on the affected side will be shown on radionuclide studies, and no renal tissue can be identified with ultrasound or CT examination.

The bladder

Bladder calcification

The most frequent cause of calcification in the bladder is calculi. Such calculi are frequently large and laminated. Calcification in the wall of the bladder is rare.

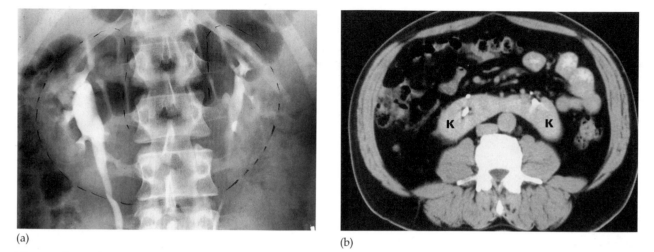

(a)   (b)

Fig. 7.43 Horseshoe kidneys. (a) The two kidneys are fused at their lower poles. The striking feature is the alteration in the axis of the kidneys: the lower calices are closer to the spine than the upper calices. The kidneys are rotated so that their pelves point forward and the lower calices point medially. The medial aspects of the lower poles cannot be identified. (b) CT scan of different patient, following i.v. contrast enhancement, showing fusion of the lower poles of the kidneys. K, kidney.

When it is seen it is due to either schistosomiasis or to calcium deposited on the surface of a bladder tumour. With the latter, once the bladder is opacified at IVU, the filling defect of the tumour is usually much more obvious than the calcification.

Bladder tumours

The bladder is the most frequent site for neoplasms in the urinary tract. Almost all are transitional cell carcinomas of varying degrees of malignancy. They vary in shape: some are delicate fronded papillary lesions, some are sessile irregular masses, and others form flat, plaque-like growths that infiltrate widely. At IVU they produce filling defects in the bladder (Fig. 7.45). The nature and extent of a tumour in the bladder is best observed at cystoscopy, so the main value of the IVU is in demonstrating ureteric obstruction. Small lesions readily identifiable at cystoscopy may be invisible on IVU. Gas and faeces in the sigmoid colon or rectum projected over the bladder outline on IVU may closely resemble a bladder neoplasm. Usually, it is possible to show on oblique views that the colonic contents lie partly outside the bladder, whereas the filling defect of a bladder tumour of necessity always lies within the bladder shadow, regardless of projection.

On CT, a tumour of the bladder is seen as a soft tissue mass projecting from the wall. Since the diagnosis is best established by cystoscopy and biopsy, the role of CT is to determine the extent of spread of the tumour (Fig. 7.46a).

Ultrasound examination (Fig. 7.46b) provides similar information to that of CT but is less accurate in detecting extravesical spread.

Bladder diverticula (Fig. 7.47)

Bladder diverticula may be congenital in origin but are usually the consequence of chronic obstruction to the bladder outflow. Because of urinary stasis, diverticula predispose to infection and stone formation and tumours may, on occasion, arise within them. Diverticula are well demonstrated at micturating cystography and after micturition during IVU, because bladder contraction is often necessary before they fill with contrast medium.

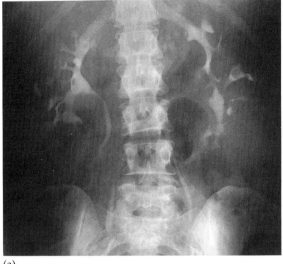

(a)

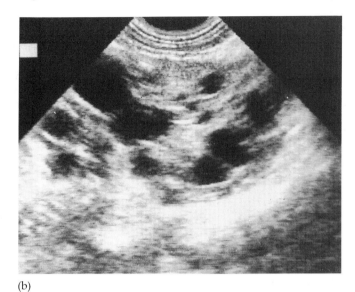

(b)

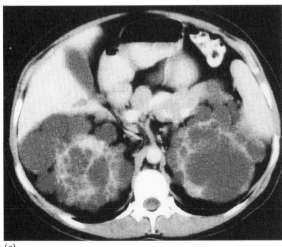

(c)

Fig. 7.44 Advanced polycystic disease in adults.
(a) IVU. The kidneys are greatly enlarged and the renal
outlines cannot be identified. The pelvicaliceal systems
are stretched and deformed by innumerable cysts.
(b) Ultrasound of a similar case showing the kidney
consists almost entirely of large cysts. The other kidney
looked the same. (c) CT scan, taken after intravenous
contrast enhancement, of similar case showing that both
kidneys are almost entirely replaced by cysts of variable
size.

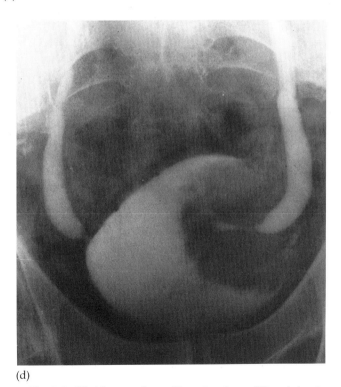

(d)

Fig. 7.45 Bladder neoplasm. There is a large filling defect in
the left side of the bladder due to a transitional cell
carcinoma.

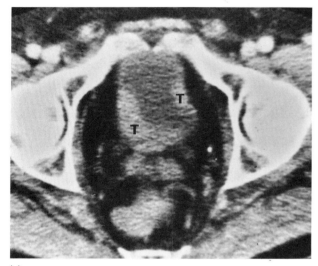

(a)

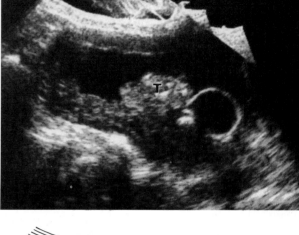

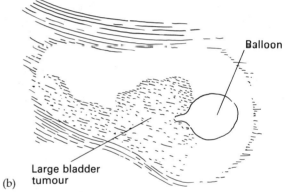

Fig. 7.46 (a) Carcinoma of bladder. CT scan showing an extensive tumour (T) involving the bladder wall but still confined to the bladder. (b) Ultrasound scan of another patient showing a large tumour (T) within the bladder.

(b)

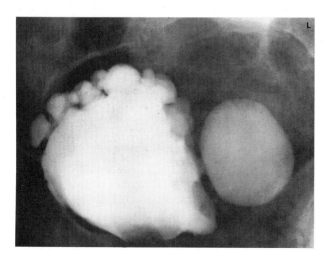

Fig. 7.47 Bladder diverticula. Cystogram showing numerous out-pouchings from the bladder with a very large diverticulum projecting to the left.

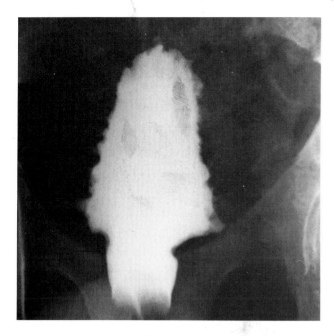

Fig. 7.48 Neurogenic bladder. The outline of the bladder is very irregular due to trabeculation of the bladder wall. The bladder has a small volume with an elongated shape. This appearance has been described as a 'fir tree bladder'. There is a balloon catheter in the dilated posterior urethra.

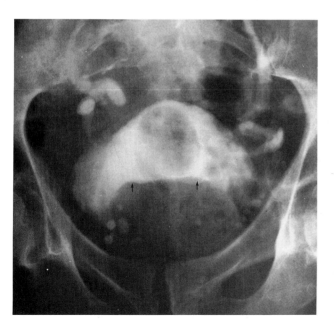

Neurogenic bladder

There are two basic types of neurogenic bladder (attempts to correlate these types with specific neurological lesions have not been satisfactory):

● The large atonic smooth walled bladder with poor or absent contractions and a large residual volume.
● The hypertrophic type, which can be regarded as neurologically induced bladder outflow obstruction. In this condition, the bladder is of small volume, has a very thick, grossly trabeculated wall and shows marked sacculation (Fig. 7.48).

The prostate

Prostatic enlargement

Prostatic enlargement is very common in elderly men. It is usually due to either benign hypertrophy or carcinoma. The diagnosis is still largely made on clinical grounds and confirmed by biopsy. The IVU provides little information about the prostate itself, although an enlarged prostate may be visible as a filling defect in the bladder base (Fig. 7.49).

Prostatic ultrasound uses a transducer designed to be introduced into the rectum. Transrectal ultrasound can show the overall size of the prostate and can diagnose relatively small masses within its substance. The ability to demonstrate masses that are impalpable led to the yet unrealised hope that ultrasound could be used as a screening test for prostatic carcinoma. Unfortunately, ultrasound cannot distinguish benign from malignant disease when confined to the prostate, except on the basis that masses in the peripheral zone are likely to be malignant and those in the central zone are more likely to be benign.

The prostate can be seen quite well at CT, but CT cannot distinguish benign from malignant disease, unless the disease has spread. However, in cases of

Fig. 7.49 Prostatic enlargement. The bladder base is lifted up and shows an impression from the enlarged prostate (arrows). The ureters are tortuous and enter the bladder horizontally. A balloon catheter is in the bladder.

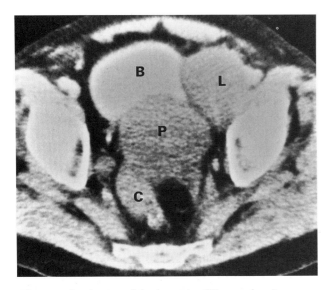

Fig. 7.50 Carcinoma of the prostate. CT scan showing massively enlarged prostate (P) indenting the bladder. The tumour has spread to involve pelvic lymph nodes. A huge lymph node mass is seen (L). B, bladder; C, colon.

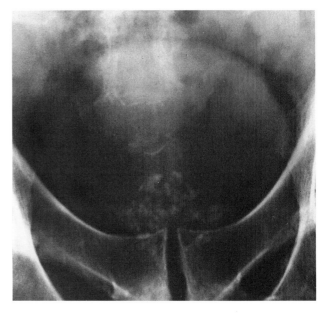

Fig. 7.51 Prostatic calcification. Numerous calculi just above the pubic symphysis are present in the prostate.

known prostatic carcinoma, it is helpful in determining the extent of local spread as well as lymph node metastases (Fig. 7.50).

Magnetic resonance imaging is a potentially promising method for imaging the prostate.

Prostatic calcification

Prostatic calcification is due to numerous prostatic calculi. It is so common that it can be regarded as a normal finding in older men. It shows no correlation with the symptoms of prostatic hypertrophy nor any relation to prostatic carcinoma. It always appears as numerous flecks of calcification of varying size, approximately symmetrical about the midline just beneath the bladder (Fig. 7.51).

Bladder outflow obstruction

The most frequent cause of bladder outflow obstruction is enlargement of the prostate. Other causes include bladder tumours, urethral strictures and, in little boys, posterior urethral valves. As discussed above, patients with neurological deficit may have neurogenic obstruction to bladder emptying. Regardless of the specific cause, the signs of bladder outflow obstruction are:

• Increased trabeculation and thickness of the bladder wall, often with diverticula formation.
• Residual urine in the bladder after micturition.
• Dilatation of the collecting systems.

Urethral stricture (Fig. 7.52)

The majority of urethral strictures are due to previous trauma or infection. Post-traumatic strictures are usually in the proximal penile urethra—the most vulnerable portion of the urethra to external trauma. Such strictures are usually smooth in outline and relatively short. Inflammatory strictures, which are usually gonococcal in origin, may be seen in any portion of the urethra, but are usually found in the anterior urethra.

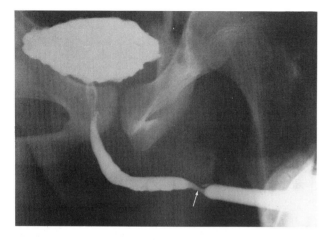

Fig. 7.52 Urethral stricture. An ascending urethrogram showing a stricture in the penile urethra (arrow). The patient had gonorrhoea.

Posterior urethral valves (Fig. 7.53)

Congenital valves may occur in the posterior urethra. They cause significant obstruction and are almost invariably discovered in boys during infancy or childhood. The IVU in such children will show hydronephrosis, hydroureter and a large, poorly emptying bladder. Urethral valves cannot be demonstrated by retrograde urethrography since there is no obstruction to retrograde flow. They are easily demonstrated at micturating cystourethrography where substantial dilatation of the posterior urethra is seen which terminates abruptly in a convex border formed by the valves. The valves are not visible at ultrasound, though the hydronephrosis and thickened bladder wall are readily demonstrated.

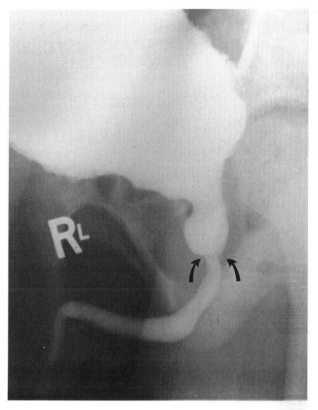

Fig. 7.53 Posterior urethral valves in a 6-year-old boy. On this micturating (voiding) cystogram the site of the valves is arrowed. The presence of the valves is recognised by dilatation of the posterior urethra. Note the irregular outline of the thick-walled bladder due to chronic obstruction.

8

Female Genital Tract

Ultrasound, computed tomography (CT) and magnetic resonance imaging (MRI) have important roles to play in gynaecological disease. Because of its ease and ready availability, ultrasound is usually the principal examination. Conventional radiology plays almost no part—the major exception being hystero-salpingography.

Normal ultrasound appearances

Ultrasound of the pelvis can be carried out two ways: either by scanning through the abdominal wall or scanning transvaginally with a specialised ultrasound probe inserted directly into the vagina. Using the transvaginal route the pelvic organs are nearer the ultrasound probe so image quality is much improved. Moreover it is not necessary for the patient to have a full bladder.

When abdominal scanning is undertaken it is essential for the patient to have a full bladder to act as a 'window' through which the pelvic structures can be seen. Scans are usually made in the longitudinal and transverse planes.

On a midline longitudinal scan the *vagina* can be recognised as a tubular structure, with a central linear echo arising from the opposing vaginal surfaces. The *uterus* lies immediately behind the bladder, and the body of the uterus can be seen to be in continuity with the cervix and vagina. The myometrium shows low level echoes, whereas the endometrial cavity gives a high amplitude linear echo (Fig. 8.1). The precise appearances of the uterus depend on the age and parity of the patient and also on the lie of the uterus. The normal *fallopian tubes* are too small to be visualised sonographically.

The *ovaries* are suspended from the broad ligament and usually lie lateral to the uterus near the side walls of the pelvis (Fig. 8.2). During the child bearing years, the ovaries measure 2.5—5 cm in greatest diameter, but after the menopause, they atrophy. The endocrine changes occurring during the menstrual cycle have a great effect on the appearance of the ovaries. During the early phase, several cystic structures are seen representing developing follicles. Around the eighth day of the cycle, one follicle becomes dominant and may reach 2—2.5 cm in diameter prior to ovulation. At

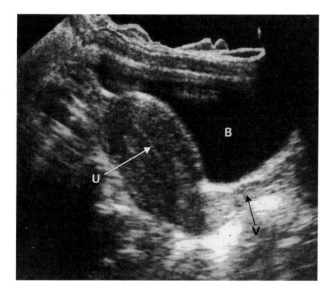

Fig. 8.1 Normal uterus and vagina. Longitudinal section, 30-year-old woman. U, central echo of uterus corresponding to endometrial cavity; the uterus itself has a homogeneous echo texture; V, vagina; B, bladder.

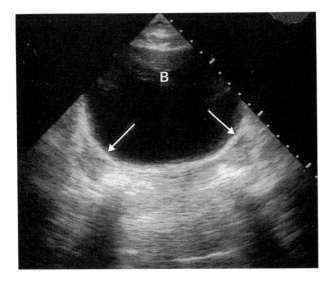

Fig. 8.2 Normal ovaries (arrows). Transverse section, 25-year-old woman. B, bladder.

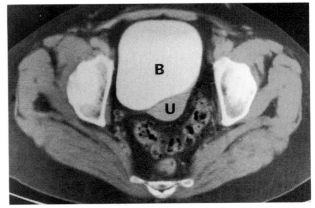

Fig. 8.3 Normal uterus, CT scan. B, bladder; U, uterus.

ovulation, the follicle ruptures and immediately decreases in size giving rise to the corpus luteum which degenerates if there is no intervening pregnancy. By observing these changes it is possible to determine whether an infertile woman is ovulating.

Normal CT appearances (Fig. 8.3)

In order to identify the *vagina*, a tampon is usually placed within it. Because of the air trapped in the tampon, it appears black on the CT images. Immediately above the tampon, the *cervix* is seen as a rounded soft tissue structure approximately 3 cm in diameter. The body of the *uterus* merges with the cervix, its precise appearance depending on the lie of the ureters. The fallopian tubes and broad ligaments are not visible and the ovaries cannot usually be identified. The parametrium is of fat density, the interface with the pelvic musculature being clearly visible. Since the peritoneal cavity extends into the pelvis, the uterus may be surrounded by loops of bowel.

Normal MRI appearances

The pelvic anatomy is very well demonstrated due to the excellent soft tissue contrast afforded by MRI. Images are usually taken in the transverse and sagittal planes but may be supplemented by coronal images, particularly for examining the ovaries. Images in the transverse plane give appearances similar to that seen on CT. The sagittal plane shows the vagina and cervix in continuity with the body of the uterus to great advantage. On a T$_2$ weighted scan the endometrium is seen, as it has a high signal. The ovaries and broad ligaments can also be identified.

Pelvic masses

Computed tomography, ultrasound and MRI will be abnormal in virtually any patient in whom a mass can be felt on physical examination. With ultrasound, it is possible to tell whether the mass is cystic or solid. Unfortunately, there is no clear association of cystic with benign disease, or of solid characteristics with malignant disease. Another limitation of both CT and ultrasound is that it is not always possible to determine from which organ the mass arises; an ovarian mass which lies in contact with the uterus may appear similar to a mass arising within the uterus and vice versa. This distinction may be possible with MRI.

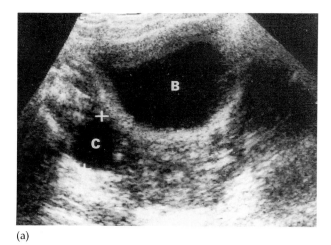

(a)

Fig. 8.4 Ovarian cyst. (a) Transverse ultrasound scan of 3 cm follicular cyst (C) in right ovary showing no internal echoes. B, bladder. (b) CT of another patient showing similar sized cyst in right ovary (arrows). Note the thin wall and uniform water density centre.

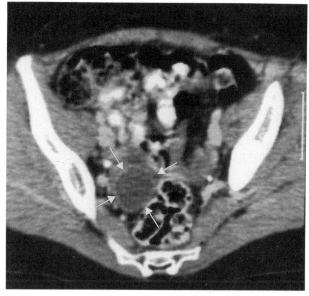

(b)

Ovarian masses

Ovarian cysts

Sometimes a follicle or corpus luteum persists as a follicular or corpus luteum cyst, both of which are easily recognised by ultrasound, CT or MRI (Fig. 8.4). Follicular cysts are mostly asymptomatic and regress spontaneously. Corpus luteum cysts are most often seen in the first trimester of pregnancy; they usually resolve, but may rupture or twist. Haemorrhage into both types of cyst may occur and gives a characteristic appearance on MRI.

Ovarian tumours

The commonest ovarian tumours are the cystadenoma and the cystadenocarcinoma. Ovarian tumours can be cystic, solid or a mixture of the two (Fig. 8.5). Those that are cystic may be multilocular. Evidence of invasion of neighbouring structures or metastasis indicates a malignant tumour. Although ultrasound, CT and MRI are reliable at showing the size, consistency

and location of an ovarian mass, it is often not possible to say whether the mass is benign or malignant unless there is evidence of local invasion or distant spread. A malignant nature is suggested if the septa are thick and there are coexisting solid nodules within, or adjacent to the cyst. With disseminated malignancy, ascites may be visible, but frequently omental and peritoneal metastases are difficult to detect due to their small size. Computed tomography, MRI and ultrasound may show hydronephrosis due to ureteric obstruction by the tumour and may also demonstrate enlarged lymph nodes and liver metastases.

A dermoid cyst can sometimes be confidently diagnosed due to the fat within it, and may contain various calcified components, of which teeth are the commonest. The findings can be recognised at ultrasound, CT or MRI and sometimes on plain radiographs (Fig. 8.6). Otherwise, only very large ovarian tumours are recognisable on plain abdominal radiographs as a soft tissue mass, occasionally containing calcium, arising from the pelvis.

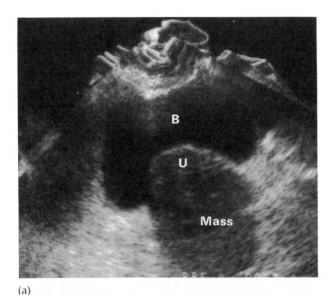

(a)

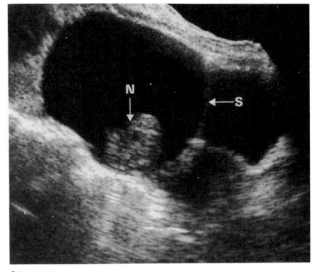

(b)

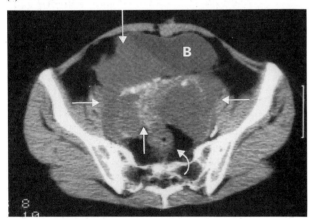

(c)

Fig. 8.5 Ovarian carcinoma. (a) Transverse ultrasound scan showing a large solid mass posterior to the uterus (U). B, bladder. (b) Longitudinal ultrasound scan showing a very large multilocular cystic tumour containing septa (S) and solid nodules (N). The lesion was a cystadenocarcinoma. (c) CT scan showing large partly cystic, partly solid ovarian carcinoma (arrows). The tumour, which contains irregular areas of calcification, has invaded the right side of the bladder (B). The rectum is indicated by a curved arrow.

Uterine tumours

Fibroid

A leiomyoma (fibroid) is the commonest gynaecological tumour. When sufficiently large, it can be seen on a plain film as a mass in the pelvis and may show multiple irregular but well defined calcifications (see Fig. 4.12, p. 141). Ultrasound and CT both show a spherical or lobular uterine mass. At ultrasound, the mass may be either sonolucent or echogenic, whereas at CT, fibroids are usually the same density as the adjacent myometrium (Fig. 8.7). Magnetic resonance imaging can readily identify fibroids as they have a different signal characteristic from the normal uterus. Degenerating and non-degenerating fibroids can also be distinguished. However, it is not possible with any technique to differentiate reliably a fibroid from a malignant tumour of the uterus.

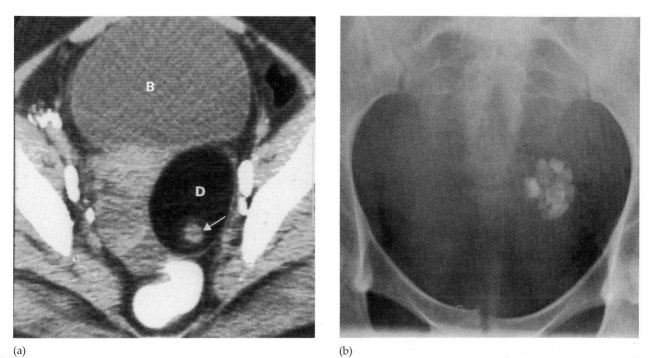

(a)   (b)

Fig. 8.6 Dermoid cyst. (a) CT scan shows oval shaped fat density of a dermoid cyst (D) containing calcified material (arrow). B, bladder, (b) Plain film of another patient showing well-developed teeth within the cyst.

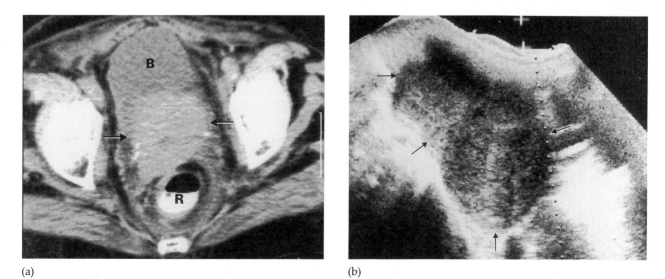

(a)   (b)

Fig. 8.7 Uterine tumour. (a) CT scan showing enlarged uterus (arrows) which was due to fibroids. It is not possible to distinguish this appearance from adenocarcinoma confined to the uterus. B, bladder; R, rectum. (b) Longitudinal ultrasound scan showing a massively enlarged fibroid uterus. Its extent is indicated by the arrows.

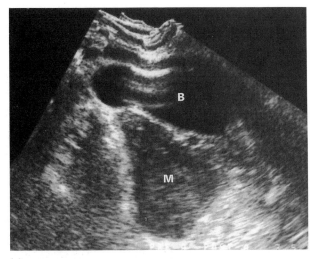

(a)

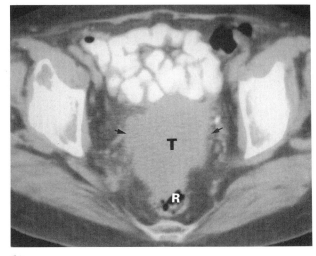

(b)

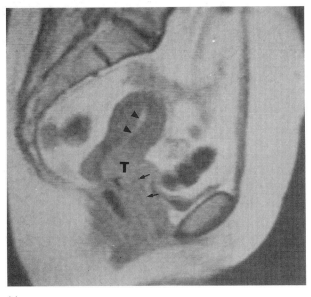

(c)

Fig. 8.8 Carcinoma of cervix. (a) Transverse ultrasound scan showing large solid mass (M) posterior to the bladder (B). The mass, which contains numerous echoes, was continuous with the uterus. (b) CT scan of another patient showing a large tumour of the cervix (T) invading the parametrium (arrows) and extending into the rectum (R) posteriorly. (c) Sagittal MRI scan showing a tumour in the cervix (T) extending into the vagina (arrows). Note the normal high signal from the endometrium (arrow heads).

Carcinoma of the cervix and body of the uterus

Neither CT, MRI nor ultrasound play much part in the initial diagnosis of these conditions, which is made by physical examination and biopsy or cytology. Computed tomography and MRI may be used to assess the extent of disease to help decide whether treatment with surgery or radiotherapy is more appropriate. With advanced disease, a mass will be seen involving the cervix or body of uterus (Fig. 8.8), which may have spread into the parametrium, pelvic lymph nodes or bladder. Distinction from fibroids may at times be impossible, particularly with endometrial carcinoma. It is important to determine whether or not the tumour has spread to involve the bone or muscles forming the pelvic side walls. The kidneys should be examined for hydronephrosis, which occurs when the tumour spreads laterally and obstructs the ureters.

Detection of intrauterine contraceptive devices

The 'lost intrauterine contraceptive device (IUCD)' is a common problem and ultrasound should be the first investigation. Different devices have characteristic appearances. They are seen as highly reflective structures and their relationship to the uterine cavity can

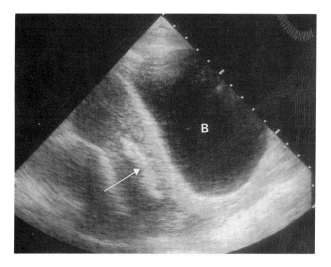

Fig. 8.9 Intrauterine contraceptive device (arrow) seen as bright echoes within the uterine cavity, shown on a longitudinal ultrasound scan. B, bladder.

be determined (Fig. 8.9). If the IUCD cannot be located in the pelvis, then a plain film of the abdomen should be taken in case the device has migrated through the uterus. If there is a coexisting pregnancy, it becomes very difficult to locate the IUCD by ultrasound after the first trimester.

Pelvic inflammatory disease

Pelvic inflammatory disease may be due to venereal infection, commonly gonorrhoea, which in the acute stages gives rise to a tubo-ovarian abscess. Pelvic inflammation and abscess formation may also occur following pelvic surgery, childbirth or abortion and may be seen in association with intrauterine contraceptive devices, appendicitis or diverticular disease. The usual imaging technique is ultrasound. Irrespective of the cause of the infection, ultrasound will show a hypoechoic or complex mass in the adnexal region or pouch of Douglas (cul-de-sac) (Fig. 8.10). Blockage of the fallopian tubes may cause a hydrosalpinx which can be recognised as a hypoechoic adnexal mass, which is often tubular in shape.

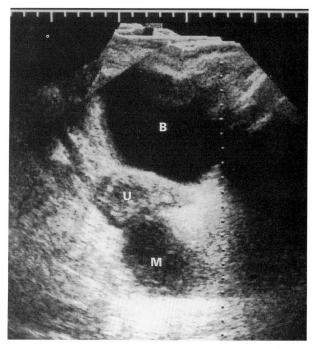

Fig. 8.10 Pelvic abscess. Transverse ultrasound scan showing a hypoechoic mass (M) behind the uterus (U). B, bladder.

The appearance of pelvic inflammatory disease may be indistinguishable from endometriosis and ectopic pregnancy (p. 282), conditions which all occur in women of reproductive years.

Endometriosis

In endometriosis, there is endometrial tissue outside the uterus, most commonly confined to the pelvis. At ultrasound, endometriosis is usually seen as a cystic or hypoechoic mass in the adnexal region and/or pouch of Douglas corresponding to the chocolate cysts found on pathological examination. Because of the recurrent haemorrhage in these endometriomas they often have a characteristic appearance on MRI (Fig. 8.11). If the endometriosis has bled into the peritoneal cavity, as it commonly does at the time of menstruation, fluid may be detectable in the pouch of Douglas.

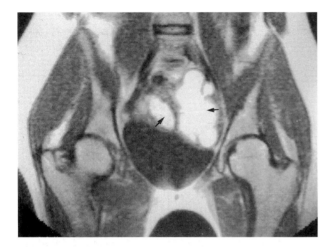

Fig. 8.11 Endometriosis. Coronal MRI showing haemorrhagic cysts in the pelvis (arrows) which give a high signal on this T_1-weighted sequence.

Hysterosalpingography

Hysterosalpingography is performed in selected cases in the investigation of infertility in order to assess the patency of the fallopian tubes. A catheter with a seal to prevent leakage from the external cervical os is inserted into the uterus. Sufficient contrast is then injected under fluoroscopic control to fill the uterus and fallopian tubes (Fig. 8.12). If the fallopian tubes are patent, there is free spill into the peritoneum, recognised by the demonstration of contrast between loops of bowel. Congenital variations in uterine morphology which may prevent maintenance of pregnancy can also be assessed.

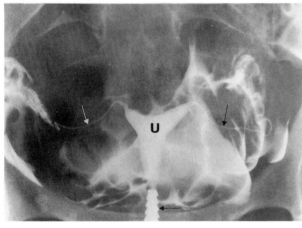

(a)

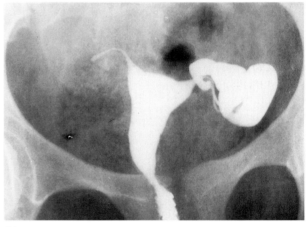

(b)

Fig. 8.12 Hysterosalpingogram. (a) Normal. Contrast has been injected to fill the uterus (U) and both fallopian tubes (vertical arrows). Free spill into the peritoneum has occurred to outline loops of bowel. Note the cannula in the cervical canal (horizontal arrow). (b) Hydrosalpinx. Both fallopian tubes are obstructed and dilated, the left one massively. There is no spill of contrast into the peritoneum.

Obstetrics

Ultrasound of the pregnant patient is simple to perform and has proved reliable in examining the fetus and in detecting the complications of pregnancy. Unlike x-ray examination (see p. 13 for discussion of radiation hazards) no biological damage has yet been attributed to ultrasound examination as currently used in obstetric practice. No fetal abnormalities have been attributable to ultrasound during pregnancy over the three decades that the technique has been in use.

The developing fetus

Ultrasound in the first trimester

Ultrasound examination during early pregnancy may be undertaken using a probe placed on the abdomen. The patient should have a full bladder, in order to lift the small bowel out of the pelvis and to act as a window to provide better visualisation of the uterus. Alternatively, transvaginal scanning may be carried out, which produces superior images and moreover a full bladder is not necessary.

The normal gestational sac is seen as a small cystic structure lying within the uterus. It first appears at the fifth week of amenorrhoea*. By the sixth week, internal echoes representing the developing fetus are seen within the gestational sac and by the seventh week movement of the fetal heart should be visible (Fig. 9.1). In the early stages, the volume of the gestational sac can be used to estimate gestational development. Later, as fetal echoes become visible, the pregnancy

* In this book the gestational age is always expressed as weeks from the last menstrual period.

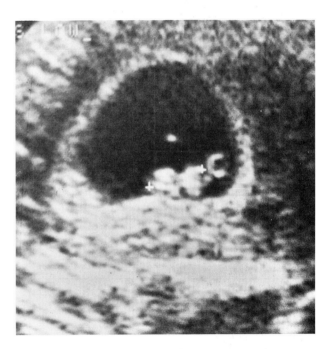

Fig. 9.1 Intrauterine gestational sac containing a 7 week fetus. The small white crosses indicate the crown rump length (10 mm). The C-shaped structure adjacent to the fetus is the yolk sac.

can be dated by measuring the crown rump length (Fig. 9.2), i.e. the longest demonstrable length of the fetus within the gestational sac. This length is a highly reliable method of dating from the seventh to twelfth weeks of pregnancy. Multiple pregnancies can be recognised by the presence of two or more gestation sacs.

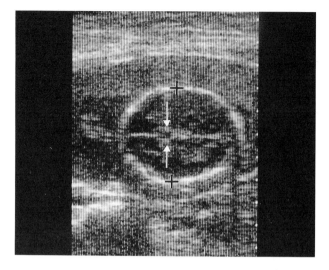

Fig. 9.3 Biparietal diameter in an 18 week fetus. The midline echo is interrupted by the box-like cavum septum pellucidum (arrows). At this level the head appears oval rather than round. The crosses indicate the measurement points for the biparietal diameter.

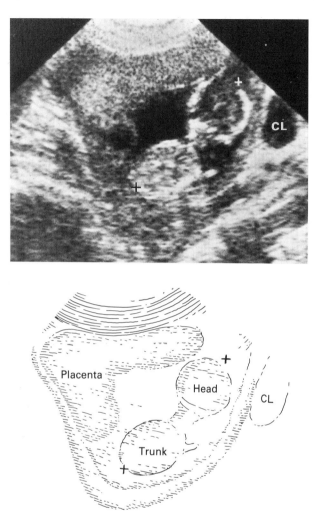

Fig. 9.2 Ten week fetus. The crown rump length is indicated by the crosses. A small corpus luteum cyst (CL) is seen in the left adnexal region.

Ultrasound in the second and third trimesters

After the first trimester, fetal maturity can be assessed by measuring both the biparietal diameter and the femur length, both of which can be precisely defined. The apposition of the two cerebral hemispheres adjacent to the falx gives a well defined midline echo. A small 'box like' structure, the cavum septum pellu-cidum, interrupts the midline echo one-third of the way between the sinciput and occiput (Fig. 9.3). This structure identifies the position, at the level of the thalami, where the biparietal diameter should be measured. By comparing the measurements with a standard growth chart an estimate of gestational age can be obtained. The chart for the biparietal diameter (Fig. 9.4) shows that there is a greater deviation from the mean in late pregnancy than in the early stages, which means that accurate dating based on the biparietal diameter must be carried out before 24–26 weeks. The femur length is measured by directing the ultrasound beam down the long axis of the femur; this length can then be compared with a standard growth chart.

At 18–20 weeks gestation the fetus is well formed and this is an appropriate time to obtain an accurate biparietal diameter to estimate fetal maturity. Also, 18–20 weeks is a suitable time to examine the fetus for fetal abnormalites, so enabling a therapeutic abortion to be performed if appropriate. Accurate dating is

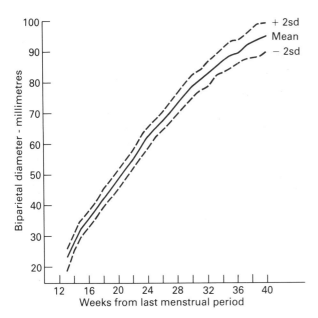

Fig. 9.4 Growth chart of biparietal diameter against gestational age, showing the mean and two standard deviations from the mean.

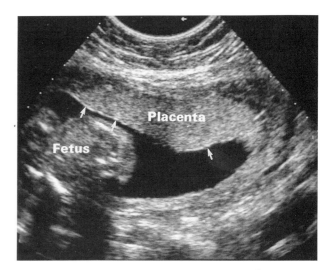

Fig. 9.5 Placenta seen on a longitudinal scan at 18 weeks gestation. The chorionic plate is seen as a thin line of bright echoes (arrows).

very helpful if problems arise in late pregnancy, as the obstetrician then knows the maturity of the fetus should induction or caesarian section become necessary.

Obtaining serial biparietal diameters and comparing them with growth curves permits observation of fetal growth. However, growth retardation may be first manifested by lack of growth of the fetal body. To detect this, the abdominal circumference is measured at the level of the umbilical vein, as it passes through the liver (see Fig. 9.12, p. 277).

Identification of the sex of the fetus is frequently possible. Though parents often like to know the sex, its medical importance is confined to those situations where there is a risk of sex-linked inherited disease. Sexual differentiation is most reliable in the third trimester, when the penis and scrotum can usually be defined.

The placenta

The placenta is easily evaluated sonographically. By the ninth week, it is seen as a well defined intrauterine structure lining the inner wall of a portion of the uterine cavity. The surface of the placenta, the chorionic plate, may be recognised as a thin line of bright echoes (Fig. 9.5). As the placenta matures it undergoes successive changes in texture but these changes are not thought to be of clinical significance.

Haemorrhage from placenta previa, the condition in which the placenta encroaches on the lower uterine segment, is a common cause of bleeding in the third trimester, occurring in about 0.5% of pregnancies. Sonography permits accurate delineation of the placental position and its relationship to the presenting part of the fetus (Fig. 9.6). Although the internal cervical os cannot always be identified as such; the position of the cervix can usually be inferred from the position of other structures.

During the second trimester, a third to a half of all placentas are low lying, thus raising the question of placenta previa. However, when followed through to

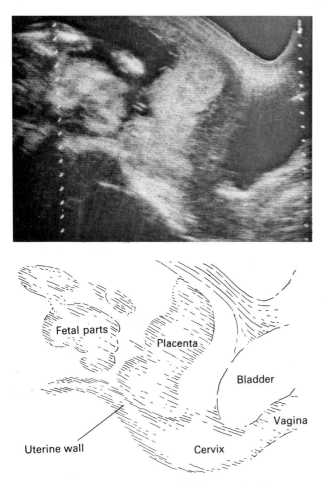

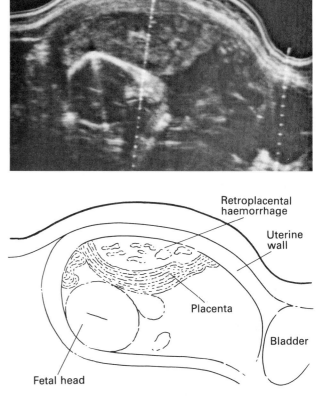

Fig. 9.7 Retroplacental haemorrhage (abruptio placentae). Longitudinal scan at 36 weeks showing separation of the placenta from the uterine wall by a retroplacental blood clot.

Fig. 9.6 Placenta previa. Longitudinal scan. The placenta is in the lower uterine segment and covers the position of the internal cervical os.

term the vast majority of these do not turn out to be true placenta previa. This is because of the differential growth rate of the uterus during pregnancy the lower uterine segment grows more than the rest of the uterus and, therefore, as pregnancy progresses, placental tissue is carried towards the fundus and away from the cervical os. Consequently, the diagnosis of a marginal placenta previa before the thirty-sixth week should always be confirmed with a repeat scan before delivery.

Abruptio placentae (accidental haemorrhage) occurs in approximately 1–2% of pregnancies. The majority of cases present with vaginal bleeding, but some are concealed. Ultrasound can be of help in making this diagnosis, if a collection of blood is seen separating the amniotic membranes from the uterine surface (Fig. 9.7). However, frequently there is no such collection, as the blood has drained into the amniotic cavity or out through the vagina.

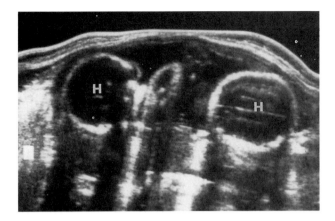

Fig. 9.8 Twins. Two heads (H) are seen on the same scan.

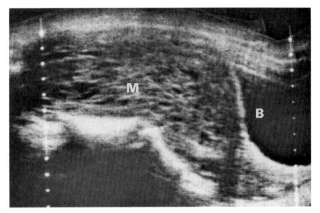

Fig. 9.9 Hydatidiform mole. Longitudinal scan showing multiple irregular vesicular structures within an enlarged uterus. M, mole; B, bladder.

'Large for dates' uterus

A common problem in obstetric care is the patient whose uterus is larger than expected. Often the cause is a false estimate of the gestational age, usually due to a mistake in calculating the date of conception. By utilising the methods outlined earlier in this chapter, it is possible to determine the fetal age with greater accuracy.

The most common causes for a uterus larger than expected for true gestational age include:

- Multiparity.
- Trophoblastic disease.
- Associated ovarian or uterine tumours, either of which may be mistaken for generalised enlargement of the uterus.
- Polyhydramnios.

Multiparity is readily diagnosed by sonography (Fig. 9.8). More than one gestational sac is seen early on. Later, two or more fetal heads and bodies can be identified and the biparietal diameters can be measured. Ultrasound is helpful to detect any fetal abnormalities, which are more frequent in multiple pregnancies. Because of the risks associated with multiple pregnancies, fetal growth is subsequently monitored throughout pregnancy.

Trophoblastic disease is a spectrum of pathology ranging from the relatively benign hydatidiform mole to the malignant choriocarcinoma. The enlarged uterus is filled with multiple vesicular (cystic) structures within a background of echoes of varying densities (Fig. 9.9). In most cases no fetal parts will be identified, but very rarely trophoblastic disease may coexist with a living pregnancy. Although it is occasionally possible to identify invasion of the myometrium by malignant trophoblastic disease, benign and malignant forms are in general indistinguishable on ultrasound examination. In about a third of cases multilocular ovarian cysts, called theca lutein cysts, may be identified. They are caused by the high output of FSH by the disordered pregnancy.

Uterine tumours are present in about 1% of pregnant patients, the most common variety being the leiomyoma (fibroid) which can increase in size under the hormonal influences of pregnancy (Fig. 9.10). Usually they arise in the body or fundus but when situated low in the uterus they can obstruct labour.

Ovarian tumours may be confused clinically with uterine enlargement. Those associated with pregnancy are usually corpus luteum cysts. At ultrasound they are seen as simple cysts adjacent to, but separate from, the gravid uterus; they frequently involute as the pregnancy progresses.

Polyhydramnios is defined as twice the volume of

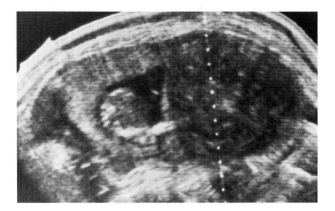

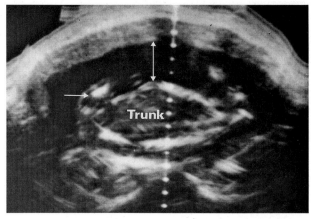

Fig. 9.11 Polyhydramnios. Transverse section showing a large echo-free space (arrowed) due to fluid anterior to the fetal trunk. This 22 week fetus was anencephalic. The horizontal arrow points to the skull base—no cranial vault was present.

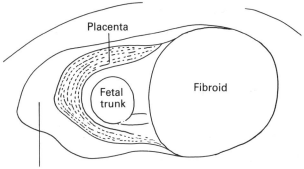

Fig. 9.10 Uterine fibroid. Transverse section in a pregnant patient with a large fibroid.

amniotic fluid expected for the period of gestation. Although mathematical formulae exist, in practice a visual estimate is usually made (Figs 9.11 and 9.16). Polyhydramnios is associated with maternal abnormalities such as diabetes and with a number of fetal conditions. The fetal abnormalities include neural tube defects, in which the hydramnios is probably due to excessive production of cerebrospinal fluid, and obstruction of the alimentary tract, e.g. oesophageal or duodenal atresia, where the hydramnios is due to an impaired circulation of swallowed amniotic fluid. Polyhydramnios also occurs with normal multiple pregnancies.

'Small for dates' uterus: intrauterine growth retardation

An important cause for a fetus that is small for dates is intrauterine growth retardation, which carries a greatly increased risk of perinatal death and will alter obstetrical management. However, it is important not to misdiagnose a fetus as being small for dates because of an error in calculating the age from the menstrual history: hence the need for accurate dating early in pregnancy.

Growth retardation can be divided into two groups. Symmetrical growth retardation affects the head and body equally and is associated with congenital abnormalities and intrauterine infections. Asymmetrical growth retardation affects growth of the fetal body (Fig. 9.12) before that of the fetal brain. Therefore, measurements of the biparietal diameter may not detect any abnormality early on. Asymmetrical growth retardation occurs in the third trimester and is associated with placental insufficiency, either primary disease of the placenta, or due to maternal causes such as hypertension or diabetes. Standards are available for biparietal diameter and abdominal circumference in

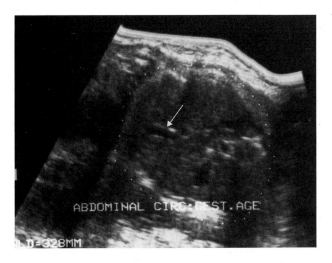

Fig. 9.12 Trunk circumference. Transverse section taken through the fetal trunk at the level of the umbilical vein (arrow). The circumference is measured electronically by indicating the measurement points with a light pen.

order that fetal growth may be assessed. In some centres, scans are performed routinely around 32 weeks in order to diagnose intrauterine growth retardation.

Fetal monitoring

In those fetuses with intrauterine growth retardation or at risk from any cause, ultrasound can be used to assess fetal well-being and may influence the decision to effect early delivery of the baby.

Doppler ultrasound of the umbilical artery enables the blood flow in the placental circulation to be studied. In normal pregnancy, placental resistance is low and a large proportion of the fetal cardiac output flows through the placenta. There is, therefore, a high diastolic flow shown by the flow velocity waveform in the umbilical artery. In conditions such as intrauterine growth retardation and maternal hypertension, the placental resistance increases so the diastolic flow in the umbilical artery is reduced or in extreme cases may be absent (Fig. 9.13).

Fetal abnormalities

It is important to recognise fetal abnormalities as early as possible during the pregnancy so that the appropriate management can be instituted. The commonest abnormalities detected by ultrasound are neural tube defects particularly spina bifida and anencephaly. Both should be identified by 18 weeks, at a time when therapeutic abortion is still an option. These conditions are associated with elevated serum and amniotic alpha fetoprotein levels.

Many of the anomalies which result in structural deformity of the fetus can be detected *in utero* during the second trimester. An indication of fetal abnormality is polyhydramnios, since polyhydramnios is due to fetal anomaly in 20% of cases.

The head

The two common cranial anomalies that can be identified are hydrocephalus and anencephaly.

The lateral ventricles are easily visualised from 16 weeks onwards. The walls of the ventricles are seen as white lines. Abnormal dilatation of the lateral ventricles precedes excessive enlargement of the calvarium in most cases. Hydrocephalus is diagnosed sonographically when the distance between the lateral walls of the lateral ventricles are greater than 50% of the biparietal diameter. Hydrocephalus frequently accompanies spina bifida.

The echo-dense choroid plexuses occupy the posterior parts of the lateral ventricles. Cysts within the choroid plexuses are a fairly common finding but these cysts are usually of no significance.

Anencephaly may be diagnosed after the twelfth week by the absence of a visible skull vault (Fig. 9.11). Echoes from the skull base and face may be seen however. The fetal body is usually well formed and moves actively.

The spine

Spina bifida is due to incomplete closure of the neural tube. It is recognised at ultrasound as an absence or a

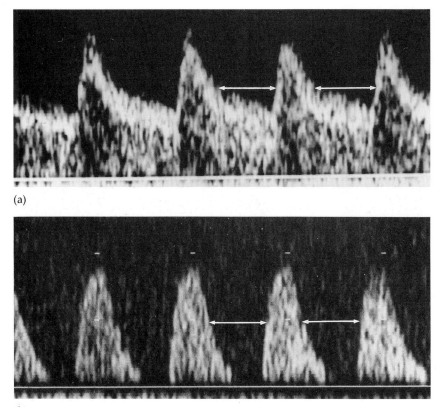

(a)

(b)

Fig. 9.13 Doppler flow velocity waveform of the umbilical artery. The peaks represent systolic flow. The arrows indicate the period of the diastolic flow. (a) Normal—note the flow during diastole. (b) Abnormal—there is an absence of flow during diastole in this fetus at risk because of maternal hypertension.

widening of the paired echoes that represent the normal fetal spine (Fig. 9.14). Severe cases are associated with meningocele or meningomyelocele, which are recognised as a sac arising from the back at the level of the widened canal. Limb motion may be absent, but even if the limbs are moving, there may be significant neurological impairment.

Tumours associated with the spine can also be diagnosed *in utero*. The most common of these is the sacral teratoma (Fig. 9.15). They may be solid, cystic or complex and may contain calcifications. Cystic hygromas, when located low on the trunk, are quite difficult to distinguish from sacral teratomas and meningomyeloceles. Since teratomas and hygromas may be curable by surgery, the distinction can be of importance.

The chest

The size and configuration of the chest may aid in the diagnosis of syndromes associated with pulmonary hypoplasia. Congenital diaphragmatic hernia is the commonest abnormality and in this condition the stomach and intestines herniate into the chest and compress the lungs.

The heart is readily seen and it is now possible to diagnose several cardiac anomalies *in utero*.

Gastrointestinal tract

The commonest congenital anomalies of the gastrointestinal tract to be diagnosed *in utero* are duodenal atresia, omphalocele and gastroschisis. Oesophageal atresia may be associated with polyhydramnios but cannot be directly demonstrated.

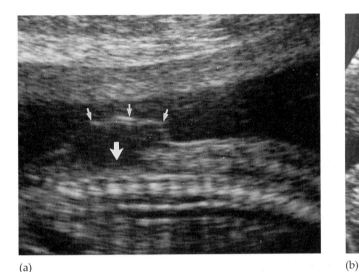

(a)

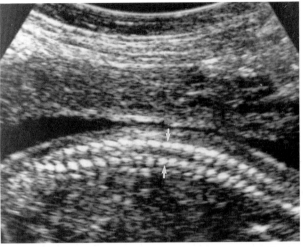

(b)

Fig. 9.14 Spina bifida. (a) There is a defect in the lumbar spine (large arrow) with a mass projecting from the baby's back representing a meningomyelocele (small arrows). (b) Normal for comparison showing the parallel paired echoes (arrows) of the normal thoracic and lumbar spine.

In duodenal atresia, two round cystic structures are seen representing the distended stomach and duodenum (Fig. 9.16).

Omphalocele and gastroschisis are diagnosed by the presence of loops of bowel or liver outside the abdominal cavity (Fig. 9.17).

The urinary tract

The kidneys contribute significantly to the amniotic fluid volume. The presence of profound oligohydramnios, although most frequently due to premature rupture of the membranes, should raise the possibility of a renal abnormality. The normal kidneys are seen as circles of diminished echoreflectivity on either side of the fetal spine. The kidneys may fail to develop at all (agenesis) or be severely dysplastic. At times, even in the normal, it may be difficult to visualise the kidneys. Therefore, an attempt is made to find the fetal bladder, since the presence of urine in the bladder indicates functioning renal tissue. However, it should be realised that the bladder may be empty at any given moment, due to fetal voiding.

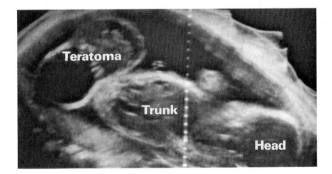

Fig. 9.15 Sacral teratoma. Longitudinal scan. Complex mass showing both cystic and solid components arising from the sacral region. The very bright echoes in the teratoma are due to calcifications.

The commonest identifiable abnormalities are hydronephrosis and the dysplastic condition, multicystic kidney (Fig. 9.18). They are difficult to distinguish from each other with ultrasound. Both are usually unilateral conditions showing multiple fluid-filled rounded spaces within the kidney. If the opposite kidney is normal, as is often the case, oligohydramnios is absent.

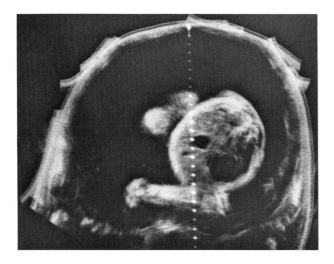

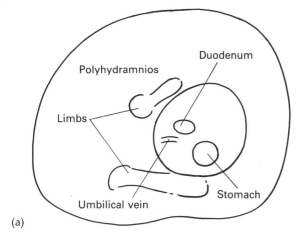

(a)

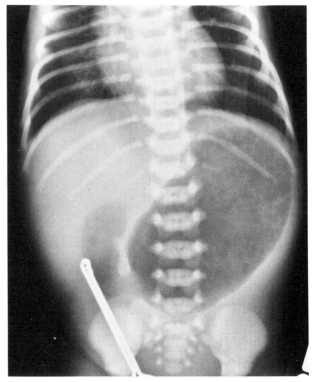

(b)

Fig. 9.16 Duodenal atresia. (a) Transverse section through fetal abdomen showing dilated fluid-filled stomach and duodenum. Massive polyhydramnios is present. (b) Plain abdominal film after birth of baby, showing dilated air filled stomach and duodenum, with no gas in the rest of the bowel.

Chronic bladder outlet obstruction, the usual cause of which is posterior urethral valves, can lead to bilateral hydronephrosis and hydroureters and a massively dilated thick-walled bladder.

The skeleton

Skeletal anomalies giving rise to dwarfism can be recognised by the presence of short limbs. The lethal forms are usually associated with polyhydramnios.

Ultrasound for karyotyping

There are three main techniques for fetal karyotyping, which all require ultrasound to guide the needle to the required position:
- Chorion villus sampling which is usually carried out between 8 and 12 weeks gestation and involves taking a sample of placental tissue.
- Amniocentesis, which is usually carried out at 16 weeks gestation and involves passing a needle through the maternal abdominal wall to withdraw a sample of amniotic fluid. In addition to analysis for chromosome

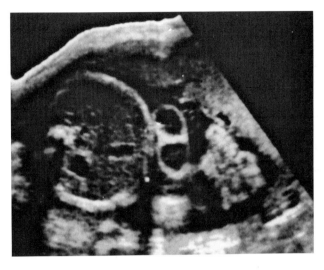

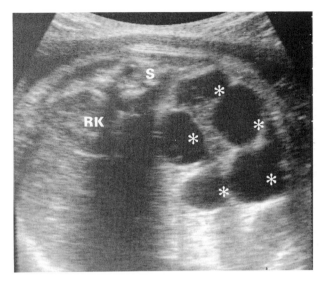

Fig. 9.18 Multicystic kidney. Transverse scan through the fetal abdomen at 36 weeks gestation showing a normal right kidney (RK) and a number of large cysts in the left kidney (asterisks). S, spine.

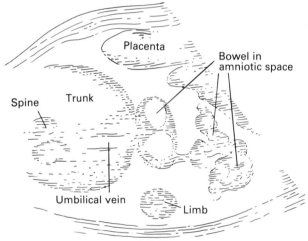

Fig. 9.17 Gastroschisis. Transverse scan through fetal trunk showing loops of bowel outside the fetal abdomen floating in the amniotic fluid.

abnormalites the alpha fetoprotein level in the amniotic fluid may be measured.

● Cordocentesis involves puncturing the umbilical vein to obtain a sample of fetal blood.

Amniocentesis is the simplest technique but it may take up to 2 weeks for karyotyping. With chorion villus sampling or cordocentesis the results may be available within 2−3 days.

Fetal death

With ultrasound it is possible to see the heart beating and observe fetal movement from the seventh week of pregnancy onward. Failure to observe these phenomena suggests fetal death, but in the early stages of pregnancy one must be careful that the gestational age has been calculated correctly. It is, therefore, important to repeat the scan after a suitable interval, if there is any doubt. After the ninth week, fetal death can be readily diagnosed by the absence of a visible heart beat.

A blighted ovum is diagnosed if the size of the gestational sac is greater than 3 cm in diameter but no fetal structures are seen within it (Fig. 9.19). In a twin pregnancy there may be two gestational sacs, one of which contains a live fetus and the other one being anembryonic. So long as the patient is not bleeding at the time of examination, there is a good possibility that the empty sac will resolve and a normal baby will be delivered at term.

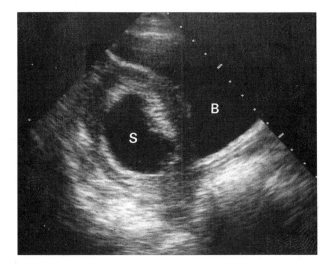

Fig. 9.19 Blighted ovum. Longitudinal scan. Nine weeks amenorrhoea, showing a gestational sac (S) with no fetal parts within it. B, bladder.

Ectopic pregnancy

Ectopic pregnancy generally presents with sudden pain due to rupture of the ectopically placed gestational sac. The ruptured ectopic pregnancy itself is not always visible. When seen sonographically, it is identified as an adnexal mass having both solid and cystic characteristics (Fig. 9.20). There should be no intrauterine pregnancy. Free fluid may be seen in the pouch of Douglas (cul de sac) due to haemorrhage. These signs, by themselves, are not enough to make the diagnosis of ectopic gestation, since pelvic inflammatory disease, rupture of adnexal cysts and various neoplasms can appear identical.

In clinical practice, if the pregnancy test is positive and no intrauterine gestation can be identified, the obstetrician may assume that there is an ectopic pregnancy.

The puerperium

Retained products of conception can readily be detected sonographically as echoes within the uterine cavity.

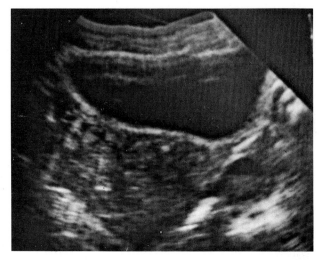

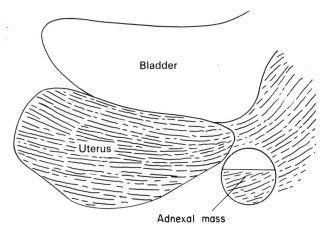

Fig. 9.20 Ectopic pregnancy. Transverse scan in a patient whose pregnancy test was positive, showing an adnexal mass and uterus containing no gestational sac.

Abdominal problems in pregnancy

The safety of ultrasound enables certain maternal abnormalities, which may coexist with pregnancy, to be examined so avoiding the dangers of radiation to the fetus. Diseases of the biliary tract and urinary tract, in particular, may be readily diagnosed.

Pelvimetry

Pelvimetry is a method used to determine the relative pelvic and fetal head dimensions. An erect lateral radiograph is taken from which the anteroposterior measurements of the pelvic inlet and outlet can be made. In some centres, a supine AP film is added so that the transverse pelvic diameters can be calculated. These diameters are of limited use because the measurements are made from bone surface to bone surface. This does not take into account the thickness of soft tissues which may be very important in determining the effective diameter available to the fetus during delivery.

10

Peritoneal Cavity and Retroperitoneum

Peritoneal cavity

The peritoneal cavity normally contains only a minute amount of fluid, which is not visualised directly by any imaging technique. However, excess fluid and tumours can be readily demonstrated by ultrasound or computed tomography (CT). Plain films, as discussed in Chapter 4, are excellent for detecting air in the peritoneal cavity and may also demonstrate substantial ascites and large abscesses, but do little else.

Ascites

Both CT and ultrasound can demonstrate ascites in amounts far below that needed for clinical detection, but neither technique can reliably distinguish the nature of the fluid, e.g. pus or ascitic fluid.

Peritoneal fluid, when free to move, collects in a predictable manner. With the patient supine, the fluid tends to fall to the most dependent portions of the peritoneal cavity, namely in the pelvis anterior to the upper rectum (known as the pouch of Douglas in females), in the space anterior to the right kidney (known as Morrison's pouch), and in the paracolic gutters. If larger amounts of fluid are present, fluid will be seen throughout the peritoneal cavity and stomach, or loops of bowel, may be seen floating in the ascites.

Computed tomography appearances in ascites (Fig. 10.1). At CT, ascites is of lower density than the liver, spleen and kidney and these organs stand out clearly compared to the adjacent fluid.

One of the easiest sites to be certain of ascites is adjacent to the liver. A uniform band of low density is readily recognisable between the liver and the diaphragm or abdominal wall. It is worth noting that ascites cannot collect posterior to the liver because of the peritoneal reflection forming the so-called bare area (Fig. 10.1b).

When loculated, ascites is seen as discrete collections of fluid partly surrounded by bands of adhesions and partly by the edges of normal abdominal structures, e.g. bowel wall or liver edge. Loculated collections of ascites cannot be distinguished from fluid in abscesses because the density of infected and uninfected fluid is identical.

Ultrasound of ascites (Fig. 10.2). Ascites is readily detected by ultrasound as echo-free regions with excellent transmission of sound. Therefore, ascites is easy to demonstrate provided no bowel gas is in the path of the ultrasound beam. Bowel dilatation with excess gas frequently accompanies all types of ascites and often limits the information available. It is almost always possible, however, to demonstrate at least some of the ascites.

Intraperitoneal abscesses

Intraperitoneal abscesses may follow a perforation of the bowel or biliary tract, either spontaneous or post-traumatic—particularly following surgery. The common locations are subphrenic, subhepatic, paracolic and pelvic. The expected site of the abscess depends on the site of perforation, e.g. duodenal leakage usually results in subhepatic or subphrenic abscess, whereas a leak from the left colon often results

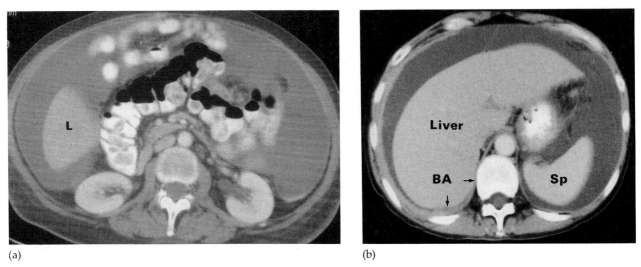

Fig. 10.1 CT scan of ascites. (a) At the level of the kidneys. The fluid is seen surrounding the lower portion of the liver (L) and the bowel loops. (b) At the level of the liver and spleen (Sp). Note that the ascites cannot collect posteromedial to the right lobe of the liver because of the peritoneal reflections of the bare area (BA).

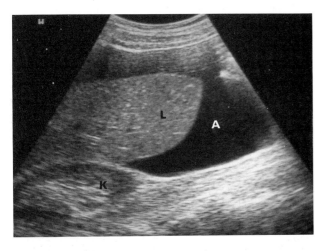

Fig. 10.2 Ultrasound of ascites. The ascites (A) appears as a transonic area. The liver is clearly seen surrounded by the ascitic fluid. K, right kidney; L, liver.

in paracolic or pelvic abscess. Multiple abscesses are not uncommon. Ascites frequently accompanies abdominal and pelvic abscesses.

Computed tomography finds most abscesses and rarely gives false positive results. Ultrasound can be just as informative, provided it is positive, and may be preferred because it is quick and simple to perform. The disadvantage of ultrasound is that gas in dilated loops of bowel can interfere with the images. Also, surgical wounds and dressings may make it impossible to place the transducer in direct contact with the skin; without such contact it is impossible to obtain images.

Ultrasound appearances. The areas best suited for ultrasound examination are the right upper quadrant and the true pelvis.

The ultrasonographer searches for any localised fluid collections lying outside the bowel (Fig. 10.3). Fluid within the bowel is recognised by observing peristaltic activity. Abscesses assume many different configurations depending on the adjacent organs. They often have slightly irregular walls and may contain internal echoes due to septations or debris. These internal echoes are not, however, specific for infection. Gas in the abscess appears echogenic and produces acoustic shadowing but gas in an abscess can be difficult to distinguish from gas within the bowel.

The major differential diagnosis is from loops of

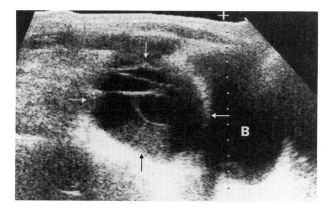

Fig. 10.3 Pelvic abscess. Ultrasound scan showing a large complex mass (arrows) just above the bladder (B). This young man had Crohn's disease.

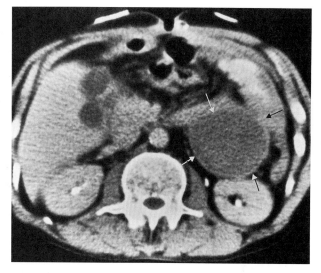

Fig. 10.4 Peritoneal abscess. CT showing a postoperative unilocular abscess (arrows) anterior to the left kidney displacing a loop of bowel. The patient had recently undergone partial small bowel resection.

bowel and loculations of ascites, blood or lymph, all of which can occur post-operatively. The distinction may require needle aspiration of the fluid.

Computed tomography appearances. The basic principles are similar to those described for ultrasound. The fluid centre of the abscess is identified as a homogeneous density surrounded by a definite wall of soft tissue lying within the peritoneal cavity but outside the bowel (Fig. 10.4). Gas within the abscess is seen in approximately half the patients and is a very useful sign since it helps distinguish infected from uninfected fluid loculations. The gas may take the form of multiple small streaks or bubbles or it may collect as one large bubble. Air–fluid levels may be present within the larger collections. The wall of the abscess often shows enhancement following intravenous contrast administration. Subphrenic abscesses (Fig. 10.5) may be difficult to distinguish from pleural empyemas at CT; the peritoneal and pleural cavities are, after all, separated only by the diaphragm, a structure that can be difficult to identify at CT. In such cases, ultrasound will usually be very helpful because it can demonstrate the abscess and also directly demonstrate the position of the diaphragm.

The major differential diagnosis of intraperitoneal abscesses at CT are:

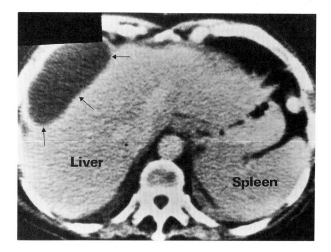

Fig. 10.5 Subphrenic abscess. CT showing abscess (arrows) anterior to liver.

- Fluid within distended or matted loops of bowel. The distinction can usually be made by opacifying the bowel. Oral Gastrografin is routinely given for this purpose before the examination in most centres.

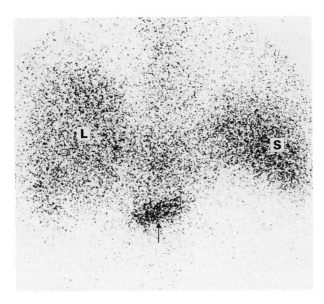

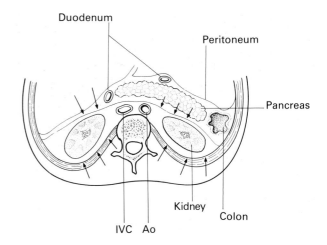

Fig. 10.7 Diagram of anterior (downward pointing arrows) and posterior (upward pointing arrows) renal fascia. Ao, aorta; IVC, inferior vena cava: K, kidney.

Fig. 10.6 Indium-111 labelled leucocyte scan of abscess. This abscess (arrow) followed small bowel surgery with subsequent anastomotic leak. Normal uptake is seen in the liver (L) and spleen (S).

● Loculated uninfected fluid. Just as with ultrasound it may not be possible to make this distinction and needle aspiration may have to be performed.

Radionuclide examinations

If CT and ultrasound have been unsuccessful in locating an abscess, then some of the patient's own white blood cells can be labelled with ^{99m}Tc or with indium-111 which will accumulate in an abscess (Fig. 10.6).

Retroperitoneum

Computed tomography, MRI and ultrasound all provide information about retroperitoneal structures. Plain films are limited to showing: very large masses or calcification within a mass; the occasional case where gas is seen in an abscess; the curvilinear calcification of an aortic aneurysm. This discussion here will be confined to: the adrenal glands; lymph nodes; aortic

aneurysms; retroperitoneal tumours, abscesses and haematomas. The urinary tract and pancreas are considered elsewhere. When considering the retroperitoneum it is useful to appreciate the anatomy of the anterior and posterior renal fascia which divides the retroperitoneum into three compartments: the anterior pararenal, the perinephric and the posterior pararenal spaces (Fig. 10.7). Infection in one of these compartments tends to be limited to that compartment.

Computed tomography

Retroperitoneal CT is particularly informative in obese subjects because fat surrounds the important structures. Indeed, retroperitoneal CT is difficult to interpret in subjects with little or no fat — children are a particular problem in this regard.

When reviewing CT scans of the retroperitoneum, the following normal features should be looked for (Figs 10.8 and 10.11):
● The complete outline of the aorta and inferior vena cava should be clearly visible throughout their lengths, except where the inferior vena cava (IVC) passes

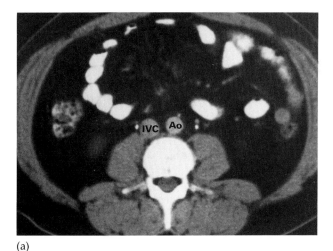

(a)

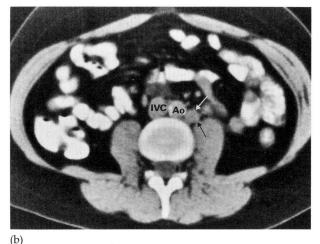

(b)

Fig. 10.8 (a) CT scan of normal retroperitoneum. Note that the aorta (Ao) and IVC are clearly outlined by fat and that there is a fat-containing space to the left of the aorta. The small white dots in the retroperitoneum are the opacified ureters. (b) An enlarged lymph node is shown to the left of the aorta (arrow).

through the liver. The aorta is round in cross-section and normally measures of 2.0–2.5 cm in diameter. The IVC varies in shape from round to oval.

- There is usually a fat-containing space to the left of the aorta, which is a good area in which to look for lymphadenopathy. The only structures other than lymph nodes to be seen in this space are the left renal vein and, on rare occasions, a loop of small bowel.
- The psoas muscles are seen as symmetrical, rounded structures outlined anteriorly by fat.
- Both adrenals are well seen in most subjects.

Magnetic resonance imaging

The place of magnetic resonance imaging (MRI) in diagnosing retroperitoneal disorders has yet to be established. With current technology, it provides few advantages over CT or ultrasound and is, therefore, rarely used. The ability to display the body in any plane gives MRI the advantage and it can localise masses with great accuracy; an advantage that may help, for instance, when deciding whether a mass has arisen in a kidney or in an adrenal gland.

Ultrasound

Retroperitoneal fat, which is very echo reflective, surrounds the various retroperitoneal structures, which are seen as relatively sonolucent areas. The aorta and inferior vena cava, as expected, are easily identified. Normal adrenal glands are rarely visible. Only the larger normal lymph nodes are identifiable.

Retroperitoneal lymphadenopathy

The normal para-aortic lymph nodes vary in size from invisible to a diameter of 1 cm. In the retrocrural area, a diameter of 6 mm is the upper limit of normal. Size is the only criterion of abnormality since normal, inflammatory and neoplastic nodes usually have the same density and texture at CT and ultrasound. Metastatic neoplasm and primary lymphoma appear identical.

Mild enlargement is seen with inflammatory as well as with neoplastic disease, whereas enlargement of over 2 cm almost always indicates neoplasm. Individually enlarged nodes may be seen (Fig. 10.8b), but not infrequently several nodes are matted together to form a lobular mass engulfing the aorta or inferior vena cava (Fig. 10.9).

Lymphography (Fig. 10.10)

Retroperitoneal lymph nodes can be opacified and then demonstrated on conventional radiographs. The technique, known as lymphography, requires can-

nulation of lymph vessels on the dorsum of the foot so that an oily contrast medium can be injected. The basic signs of abnormality are enlargement and filling defects within opacified nodes. The major use of lymphography is staging malignant lymphoma, but it has now been almost entirely replaced by CT.

Adrenal glands

The normal adrenal glands are thin, bilobed structures surrounded by fat (Fig. 10.11). The right adrenal gland is situated above the upper pole of the right kidney. The left adrenal gland is usually situated just anterior to the upper pole of the left kidney. Enlargement of the adrenal glands can be recognised at CT, ultrasound and MRI. Enlargement may be due to neoplasm, hyperplasia, cyst, abscess or haemorrhage. CT is the best routine technique for diagnosing adrenal enlargement because it consistently shows the size and shape of the glands. Both ultrasound and MRI have one advantage over CT: they can display the retroperitoneum in any plane and can, therefore, show the relationship of masses to adjacent organs. This can be of real benefit

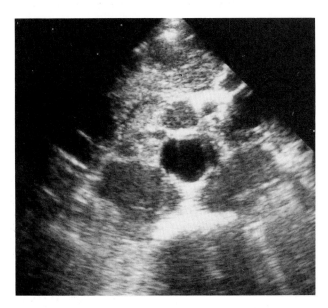

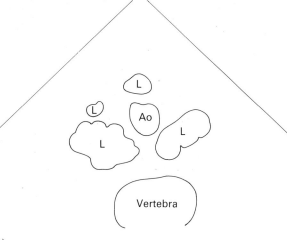

(a)

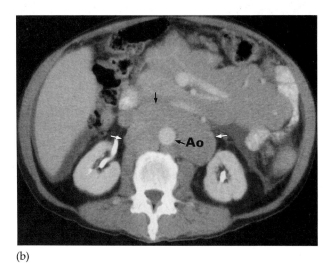

(b)

Fig. 10.9 Massive retroperitoneal lymphadenopathy (L). (a) Ultrasound showing multiple greatly enlarged lymph nodes surrounding the aorta. (b) CT scan of same patient. The arrows point to the enlarged nodes. Enlarged mesenteric nodes are also present. Ao, aorta.

when there is doubt about the origin of a mass, e.g. kidney or adrenal gland.

Functioning adrenal tumours

Patients with tumours producing an excess of hormones will have had their endocrine disorder diagnosed clinically and biochemically prior to the imaging examination and constitute a special group. CT is used in this group primarily to localise the tumour. Such tumours, which are usually benign adenomas but which may be carcinomas, cause spherical enlargement of the adrenal gland. The distinction between adrenal adenoma and adrenal hyperplasia as a cause of

Cushing's or Conn's syndromes can usually be made based on biochemical findings but, on occasions, particularly in Cushing's syndrome, the precise diagnosis can be in doubt. Adenomas giving rise to Cushing's disease are nearly always larger than 2 cm and can virtually always be localised, whereas aldosteronomas (Conn's tumour) are usually less than 1 cm

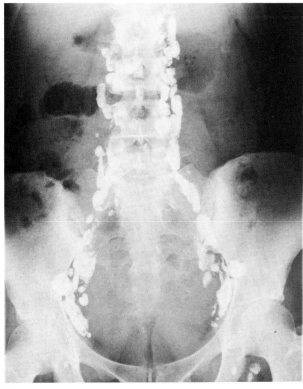

(a)

Fig. 10.10 (a) Normal lymphogram. (b) Lymphogram in a patient with malignant lymphoma, showing enlarged nodes with an abnormal (foamy) texture.

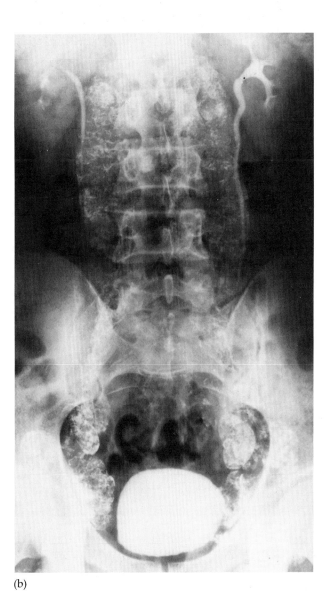

(b)

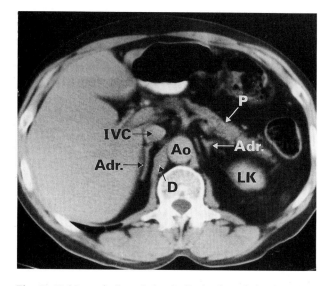

Fig. 10.11 Normal adrenal glands. Both adrenal glands (Adr.) are visible in this section. Note the different shape of the two glands. Ao, aorta; D, diaphragmatic crus; IVC. inferior vena cava; LK, left kidney; P, pancreas.

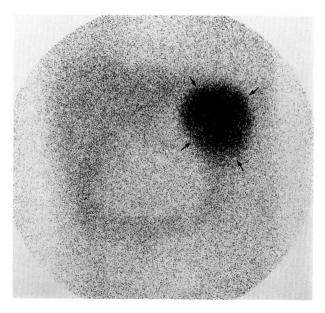

Fig. 10.13 Radio-iodine labelled MIBG scan of a phaeochromocytoma (arrows) in the left adrenal gland.

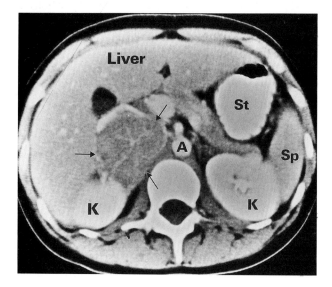

Fig. 10.12 CT scan showing large phaeochromocytoma (arrows) between right kidney, liver and spine. The inferior vena cava is compressed. A, aorta; K, kidney; Sp, spleen; St, stomach.

in size and may, on occasion, be difficult to see. Most hyperplastic glands appear normal at CT, but the glands may show uniform bilateral enlargement.

Phaeochromocytomas are frequently very large at presentation (Fig. 10.12) and virtually all are demonstrable at CT. Ten per cent of phaeochromocytomas are bilateral and, therefore, the opposite adrenal gland must be looked at carefully if a phaeochromocytoma is diagnosed. It should also be remembered that 10% of phaeochromocytomas arise outside the adrenal gland, usually in another retroperitoneal site.

Radionuclide scans can be used to localise functioning adrenal tumours. The only radionuclide in widespread use, now that CT has become the prime method of localising cortisol and aldosterone-producing tumours, is iodine-123 labelled MIBG (meta-iodo-benzyl guanidine), an agent which is concentrated by phaeochromocytomas (Fig. 10.13). As already mentioned, the great majority of phaeochromocytomas are single, but a few are multiple, either in both adrenal glands or extra-adrenal in location, and a radioiodine-labelled MIBG scan is an excellent survey technique for finding all sites of phaeochromocytoma.

Non-functioning adrenal adenomas

A small non-functioning adenoma is indistinguishable by CT or ultrasound from a small metastasis. This can pose a major dilemma for patients undergoing staging for a cancer in whom a small adrenal mass (up to 3 cm in diameter) is discovered. MRI has been investigated to see whether a distinction between non-functioning adenoma and metastasis can be made based on signal characteristics, but currently MRI cannot provide a clear answer in all cases. The technique may, however, prove to be of help in the future. In some patients, percutaneous biopsy will be needed, but as with all needle biopsy techniques it is only possible to prove, not exclude, diagnosis of cancer.

Non-functioning adenomas larger than 3 cm are very rare and, therefore, larger adrenal masses in patients being staged for the spread of cancer are assumed to be metastases, particularly if they are bilateral (Fig. 10.14).

Metastases to the adrenal gland are common; they are frequently bilateral (Fig. 10.14). Many different tumours metastasise to the adrenal glands. It is a particular feature of lung carcinoma; it is for this reason that the adrenals are frequently added to CT scans of the chest in patients being staged for bronchial carcinoma.

Both abscesses and haemorrhage are usually bilateral and are indistinguishable from one another at CT and ultrasound. The clinical features usually suggest the correct diagnosis.

Aortic aneurysm

Abdominal aortic aneurysms are readily diagnosed at ultrasound, CT and MRI, though MRI is rarely used for this purpose (Fig. 10.15). Both CT and ultrasound allow one to measure the true maximum diameter of the aneurysm and to identify separately the wall and

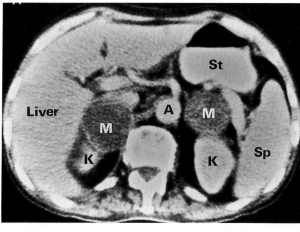

Fig. 10.14 CT scan showing large bilateral adrenal metastases (M). These masses are separate from the kidneys (K). Only the extreme top of the right kidney is visible on this particular section. A, aorta; Sp, spleen; St, stomach.

any lining thrombus. It is also relatively easy to see any retroperitoneal bleeding from an aneurysm at CT. It is generally held that aneurysms of greater than 6 cm in diameter are in serious danger of rupture, whether or not the patient has had any demonstrable retroperitoneal bleeding.

It is the thrombus, not the wall that forms the outline of the aortic lumen at angiography. Aortography is, therefore, of limited use in assessing the true diameter of an aneurysm, although it is a good technique for showing the aorta above the aneurysm as well as for showing stenoses of branches of the aorta (far better than CT or ultrasound, both of which are very poor in this regard).

Aortic aneurysms may also be recognisable in plain films of the abdomen (p. 141), but only if substantial calcification is present in the wall of the aneurysm.

Retroperitoneal tumours

The term retroperitoneal tumour covers tumours arising primarily in retroperitoneal muscles, fat or connective tissue, the commonest being liposarcoma and fibrosarcoma. All these appear as masses on CT, ultra-

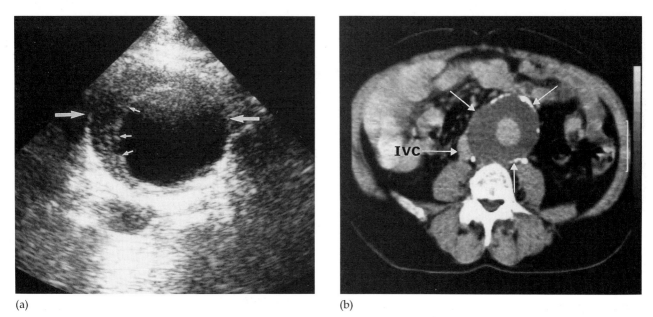

(a)   (b)

Fig. 10.15 Abdominal aortic aneurysm. (a) Ultrasound. Transverse scan showing a layer of blood clot (small arrows) within the aneurysm (large arrows). (b) CT scan with intravenous contrast enhancement. The diameter of this 7 cm aneurysm (arrows) was measured by comparison with the 5 cm bar superimposed on the left abdominal wall. The round density in the centre is the opacified blood. The lower density material surrounding the lumen is blood clot. The wall shows patches of calcification. The inferior vena cava (IVC) is displaced by the aneurysm.

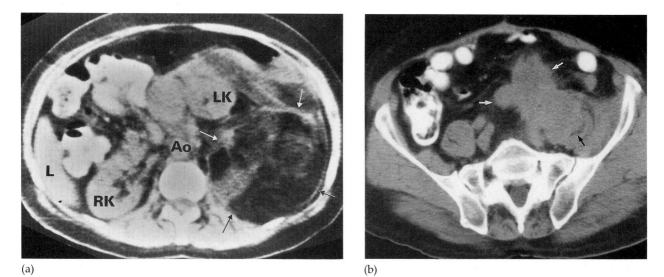

(a)   (b)

Fig. 10.16 Retroperitoneal tumours. (a) Liposarcoma. CT scan showing large partially fatty tumour (arrows) displacing the left kidney forward. The right kidney is in normal position. Ao, aorta; L, liver, LK, left kidney; RK, right kidney. (b) Malignant tumour (recurrent colon carcinoma) in left retroperitoneum (arrows). Note the asymmetry of the retroperitoneal tissues.

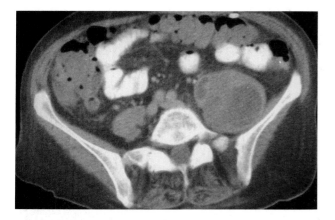

Fig. 10.17 CT scan of a large haematoma in the left iliopsoas muscle. Note the variable density, much of which is of lower density than the normal muscles.

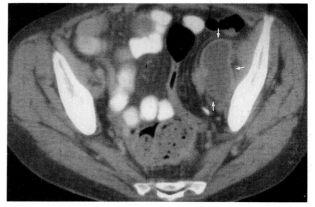

Fig. 10.18 Psoas abscess. CT scan showing left psoas abscess (arrows). Note the uniformly thick wall and the uniform low density of the contents.

sound or MRI. Sometimes, the edge of the mass is well defined, but sometimes there is invasion of the adjacent tissue. A liposarcoma (Fig. 10.16a) almost always contains significant amounts of recognisable fat interspersed between strands or masses of soft-tissue density; a combination that permits a specific diagnosis to be made at CT. Otherwise, it is usually impossible to determine the nature of the tumour (Fig. 10.16b).

Retroperitoneal haematoma

Retroperitoneal bleeding is usually due to trauma or to bleeding from an aortic aneurysm. It is occasionally spontaneous in patients with bleeding disorders or in those on anticoagulant therapy. Haematomas may have similar CT and ultrasound features to the non-fatty retroperitoneal tumours, but frequently CT numbers are higher or lower than muscle, depending on how recently the bleeding occurred (Fig. 10.17). Recent haemorrhage may show areas of high density, an appearance that can be pathognomonic, whereas older haematomas have often undergone liquefaction, the liquified areas then being of low attenuation. MRI may show the characteristic features of haematoma.

Retroperitoneal abscesses

Retroperitoneal abscesses are usually due to spread of infection from the appendix, colon, kidney, pancreas or spine. They are often found close to the organ of origin.

Retroperitoneal abscesses have many similar features to tumours and haematomas at both CT and ultrasound (Fig. 10.18). Usually, however, there is evidence of a fluid centre and then there may also be gas present within the abscess, best seen at CT. Abscesses can be confused with normal colon unless the colon is carefully identified on each image at CT. This is much easier to do if bowel opacification has been used. The wall of the abscess may enhance with contrast medium, a feature that is also seen with neoplasms. The radionuclide findings of retroperitoneal abscesses are the same as with intraperitoneal abscesses (see p. 288).

Psoas abscesses may occasionally be seen as an isolated entity. A psoas abscess will show enlargement of the psoas muscle. In order to make this diagnosis, it is helpful to compare the two psoas muscles, as they are normally symmetrical.

Retroperitoneal fibrosis

See page 239.

11

Bone Disease

The plain radiograph

Plain radiographs are the initial method of imaging the skeleton with the one exception of surveying for metastases, where radionuclide bone scanning may be used as the initial test.

The anatomical terms used to describe a normal long bone are shown in Fig. 11.1.

The radiological responses of bone to any pathological process are limited, thus similar x-ray signs occur in widely different conditions:

• *Decrease in bone density* which may be focal or

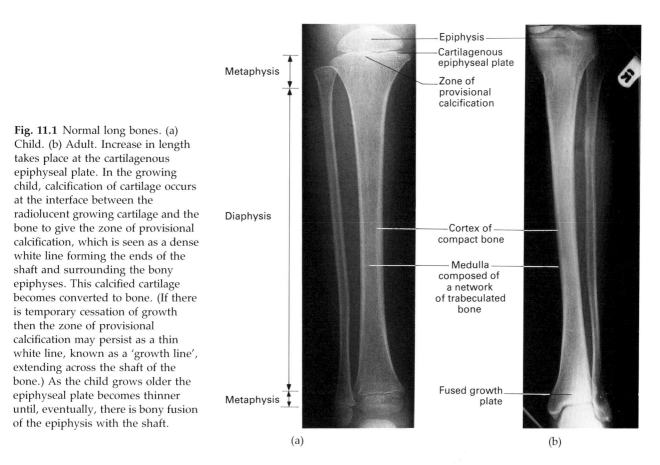

Fig. 11.1 Normal long bones. (a) Child. (b) Adult. Increase in length takes place at the cartilagenous epiphyseal plate. In the growing child, calcification of cartilage occurs at the interface between the radiolucent growing cartilage and the bone to give the zone of provisional calcification, which is seen as a dense white line forming the ends of the shaft and surrounding the bony epiphyses. This calcified cartilage becomes converted to bone. (If there is temporary cessation of growth then the zone of provisional calcification may persist as a thin white line, known as a 'growth line', extending across the shaft of the bone.) As the child grows older the epiphyseal plate becomes thinner until, eventually, there is bony fusion of the epiphysis with the shaft.

Metaphysis

Diaphysis

Metaphysis

Epiphysis
Cartilagenous epiphyseal plate
Zone of provisional calcification

Cortex of compact bone

Medulla composed of a network of trabeculated bone

Fused growth plate

(a)

(b)

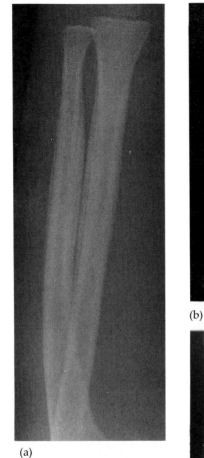

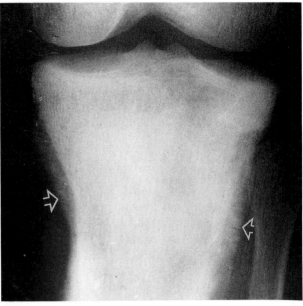

(b)

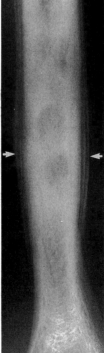

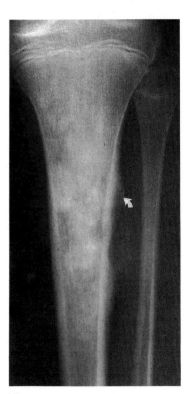

(a)

Fig. 11.2 Different types of
periosteal reactions. (a)
Smooth lamellar periosteal
reaction on the radius and ulna
in a case of non-accidental
injury. (b) Spiculated (sunray)
periosteal reaction in a case of
osteogenic sarcoma (arrows).
(c) Onion skin periosteal
reaction in a case of Ewing's
sarcoma (arrows). Here the
periosteal new bone consists
of several distinct layers.
(d) Codman's triangle in a case
of osteogenic sarcoma. At the
edge of the lesion the
periosteal new bone is lifted
up to form a cuff (arrow).

(c)   (d)

generalised. When focal, it is usually referred to as a 'lytic area' or an area of 'bone destruction'. When generalised, decrease in bone density is best referred to as 'osteopenia' until a specific diagnosis such as osteomalacia or osteoporosis can be made.

• *Increase in bone density (sclerosis)* which may also be focal, or generalised.

• *Periosteal reaction.* The periosteum is not normally visible on a radiograph. The term 'periosteal reaction' refers to excess bone produced by the periosteum, which occurs in response to such conditions as neoplasm, inflammation or trauma. Several patterns of periosteal reaction are seen (Fig. 11.2) but they do not correlate with specific diagnoses. At the edge of a very active periosteal reaction there may be a cuff of new bone known as a Codman's triangle (Fig. 11.2d). Although often seen in highly malignant primary bone tumours, e.g. osteosarcoma, a Codman's triangle is also found in other aggressive conditions.

• *Cortical thickening* also involves the laying down of new bone by the periosteum (Fig. 11.3), but here the process is very slow. The result is that the new bone, though it may be thick and irregular, shows the same homogeneous density as does the normal cortex. There are no separate lines or spicules of calcification as seen in a periosteal reaction. The causes are many, including chronic osteomyelitis, healed trauma, response to chronic stress or benign neoplasm. The feature common to all these conditions is that the process is either very slow or has healed.

• *Alteration in trabecular pattern* is a complex response usually involving a reduction in the number of trabeculae with an alteration in those that remain. Examples are osteoporosis and Paget's disease. Osteoporotic bones also show thinning of the cortex. Those trabeculae that remain appear more prominent than usual. In Paget's disease the trabeculae are thickened and trabeculation is seen in the normal compact bone of the cortex (Fig. 11.4).

• *Alteration in the shape of a bone* is another complex response with many causes. Many cases are congenital in origin; some are acquired, e.g. acromegaly and expanding bone tumours.

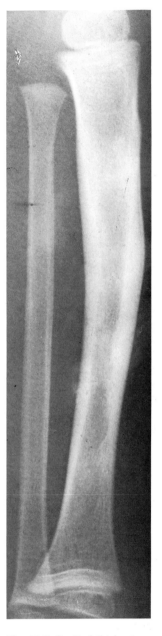

Fig. 11.3 Cortical thickening. Note the thickened cortex in the midshaft of the tibia due to old, healed osteomyelitis. Same case as in Fig. 11.15, taken 1 year later.

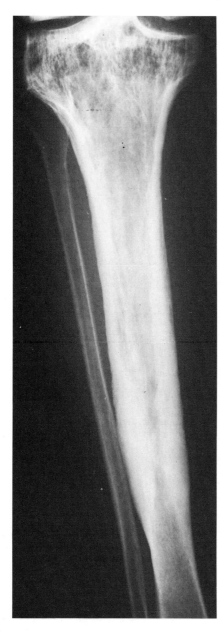

Fig. 11.4 Alteration of trabecular pattern. Paget's disease involving the upper part of the tibia leaving the lowest part of the tibia and the fibula unaffected. Note the coarse trabeculae. The other features of Paget's disease—thickened cortex and bone expansion—are also present.

• *Alteration in bone age.* The time of appearance of the various epiphyseal centres and the time when they fuse depends on the age of the child. Sets of standard films have been published which provide an indication of skeletal maturation. For the measurement of 'bone age' it is usually most convenient to take a film of the hand and wrist, but in the neonatal period films of the knee provide the most accurate assessment.

It takes time for all the above signs to develop, e.g. in adults, it takes several weeks for a periosteal reaction to be visible after trauma, and in a child with osteomyelitis, the clinical features are present 7 to 10 days before the first sign is visible on the radiograph. In general, the signs take longer to develop in adults than they do in children.

Radionuclide bone scanning

Technetium-99m (^{99m}Tc) labelled phosphate complexes given as an intravenous injection are the agents used for bone scanning. They are taken up selectively by the bones (Fig. 11.5) and also excreted in the urine. These agents may be concentrated by certain soft tissue tumours, by soft tissue calcifications and by sites of tissue damage.

Increased uptake on the bone scan is seen in conditions where there is an increased blood supply and high bone turnover. Many bone abnormalities including fractures, benign or malignant tumours, infection, infarction and Paget's disease give positive scans, so correlation with plain radiographs is frequently essential.

Indications for radionuclide bone scanning are:
• Detection of metastases.
• Detection of osteomyelitis.
• To determine whether a lesion is solitary or multifocal.
• Investigation of a clinically suspected bone lesion despite a normal radiograph. This may occur with metastases, trauma (particularly stress injury), osteoid osteoma or early osteomyelitis (Fig. 11.6a).
• To decide, in equivocal cases, whether an abnor-

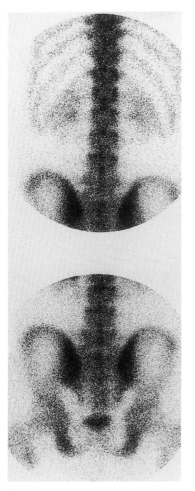

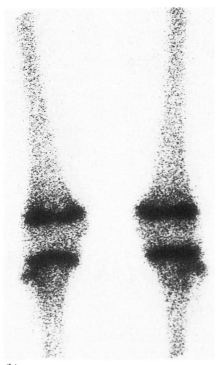

(b)

Fig. 11.5 Normal radionuclide bone scan.
(a) Adult. Posterior scans of thorax,
abdomen and pelvis. Note the radionuclide
in the bladder. (b) Child. Scan of lower
thighs and knees. Note the bands of
increased uptake in the epiphyseal plates
where bone growth is occurring.

(a)

mality seen on the radiograph is significant or not. A positive bone scan makes it likely that a true lesion exists and a negative one reduces the probability of disease considerably.

● Investigation of painful hip prostheses.

Computed tomography in bone disease

Plain radiographs are usually very informative so that computed tomography (CT) is only needed in selected cases. For specific bone details, special settings are needed. Routine settings as used for the brain, chest and abdomen, though clearly not optimal, should nevertheless be carefully scrutinised for skeletal abnormalities.

The indications for bone CT are the evaluation of:

● Disc herniation and spinal stenosis.

● Complex shaped bones, such as the spine and pelvis where plain films are frequently very difficult, or even impossible, to interpret. The transaxial display is particularly useful in diagnosing the presence and extent of fractures of these bones (see Fig. 14.13, p. 381). With more advanced scanners a three-dimensional reconstruction can be made. This is particularly useful for

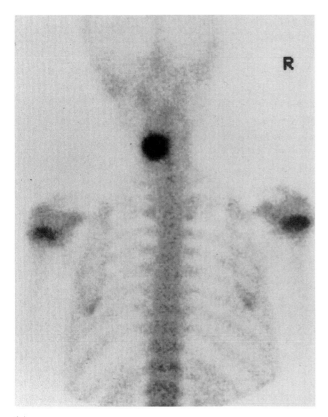

(a)

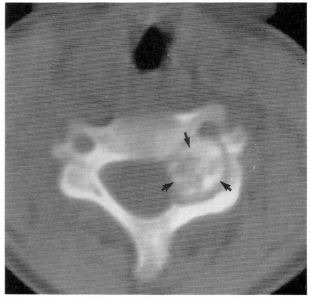

(b)

Fig. 11.6 Giant osteoid osteoma (osteoblastoma) which was difficult to appreciate on plain films. (a) Bone scan (posterior view) showing a focal area of intense increased uptake in the cervical spine. (b) CT of the cervical spine demonstrates the tumour arising from the pedicle (arrows).

appreciating fractures and planning corrective surgery in the pelvis and faciomaxillary region.

• The extent of bone tumours both within the bone and adjacent soft tissues, where this information will materially affect management, e.g. most pelvic and spinal tumours and those peripheral tumours where conservative surgery is a possibility (Fig. 11.6b).

Magnetic resonance imaging in bone disease

Calcified tissues produce no signal with magnetic resonance imaging (MRI) and it is the bone marrow that is imaged. Magnetic resonance imaging is also particularly good at showing soft tissue abnormalities.

The major indications for musculoskeletal MRI are:
• disc herniation and spinal cord compression
• to show the extent of primary bone tumours and to demonstrate bone metastases, myeloma and lymphoma
• to image soft tissue tumours
• to diagnose avascular necrosis and other joint pathologies
• to image injury to joint cartilages, ligaments and other soft tissues.

BONE DISEASES

For *diagnostic purposes* bone diseases can be divided into:
• solitary lytic or sclerotic lesions
• multiple focal lesions, i.e. several discrete lytic or sclerotic lesions in one or more bones
• generalised lesions where all the bones show diffuse increase or decrease in bone density

- processes which alter the trabecular pattern
- entities which change the shape of the bone.

Solitary lesions (for fractures see Chapter 14)

The common solitary lesions are localised areas of lysis or sclerosis, or a combination of the two. They may be accompanied by a periosteal reaction or a fracture and are usually one of the following:

1 Bone tumours
- malignant (primary or secondary)
- benign.

2 Osteomyelitis.

3 Bone cysts, fibrous dysplasia or other non-neoplastic defects of bone.

4 Conditions of uncertain nature such as histiocytosis X and osteoid osteoma.

The radiological diagnosis of a localised bone lesion can be a problem. Some conditions are readily diagnosed, but in others, even establishing which broad category of disease is present can be difficult. The initial radiological decision is usually to try and decide whether the lesion is benign, i.e. stationary or very slow growing, or whether it is aggressive, i.e. a malignant tumour or an infection. This decision is easier in primary bone lesions than in metastatic disease because some metastatic cancers and myeloma have radiological features in common with benign lesions. In these cases, the presence of a known primary tumour or multiple lesions will usually prevent the erroneous diagnosis of a benign lesion.

It is always important to know the age of the patient since certain lesions tend to occur in a specific age range.

The signs to look for on plain radiographs and CT when trying to decide the nature of a localised bone lesion are:

1 *The edge.* The edge of any lytic or sclerotic lesion should be examined carefully to see whether it is well demarcated or whether there is a wide zone of transition between the normal and the abnormal bone. There are two extremes: a lesion with a well-defined sclerotic edge is almost certainly benign, e.g. a fibrous cortical defect (Fig. 11.7a) or a bone island (Fig. 11.7b), whereas a lytic or sclerotic area with an ill-defined edge is likely to be aggressive (Fig. 11.7c). In the middle of this spectrum lies the lytic area with no sclerotic rim, which may be a benign or malignant lesion. Metastases and myeloma (Fig. 11.7d) are a frequent cause of this pattern.

2 *The adjacent cortex.* Any destruction of the adjacent cortex indicates an aggressive lesion such as a malignant tumour or osteomyelitis (Fig. 11.7e).

3 *Expansion.* Bone expansion with an intact well-

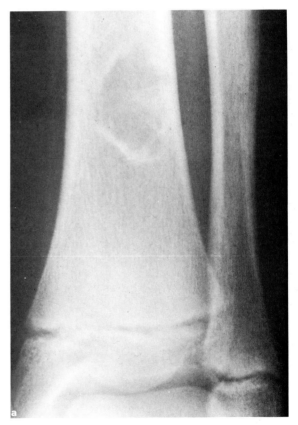

(a)

Fig. 11.7 The localised lesion. (a) With a well-defined sclerotic edge indicating a benign lesion—a fibrous cortical defect.

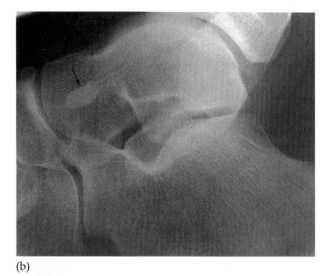

(b)

formed cortex usually indicates a slow growing lesion such as an enchondroma or fibrous dysplasia (Fig. 11.7f).

4 *Periosteal reaction.* The presence of an active periosteal reaction in the absence of trauma usually indicates an aggressive lesion (Fig. 11.7g). The causes of localised periosteal reactions are:

- osteomyelitis
- malignant bone tumour, particularly Ewing's sarcoma and osteosarcoma
- occasionally metastasis, particularly neuroblastoma
- histiocytosis X.

A periosteal reaction following trauma may lead to an erroneous impression of an aggressive process.

5 *Calcific densities within the lesion.* Calcification of the

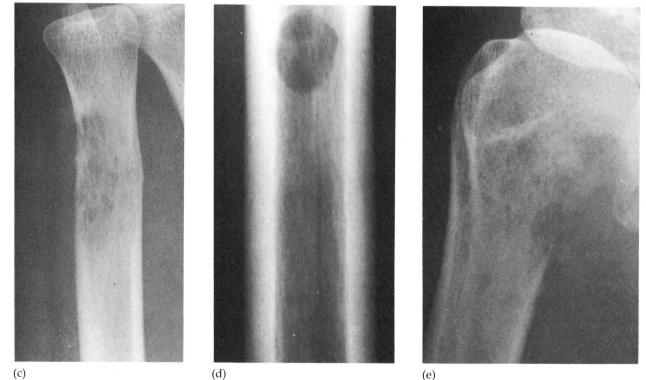

(c)   (d)   (e)

Fig. 11.7 (Continued) (b) Bone island. There is a small, well-defined area of compact bone in the talus (arrow). This common finding is without significance. (c) With an ill-defined edge—in this case a metastasis; this type of bone destruction is known as permeative. (d) With a well-defined edge—a metastasis in the shaft of the femur. (e) With destruction of the cortex indicating an aggressive lesion—another metastasis.

matrix occurs in specific conditions, e.g. patchy calcification of a popcorn type usually indicates a cartilage tumour (Fig. 11.7h), whereas diffuse ill-defined calcification suggests osteoid formation and indicates an osteosarcoma.

6 *Soft tissue swelling.* The presence of a soft tissue mass suggests an aggressive lesion; the better defined it is, the more likely it is that the lesion is a neoplasm. Ill-defined soft tissue swelling often indicates oedema, due to infection. Sometimes a tumour arising primarily in the soft tissues may be responsible for the bone lesion by pressure erosion or direct invasion.

7 *Site.* The site of a lesion is important since certain lesions tend to occur at certain sites, e.g. osteomyelitis characteristically occurs in the metaphyseal areas particularly of the knee and lower tibia, whereas a giant cell tumour is subarticular in position.

Bone tumours

The precise diagnosis of a bone tumour is often notoriously difficult both for the radiologist and the pathologist. Bone tumours may be primary or secondary. Metastatic malignant tumours are by far the commonest, outnumbering many times primary malignant tumours. They are discussed on page 312.

Primary malignant tumours

On plain films and CT, primary malignant tumours usually have poorly defined margins, often with a wide zone of transition between the normal and abnormal bone. The lesion may destroy the cortex of the bone. A periosteal reaction is often present and a soft tissue mass may be seen.

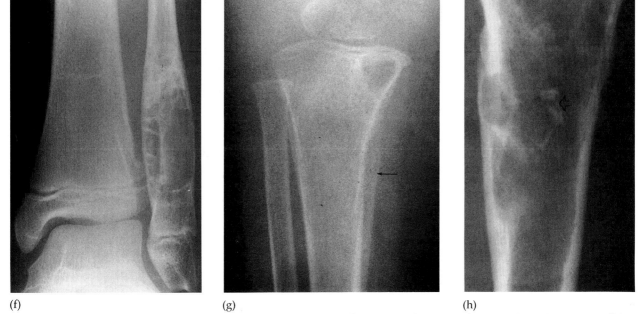

(f) (g) (h)

Fig. 11.7 (Continued) (f) With expansion of the cortex—fibrous dysplasia. (g) With periosteal reaction (arrow)—osteomyelitis. (h) Containing calcium (arrow)—a cartilage tumour, in this case a chondrosarcoma.

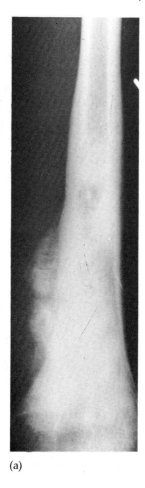

(a)

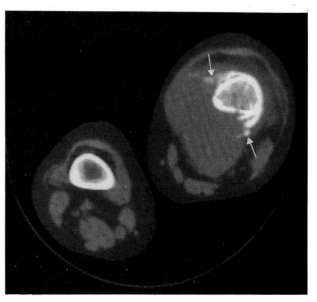

(b)

Fig. 11.8 Osteogenic sarcoma. (a) Radiograph showing patchy bone destruction with marked sclerosis and spiculated periosteal reaction. (b) Osteosarcoma. CT scan (different patient) showing a tumour arising from and destroying the femur. The size and extent of soft tissue mass is clearly demonstrated. Bone formation in the tumour is seen (arrows). The opposite thigh is normal.

Radionuclide bone scans invariably show substantially increased activity in the lesion. The adjacent bone and soft tissues may also show some increased activity, in many cases due to the accompanying hyperaemia. It is for this reason that radionuclide scanning has not proved very useful in determining the extent of tumour involvement.

Although CT is no better than plain radiographs at making a diagnosis, CT scans are used to show the extent of a tumour. Extension within the marrow cavity can be recognised by increased density of what should normally be a density close to that of fat. Extension into the soft tissue can be accurately defined, as can the relationship to important nerves and arteries.

Similar information may be obtained using MRI with the advantage that images may be produced in the sagittal or coronal planes and bone marrow and soft tissue involvement is more acurately predicted.

Osteosarcoma (osteogenic sarcoma) (Fig. 11.8) occurs mainly in the 5–20 year old age group, but is also seen in the elderly following malignant·change in Paget's disease. The tumour often arises in the metaphysis, most commonly around the knee. There is usually bone destruction with new bone formation and typically a florid spiculated periosteal reaction is present ('sunray appearance'). The tumour may elevate the periosteum to form a Codman's triangle.

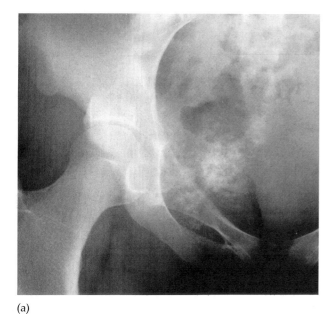

(a)

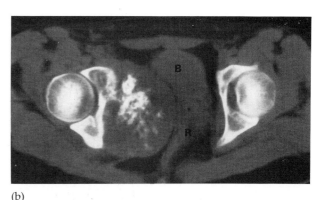

(b)

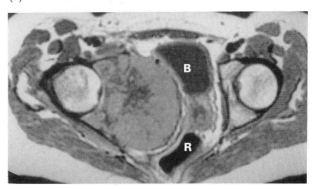

(c)

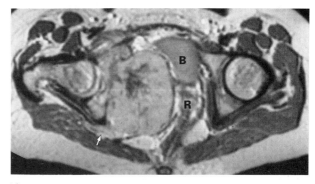

(d)

Chondrosarcoma occurs mainly in the 30−50 year old age group, most commonly in the pelvic bones, scapulae, humeri and femora. A chondrosarcoma produces a lytic expanding lesion containing flecks of calcium, a sign that indicates its origin from cartilage cells. It can be difficult to distinguish from its benign counterpart, the enchondroma, but a chondrosarcoma is usually less well defined in at least one portion of its outline and it may show a periosteal reaction (Fig. 11.9). A chondrosarcoma may arise from malignant degeneration of a benign cartilagenous tumour.

Fibrosarcoma and malignant fibrous histiocytoma are rare bone tumours with similar histological features. Radiographically, they are indistinguishable from one another. They most often present in young and middle-aged adults, usually around the knee. The features on plain radiographs are an ill-defined area of lysis with periosteal reaction. Frequently the cortex is breached. There are no features that distinguish these tumours from metastases or histiocytic lymphoma.

Fig. 11.9 Chondrosarcoma. (a) Plain film shows a large mass containing calcification arising from the pubic ramus. (b) CT shows the large mass containing calcium. There is also displacement of the bladder (B) and rectum (R). (c) Axial MRI T_1-weighted scan at the same level. Note that the calcification gives no signal. (d) MRI balanced scan at a lower level showing the tumour extending into the gluteal muscles (arrow).

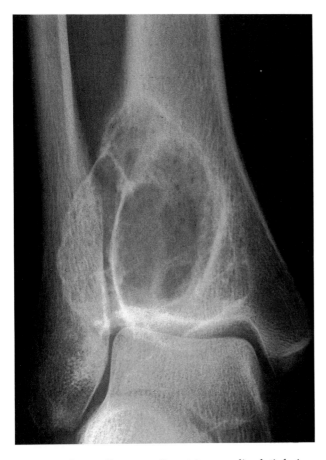

Fig. 11.10 Giant cell tumour. Eccentric expanding lytic lesion crossed by strands of bone which has thinned the cortex. The subarticular position is characteristic of this tumour.

Ewing's tumour is a highly malignant tumour, commonest in children, arising in the shaft of long bones. It produces ill-defined bone destruction with periosteal reaction that is typically 'onion skin' in type, (Fig. 11.2c, p. 298).

Giant cell tumour has features of both malignant and benign tumours. It is locally invasive but rarely metastasises. It occurs most commonly around the knee and at the wrist after the epiphyses have fused. It is an expanding destructive lesion which is subarticu-

lar in position (Fig. 11.10). The margin is fairly well defined but the cortex is thin and may in places be completely destroyed.

Benign tumours and tumour-like conditions

Under this heading are included benign tumours such as enchondroma, certain benign conditions similar to, but not strictly tumours, such as fibrous dysplasia and some abnormalities which are difficult to classify, such as osteoid osteoma and histiocytosis X. Benign lesions usually have an edge which is well demarcated from the normal bone by a sclerotic rim. They cause expansion but rarely breach the cortex. There is no soft tissue mass and a periosteal reaction is unusual unless there has been a fracture through the lesion.

Radionuclide scans in benign tumours usually show little or no increase in activity, provided no fracture has occurred. CT and MRI scanning are rarely needed in the evaluation of benign tumours.

An enchondroma is seen as a lytic expanding lesion, most commonly in the bones of the hand (Fig. 11.11). It often contains a few flecks of calcium.

Fibrous cortical defects (non-ossifying fibromas) are common chance findings in children and young adults. They are well-defined lucent areas in the cortex of long bones (Fig. 11.7a, p. 303).

Fibrous dysplasia may affect one or several bones. It occurs most commonly in the long bones and ribs as a lucent area with a well-defined edge and may expand the bone (Fig. 11.7f, p. 305). There may be a sclerotic rim around the lesion.

A bone cyst has a wall of fibrous tissue and is filled with fluid. It occurs in children, most commonly in the humerus and femur. It appears as a lucency across the width of the shaft of the bone, with a well-defined edge. The cortex may be thin and the bone expanded (Fig. 11.12). Often a pathological fracture draws attention to it.

Fig. 11.11 Enchondromas in the metacarpal, proximal and middle phalanges showing lytic areas that expand but do not breach the cortex.

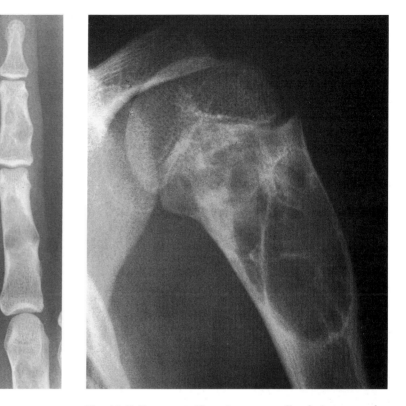

Fig. 11.12 Bone cyst. There is an expanding lesion crossed by strands of bone in the upper end of the humerus in a child. The lesion extends to but does not cross the epiphyseal plate.

An osteoid osteoma is a painful condition occurring most commonly in the femur and tibia in young adults, with a characteristic radiological appearance. There is a small lucency known as a nidus surrounded by dense sclerotic rim and a periosteal reaction may be present as well (Fig. 11.13). The nidus may contain a small speck of calcification. CT may also be used to show these features.

Histiocytosis X occurs in children and young adults and produces lytic lesions which may be single or multiple, most frequently in the skull, pelvis, femur and ribs. In the skull the lesions may be extensive giving the so-called 'geographical skull' (see Fig. 15.9, p. 391). In the long bones there is bone destruction which may be well defined or ill defined and may have a sclerotic rim. A periosteal reaction is sometimes seen. Histiocytosis X of the spine is discussed on page 353.

Osteomyelitis

Osteomyelitis is most often caused by *Staphylococcus aureus* and usually affects infants and children. The initial radiographs are normal as bone changes are not visible until 7−14 days after the onset of the infection but the ^{99m}Tc radionuclide bone scan shows increased uptake after 2−3 days. Gallium, or indium-labelled white cells can be used for confirmation. Radionuclide bone scanning has thus replaced radiography in the diagnosis of early osteomyelitis. Increased activity on the early (blood pool) images occurs in cellulitis as well as in osteomyelitis, reflecting the hyperaemia common to both conditions. However, the delayed images are normal with cellulitis but show persistent

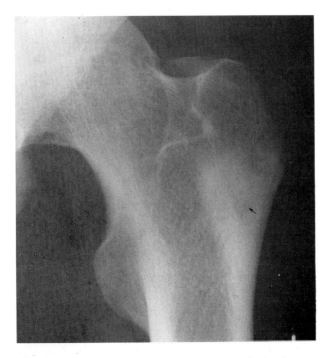

Fig. 11.13 Osteoid osteoma. There is an area of sclerosis in the upper end of the femur containing a central lucency (arrow) known as a nidus.

increased activity if osteomyelitis is present (Fig. 11.14).

The earliest sign on plain radiographs is bone destruction in the metaphysis with a periosteal reaction, which eventually may become very extensive and surround the bone to form an involucrum (Fig. 11.15). A part of the original bone may die and form a separate dense fragment known as a sequestrum (Fig. 11.16a).

In chronic osteomyelitis, the bone becomes thickened and sclerotic with loss of differentiation between the cortex and the medulla. Within the bone there may be sequestra and areas of bone destruction. Such a bone abscess is known as a Brodie's abscess (Fig. 11.16b). Computed tomography is used in selective cases to show sequestra.

Distinction of neoplasm from osteomyelitis

It is not always possible using imaging tests to distinguish osteomyelitis from a bone tumour and biopsy is then needed. The clinical history is clearly important. With malignant bone tumours, the radiographs

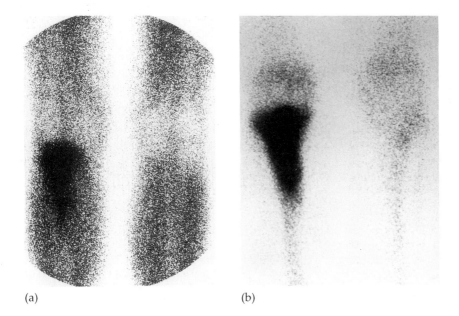

(a)   (b)

Fig. 11.14 Osteomyelitis. Radionuclide scans of knees. (a) The blood pool scan taken 1 minute after injection of radionuclide shows increased uptake in the upper part of the leg due to hyperaemia. (b) The delayed scan taken 3 hours later shows substantially increased uptake in the bone itself.

are usually abnormal when the patient first presents, whereas with osteomyelitis the initial films are often normal. But if early films are not available, difficulties may arise in distinguishing acute osteomyelitis from a highly malignant tumour such as Ewing's tumour or osteosarcoma. Chronic osteomyelitis may simulate a benign bone tumour on imaging examinations, but the presence of fever, and sometimes of discharging sinuses, usually helps to diagnose an infective lesion.

The ^{99m}Tc bone scan is positive in both osteomyelitis and malignant tumours and cannot be used in differentiation.

Bone infarction

Bone infarction occurs most often in the intra-articular portions of the bones and is therefore described in the chapter on joint disease (p. 342). However, infarcts can occur in the medulla in several diseases including caisson disease, sickle cell disease or following radiation therapy. Though infarcts are usually solitary, they may be multiple. Sometimes, they are found

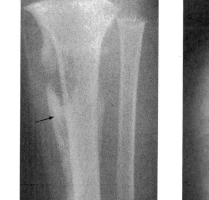
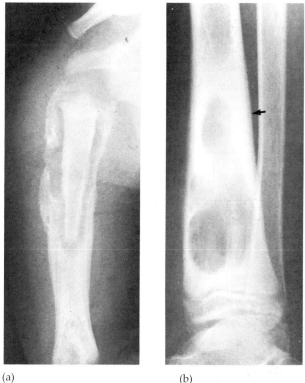

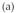 (a)    (b)

Fig. 11.15 Osteomyelitis. (a) Initial films reveal no abnormality. (b) Films taken 3 weeks later show some destruction of the upper end of the tibia and an extensive periosteal reaction along the tibia, particularly the medial side (arrow).

(a)   (b)

Fig. 11.16 (a) Late acute osteomyelitis. The upper part of the humerus has separated to form a sequestrum. It is surrounded by an extensive periosteal reaction to form an involucrum. (b) Chronic osteomyelitis (Brodie's abscess) showing a lucency surrounded by substantial sclerosis. A faint periosteal reaction is present (arrow).

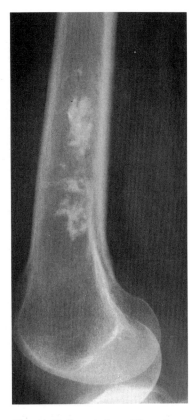

Fig. 11.17 Bone infarct. There is calcification in the medulla of the lower end of the femur.

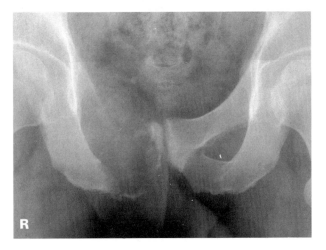

incidentally in older people with no known cause. In the acute phase no abnormality is visible, except occasionally periosteal reaction. Once healed, they appear as irregular calcification in the medulla of a long bone (Fig. 11.17).

Multiple focal lesions

Metastases

Metastases are by far the commonest bone tumour, outnumbering many times primary malignant bone tumours. Metastases may be sclerotic, lytic or a mixture of lysis and sclerosis. Those bones containing red marrow are the ones most commonly affected, namely the spine, skull, ribs, pelvis, humeri and femora.

Many tumours metastasise to bone but lytic metastases in adults most commonly arise from a carcinoma of the bronchus, breast, kidney or thyroid and in children from neuroblastoma or leukaemia. Lytic metastases give rise to well-defined or ill-defined areas of bone destruction without a sclerotic rim. The lesions vary from small holes to large areas of bone destruction (Fig. 11.18). In the long bones metastases usually arise in the medulla and as they grow they enlarge and destroy the cortex. Metastases and myeloma are virtually the only causes of multiple lytic lesions in bone. Expansion of the bone is uncommon with metastases but, when present, suggests secondary deposits from a thyroid or renal carcinoma.

Sclerotic metastases appear as ill-defined areas of increased density of varying size with ill-defined margins. In men, they are most commonly due to metastases from carcinoma of the prostate (Fig. 11.19), and in women from carcinoma of the breast.

Mixed lytic and sclerotic metastases are not uncommon. They are often seen with carcinoma of the breast (Fig. 11.20).

Fig. 11.18 Metastasis from a carcinoma of the kidney causing a large area of bone destruction with an ill-defined edge in the right superior and inferior pubic rami.

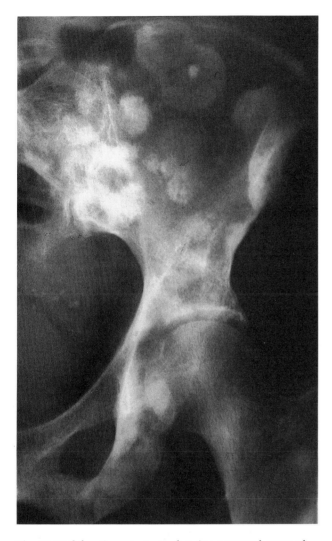

Fig. 11.19 Sclerotic metastases showing scattered areas of increased density.

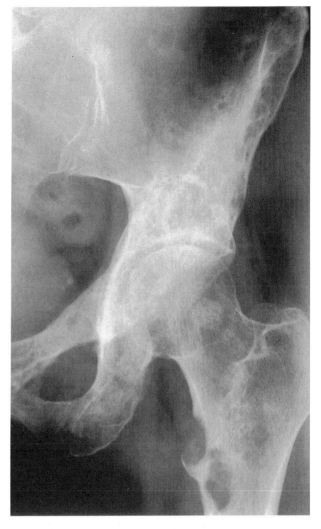

Fig. 11.20 Multiple metastases from carcinoma of the breast showing both lytic and sclerotic areas.

A periosteal reaction is uncommon with metastases, except in neuroblastoma (Fig. 11.21).

A radionuclide bone scan is much more sensitive in detecting metastases than are plain films. Not only are more lesions detected, it is also an easier examination for the patient than a radiographic skeletal survey, which involves taking numerous films. Approximately 30% of metastases seen on a bone scan will not be visible on plain films. Increased uptake on the scan of a patient with a known primary tumour but otherwise normal radiographs suggests metastases. If numerous areas of increased activity are seen in a patient with a known primary carcinoma, then the diagnosis of metastases is virtually certain (Fig. 11.22). If only one, or a few, areas of increased activity are present, radiographs will be needed to exclude the possibility of a benign condition such as degenerative change or fracture being responsible for the increased uptake of the radionuclide. If the bone scan is normal, it is most unlikely that radiographs will show metastases.

Radionuclide bone scanning can be used to examine the whole skeleton with one procedure whereas a whole skeletal survey using MRI is extremely time-consuming and very expensive. This means that MRI is only used in selected cases, although MRI is better than radionuclide scanning for the detection of metastases (Fig. 11.23). Computed tomography has little to offer for detecting metastases as it is less sensitive than MRI and is unsuitable for surveying large portions of the skeleton.

Multiple myeloma

Although myeloma deposits may be found in any bone, they are most frequently seen in bones with active haemopoiesis. The bone lesions may resemble lytic metastases in every way (Fig. 11.24) but are often

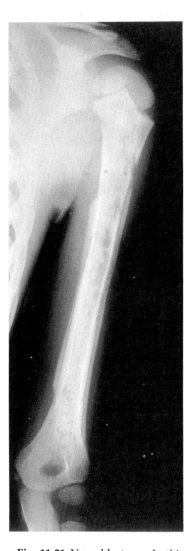

Fig. 11.21 Neuroblastoma. In this child's humerus there are several lytic areas and a florid periosteal reaction.

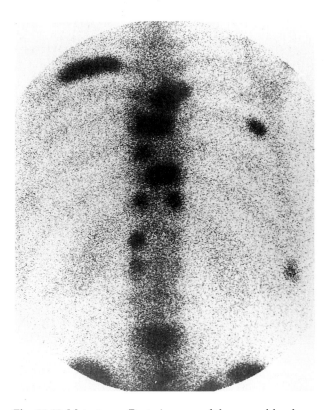

Fig. 11.22 Metastases. Posterior scan of thorax and lumbar region showing numerous discrete areas of increased uptake due to metastases from carcinoma of the prostate.

better defined and may cause expansion of the bone. Diffuse marrow involvement may give rise to generalised loss of bone density, producing a picture similar to that of osteoporosis.

Most myeloma deposits show increased activity on radionuclide bone scans. In some instances, however, even large areas of bone destruction, which are clearly visible on plain radiographs, show no abnormality on the scan. Nevertheless, it is rare for all the lesions in a particular patient to be invisible, so bone scanning is still used for survey purposes, with radiographic skeletal surveys held in reserve. The limited role of CT and MRI for detecting metastases applies also to multiple myeloma.

Malignant lymphoma

Malignant lymphoma involving bone may give rise to lytic or sclerotic lesions closely resembling metastases on all imaging modalities.

Multiple periosteal reactions

Multiple periosteal reactions are seen in conjunction with other signs in:
- Non-accidental injury.

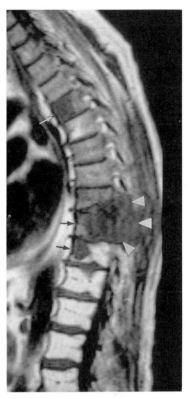

Fig. 11.23 Metastases from carcinoma of the prostate. Sagittal MRI scan showing low signal intensity in several vertebral bodies (arrows). Note the metastases also involve the posterior elements of two adjacent vertebrae (arrow heads).

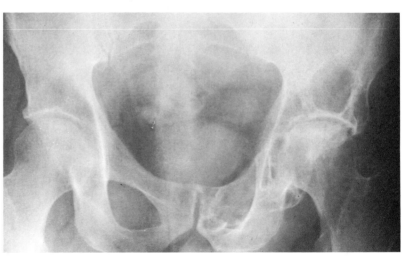

Fig. 11.24 Localised myeloma deposits causing lysis and expansion of bone.

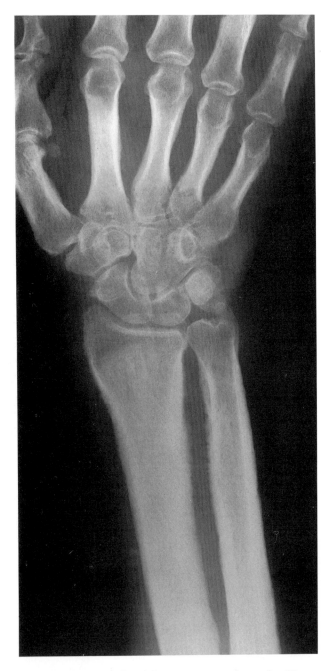

Fig. 11.25 Hypertrophic pulmonary osteoarthropathy. There is a periosteal reaction which was present bilaterally along the shafts of the radius and ulna and the metacarpals. In this case it was associated with a bronchial carcinoma.

- Scurvy.
- Widespread bone infection, e.g. congenital syphilis, neonates with infected intravenous catheters.
- Venous stasis and ulceration of the legs, where low-grade periosteal reaction and cortical thickening of the tibia and fibula may be encountered.
- Hypertrophic pulmonary osteoarthropathy. In this condition, there is widespread periosteal reaction around the bones of the forearms and lower legs which, when severe, extends to involve the hands and feet (Fig. 11.25). Finger clubbing is invariably present. Hypertrophic pulmonary osteoarthropathy is seen in a number of conditions, mostly intrathoracic, of which carcinoma of the bronchus is by far the commonest.

Generalised decrease in bone density (osteopenia)

The radiographic density of bone is dependent on the amount of calcium present in the bones. Calcium content may be reduced due to a disorder of calcium metabolism, as in osteomalacia or hyperparathyroidism, or to a reduction in protein matrix, as in osteoporosis. The radiological diagnosis of decreased bone density is often difficult, especially as the appearances of the bones are markedly affected by radiographic exposure factors. Before deciding that the bone density is reduced, the exposure should be assessed by looking at the soft tissues.

The main causes of generalised decrease in bone density are:
- osteoporosis
- osteomalacia
- hyperparathyroidism
- multiple myeloma, which may cause generalised loss of bone density, with or without focal bone destruction.

Each of these conditions may have other radiological features which enable the diagnosis to be made, but when they are lacking, as they frequently are in osteoporosis and osteomalacia, it becomes very difficult to distinguish between them radiologically.

Osteoporosis

Osteoporosis is due to a deficiency of the protein matrix (osteoid). Because the matrix is reduced in quantity there is necessarily a reduction in calcium content.

The causes of osteoporosis are:
- Idiopathic—often subdivided according to age of onset, e.g. juvenile, postmenopausal, senile. Senile osteoporosis is the commonest form.
- Cushing's syndrome and steroid therapy.
- Osteogenesis imperfecta.
- Disuse.
- Scurvy.

A radiological diagnosis of osteoporosis is only made after other diseases have been excluded. Bone destruction, which would indicate metastatic carcinoma, and evidence of hyperparathyroidism and osteomalacia should be sought, since these conditions can closely resemble osteoporosis.

The changes of osteoporosis are best seen in the spine (Fig. 11.26). Although there is an overall decrease in bone density the cortex stands out clearly, as if pencilled in. An important feature is collapse of the vertebral bodies. These are compression fractures which result in the vertebral bodies appearing wedged or biconcave. Several vertebrae may be involved and the disc spaces often appear widened.

The long bones have thin cortices. Many of the trabeculae are resorbed but those that remain stand out clearly.

In *Cushing's disease* and in patients on *steroid therapy*, the appearances are similar to idiopathic osteoporosis but may show the additional feature of florid callus around fractures.

Osteogenesis imperfecta is a dysplasia of bone. There is generalised osteoporosis and the bones are so fragile that they bend and fracture easily: the resulting deformity can be considerable (Fig. 11.27). An important diagnostic feature is the presence of a large number of Wormian bones in the skull.

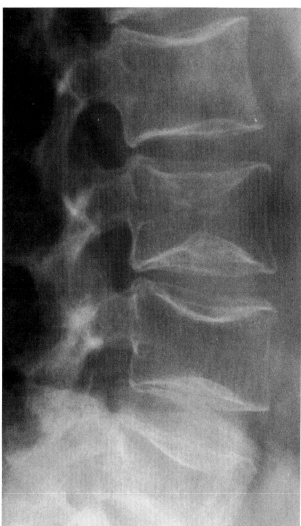

Fig. 11.26 Senile osteoporosis. There is decreased bone density but the edge of the vertebral bodies are well demarcated. Note the partial collapse of several of the vertebral bodies and the widening of the disc spaces.

Disuse osteoporosis. Osteoporosis can occur with disuse, the commonest causes being pain or immobilisation of a fracture (Fig. 11.28). Besides a reduction in density and thinning of the cortex, the bone may have a spotty appearance.

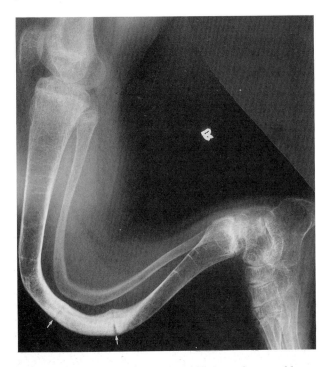

Fig. 11.27 Osteogenesis imperfecta. There is decreased bone density with a gross deformity of the leg. Old fractures can be seen in the tibia (arrows).

Sudeck's atrophy (reflex sympathetic dystrophy syndrome) is a disorder of the sympathetic nervous system where there is severe osteoporosis and oedema of the soft tissues following a fracture. The degree of osteoporosis is disproportionate to the trauma or the degree of disuse.

Scurvy is due to lack of vitamin C, which results in a deficiency of the protein matrix in the bone. Calcification of cartilage is not affected and therefore the zone of provisional calcification is seen as a relatively dense white line. Similarly, the outline of the epiphyseal centres shows a dense ring of calcification. Transformation of calcified cartilage to bone is impaired, resulting in a radiolucent zone. Due to the weakened bone, fractures may occur, usually through the metaphyses (Fig. 11.29).

In the active stage of the disease, large subperiosteal haemorrhages may form which calcify during the healing stage.

Screening for osteoporosis

Although established osteoporosis is difficult to treat,

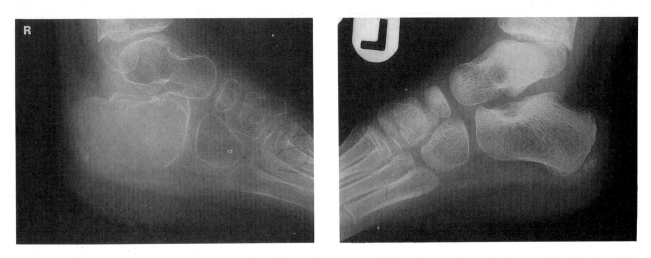

Fig. 11.28 Disuse osteoporosis due to osteomyelitis of the right calcaneum. The calcaneum is partly destroyed by infection. The remaining bones of the right foot show a marked reduction in bone density with well-defined cortex. Compare these bones with those in the normal left foot.

hormone replacement therapy may prevent the loss of bone mass that occurs after the menopause and so can prevent osteoporosis and particularly the fractures that are the major cause of symptoms.

Bone density can be measured. Conventional x-ray films are too imprecise for this purpose, so absorption bone densitometry techniques have been devised to assess the mineral content of bone. This involves measuring the attenuation by the bones of radiation from either a radionuclide source or an x-ray beam. For population screening, the hips and lumbar spine are examined. Bone density can be accurately and reproducibly measured but it is not yet clear how useful bone densitometry will prove to be in selecting patients for preventive therapy on a population-wide basis.

Rickets and osteomalacia

In these conditions there is lack of calcium in the body tissues with poor mineralisation of osteoid. If this occurs before epiphyseal closure, the condition is known as rickets—in adults it is known as osteomalacia.

The main causes of rickets and osteomalacia are:
1 Dietary deficiency of vitamin D, or lack of exposure

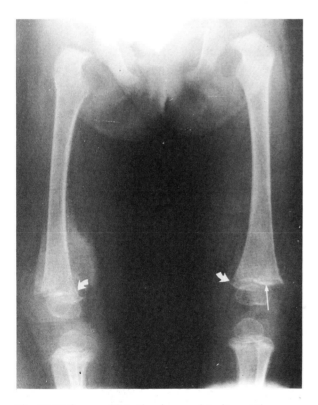

Fig. 11.29 Scurvy. Note the dense white line at the metaphysis (arrow), metaphyseal fractures (curved arrows) and calcifying subperiosteal haematoma. Reduction in bone density is not marked in this case.

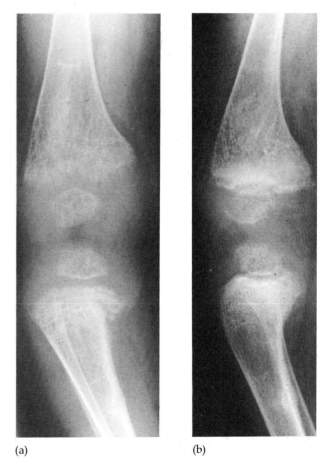

(a)   (b)

Fig. 11.30 (a) Rickets. Dietary rickets showing widening and irregular mineralisation of the metaphyses which have a frayed appearance. There is reduced bone density and bowing of the limbs. (b) After commencement of vitamin D treatment mineralisation of the metaphyses has occurred.

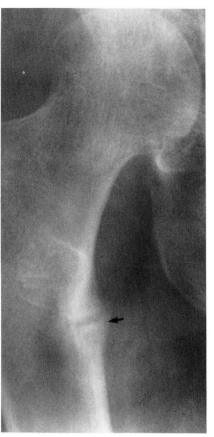

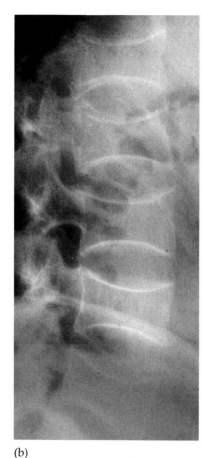

(a)   (b)

Fig. 11.31 Osteomalacia. (a) Looser's zone showing the horizontal lucent band with sclerotic margins running through the cortex of the medial side of the upper femur (arrow). (b) There is decreased bone density and partial collapse of all the vertebral bodies to approximately the same extent.

to sunlight, resulting in decreased production of endogeneous vitamin D.

2 Malabsorption, resulting in impaired absorption of calcium or vitamin D.

3 Renal disease, where rickets develops despite normal amounts of vitamin D in the diet, hence the term 'vitamin D-resistant rickets'.

- tubular defects: hypophosphataemia, Fanconi syndrome and renal tubular acidosis
- chronic renal failure: impaired ability to activate vitamin D.

Regardless of the cause of the osteomalacia or rickets, the bone changes are similar. When it is due to chronic renal failure, the changes of hyperparathyroidism may also be present.

In *rickets* the changes are maximal where bone growth is occurring, so they are best seen at the knees, wrists and ankles. The zone of provisional calcification is deficient and the metaphyses are irregularly mineralised, widened and cupped (Fig. 11.30). This results in an increased distance between the visible epiphysis and the calcified portion of the metaphysis. The generalised decrease in bone density, however, may not be very obvious. There is retardation of growth. Deformities of the bones occur because the under-mineralised bone is soft. Greenstick fractures are common.

In *osteomalacia* the characteristic features are loss of bone density, thinning of the trabeculae and the cortex, and Looser's zones (pseudofractures) (Fig. 11.31a).

Looser's zones are short lucent bands running through the cortex at right-angles, usually going only part way across the bone. They may have a sclerotic margin making them more obvious. They are commonest in the scapulae, medial aspects of the femoral necks and in the pubic rami.

Bone deformity, consequent upon bone softening, is an important feature. In the spine, the vertebral bodies are biconcave (Fig. 11.31b), the femora may be bowed and in severe cases the side walls of the pelvis may bend inwards, giving the so-called 'triradiate pelvis'.

Hyperparathyroidism

Excess parathyroid hormone secretion mobilises calcium from the bones, resulting in a decrease in bone density.

Hyperparathyroidism may be primary, due to hyperplasia or to a tumour of the parathyroid glands, or secondary to chronic renal failure.

Many patients with primary hyperparathyroidism present with renal stones and only a small minority have bone changes radiologically.

The signs of hyperparathyroidism in the bones are:
• A generalised loss of bone density, with loss of the differentiation between cortex and medulla. The trabecular pattern may have a fine lacework appearance.
• The hallmark of hyperparathyroidism is subperiosteal bone resorption (Fig. 11.32a), which occurs particularly in the hands on the radial side of the middle phalanges and at the tips of the terminal phalanges. There may also be resorption of the outer ends of the clavicles.
• Soft tissue calcification, vascular calcification and chondrocalcinosis sometimes occur. With advanced disease there may be marked deformity of the skeleton.
• 'Brown tumours' are occasionally present. These are lytic lesions, which may be single or multiple. They are of varying size and may expand the bone. They occur most commonly in the mandible and pelvis but any bone may be involved (Fig. 11.32b).

The bone changes in primary and secondary hyper-

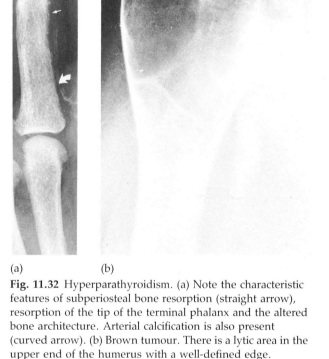

(a)　　　(b)

Fig. 11.32 Hyperparathyroidism. (a) Note the characteristic features of subperiosteal bone resorption (straight arrow), resorption of the tip of the terminal phalanx and the altered bone architecture. Arterial calcification is also present (curved arrow). (b) Brown tumour. There is a lytic area in the upper end of the humerus with a well-defined edge.

parathyroidism are similar except that 'brown tumours' are much rarer and vascular calcification is commoner in secondary hyperparathyroidism.

Renal osteodystrophy

Three distinct bone lesions can occur, often together, in patients with chronic renal failure:
1 Osteomalacia in adults; rickets in children.
2 Hyperparathyroidism.
3 Sclerosis is an infrequent feature. It may be seen in

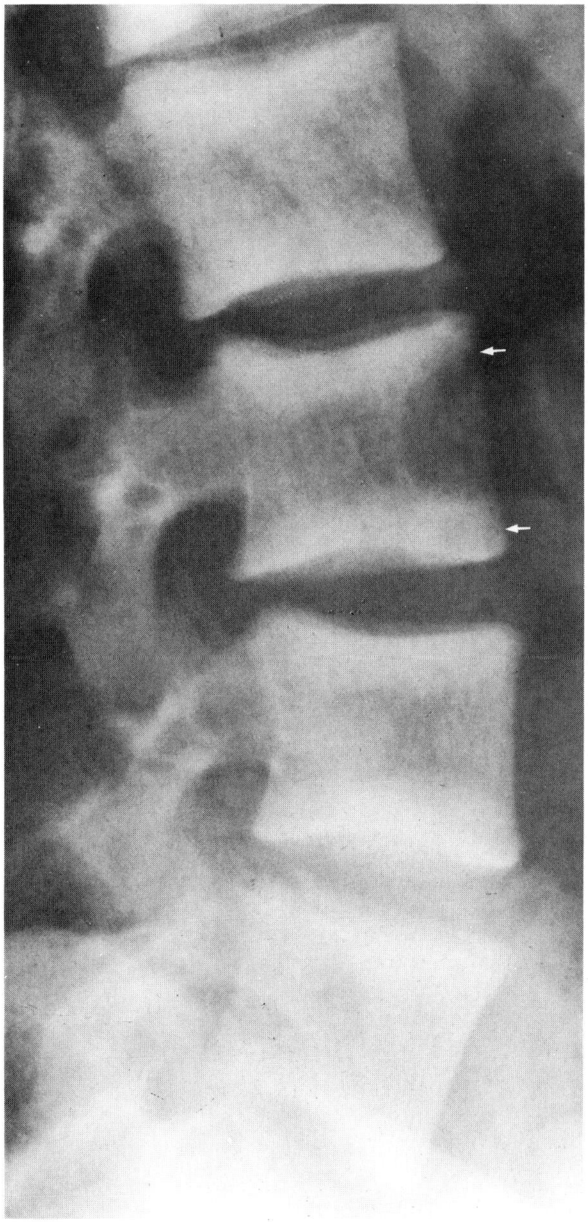

Fig. 11.33 Rugger jersey spine (renal osteodystrophy). There are sclerotic bands running across the upper and lower ends of the vertebral bodies of the lumbar spine (arrows).

the spine as bands across the upper and lower ends of the vertebral bodies, giving the so-called 'rugger jersey' spine (Fig. 11.33) or at the metaphyses of the long bones.

Generalised increase in bone density

Several conditions can cause a generalised increase in bone density. They include:

• *Sclerotic metastases*, particularly from prostatic or breast carcinoma. These may diffusely affect the skeleton (Fig. 11.34).

• *Osteopetrosis (marble bone disease)*. In this congenital disorder of bone formation the bones are densely sclerotic because most of the bone is in the form of compact bone rather than trabecular bone and, therefore, there is no differentiation between cortex and medulla (Fig. 11.35). The bones are brittle and may fracture readily but if fractured they heal easily.

• *Myelosclerosis* is a form of myelofibrosis in which, in addition to the replacement of bone marrow by fibrous tissue, the process extends to lay down extra-trabecular bone, usually in a rather patchy fashion (Fig. 11.36). The spleen is invariably enlarged due to it becoming the site of haemopoiesis. It may reach a very large size and forms an important sign on abdominal radiographs.

Alteration of trabecular pattern

Paget's disease

The incidence of Paget's disease varies greatly from country to country, being common in the UK but rare in the USA. It is usually a chance finding in an elderly patient. One or more bones may be affected, the usual sites being the pelvis, spine, skull and long bones.

Although there is a rare lytic form of Paget's disease, e.g. osteoporosis circumscripta of the skull, the cardinal features are thickening of the trabeculae and of the cortex, leading to loss of corticomedullary differentiation and increased bone density, together with enlargement of the affected bone (Fig. 11.37a).

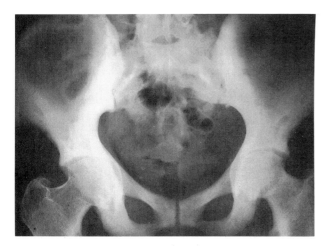

Fig. 11.34 Metastases from carcinoma of the breast causing a widespread increase in bone density.

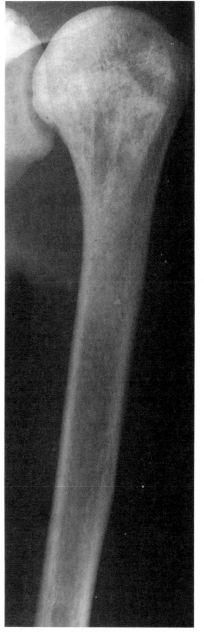

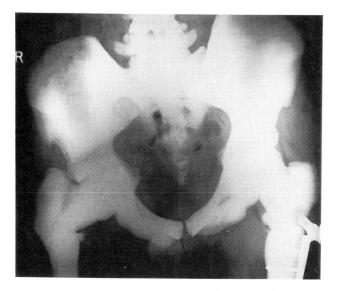

Fig. 11.35 Osteopetrosis. There is a marked generalised increased bone density affecting all bones. There are multiple healed fractures, with a pin and plate in the left femur.

Fig. 11.36 Myelosclerosis. Patchy increase in bone density in the humerus is seen. In this condition the bone marrow becomes replaced with bone.

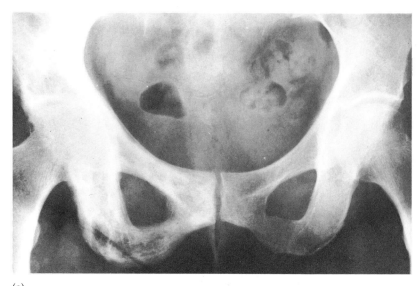

(a)

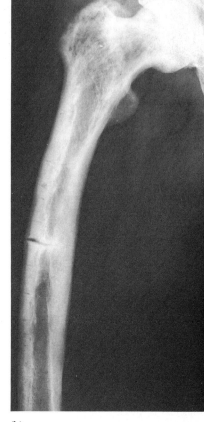

Fig. 11.37 Paget's disease. (a) There is sclerosis with coarse trabeculae in the right pubic and ischial rami. Note that the width of the affected bones is increased. (b) Incomplete fractures, known as infractions, of the lateral aspect of the femur. Note the marked thickening of the cortex and bowing of the femur.

(b)

In the skull there are many circumscribed areas of sclerosis scattered in the skull vault giving a mottled appearance which has been likened to cotton wool. An increased thickness of the calvarium is a particularly obvious feature (Fig. 15.12, p. 393).

These changes of sclerosis, cortical thickening, coarse trabeculae and most particularly, increase in the size of the bone, distinguish Paget's disease from metastases due to prostatic or breast carcinoma, which are also common in the elderly.

Bone softening causes bowing and deformity of the bones and basilar invagination in the skull (p. 392). Pathological fractures, often seen as incomplete or complete transverse fractures across the bone, may occur (Fig. 11.37b).

Malignant degeneration, with development of an osteosarcoma in abnormal bone is an occasional occurrence (Fig. 11.38).

There is greatly increased uptake of radionuclide at bone scanning in bones involved by Paget's disease (Fig. 11.39) which can be useful to define the extent of disease and response to treatment. Perhaps more importantly, it should be realised that Paget's disease may mimic tumours on bone scans and on plain radiographs.

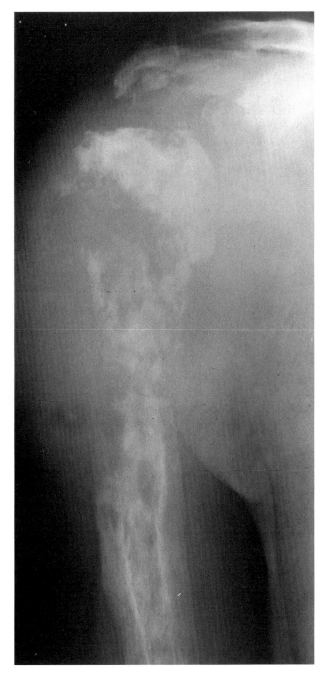

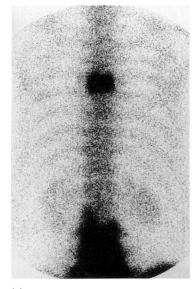

(a)

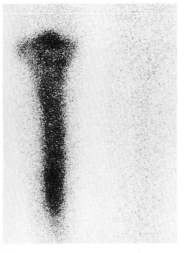

(b)

Fig. 11.38 Sarcoma in Paget's disease. There is extensive bone destruction in the humeral head and shaft. Evidence of the underlying Paget's disease can be seen.

Fig. 11.39 Paget's disease — radionuclide bone scan showing increased uptake in (a) a midthoracic vertebra, several lower lumbar vertebrae, the iliac bones and (b) the right tibia. Note the resemblance to metastases. Also note that individual lesions, e.g. in the spine are indistinguishable from malignant neoplasm.

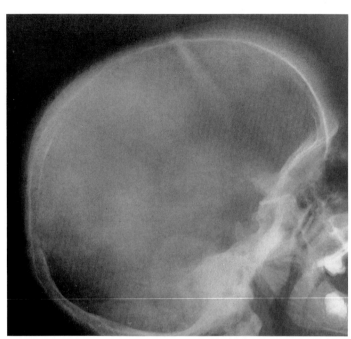

(a)

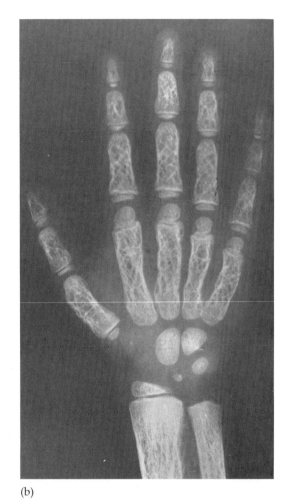

Fig. 11.40 Haemolytic anaemia—thalassaemia. (a) Skull showing thickened diploë. (b) Hand. Due to marrow expansion the bones are expanded and those trabeculae that remain are very thickened.

(b)

Haemolytic anaemia

There are several types of haemolytic anaemia but radiological changes are important in two main types, namely thalassaemia and sickle-cell disease. Both show changes of marrow hyperplasia, but sickle-cell anaemia may also show evidence of bone infarction and infection.

Marrow hyperplasia. Overactivity and expansion of the bone marrow causes thinning of the cortex and resorption of some of the trabeculae so that those that remain are thickened and stand out more clearly. Loss of bone density may be apparent. In the skull, there is

widening of the diploë and there may be perpendicular striations giving an appearance known as 'hair-on-end' (Fig. 11.40a). The ribs may enlarge and the phalanges may become rectangular (Fig. 11.40b).

Infarction and infection. Infarction at bone ends causes flattening and sclerosis of the humeral and femoral heads.

Areas of bone destruction with periosteal new bone formation, or just a periosteal reaction, may be seen in the shafts of the bones. These signs are due to bone infarction. It is not possible to determine from the radiographs whether or not these infarcts are infected.

Sarcoidosis

Sarcoidosis occasionally involves the bones. The phalanges of the hands and feet are virtually the only bones affected. The signs are either small cysts with a well-defined edge or areas of bone destruction showing a lace-like pattern (Fig. 11.41). If the bones are involved, there is invariably evidence of sarcoidosis in the chest and sarcoid skin lesions are usually present.

Changes in bone shape

Bone dysplasias

Bone dysplasias are congenital disorders resulting in abnormalities in the size and shape of the bones. There are a large number of different dysplasias; many of them are hereditary and all of them are rare. Only two of the commoner examples will be described here: achondroplasia and diaphyseal aclasia. (Osteogenesis imperfecta has been described on page 317 and osteopetrosis on page 322).

In *achrondroplasia* there is defective ossification of the bones formed in cartilage. It results in dwarfism characterised by shortening of the shafts of the long bones (Fig. 11.42a). There is reduction in the growth of the skull base, as this is formed in cartilage, and the vault is disproportionately large. A characteristic feature is that the distance between the pedicles narrows going down the lumbar spine (Fig. 11.42b). This is the reverse of what happens in the normal. The pelvis is contracted and the sacrum is set low within the pelvis.

In *diaphyseal aclasia (multiple exostoses)* there are bony projections known as oteochondromas or exostoses. They have a cartilagenous cap which may contain calcification. When osteochondromas occur on the long bones they are near the metaphyses and are directed away from the joint (Fig. 11.43).

Occasionally, a chondrosarcoma may develop in the cartilage cap. This should be suspected if there is either rapid growth, an ill-defined edge to the bone, or extensive calcification extending into the soft tissues.

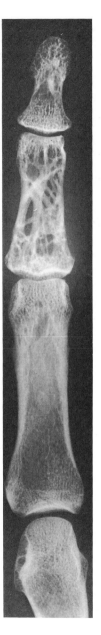

Fig. 11.41 Sarcoidosis, showing the characteristic lace-like trabecular pattern in the middle phalanx.

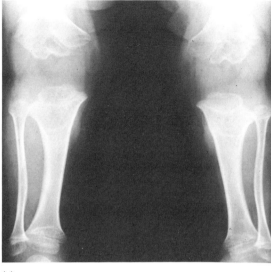

(a)

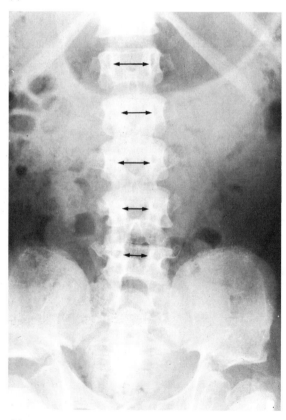

(b)

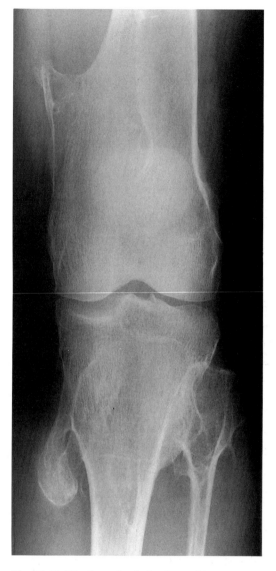

Fig. 11.43 Diaphyseal aclasia. Several bony projections (exostoses) are seen arising around the knee, directed away from the joint. The opposite knee was similarly affected.

Fig. 11.42 Achondroplasia. (a) This child shows shortening of the bones with expansion of the metaphyses. (b) The lumbar spine shows narrowing of the interpedicular distances (arrows). These distances decrease from L1 to L5 which is the reverse of normal. Note the horizontal acetabular roofs.

Gigantism and acromegaly

Both these conditions are due to overproduction of growth hormone by the anterior pituitary. When this occurs before normal growth has ceased, bony overgrowth results in gigantism; after epiphyseal closure acromegaly will develop. The bone and soft tissue overgrowth is maximal in the hands, feet and face. The tufts of the terminal phalanges enlarge and overgrowth of the articular cartilage in the hands and feet results in widened joint spaces. The outline of the bones becomes irregular (Fig. 11.44a). The changes, however, may be difficult to differentiate from a normal hand in a manual worker.

In the skull, the pituitary fossa is frequently enlarged by the growth hormone secreting adenoma responsible for the excess growth hormone. The skull vault may be thickened and the sinuses and mastoid air cells enlarged (Fig. 11.44b). A typical feature is the prognathous jaw with an increase in the angle between the body and ramus of the mandible.

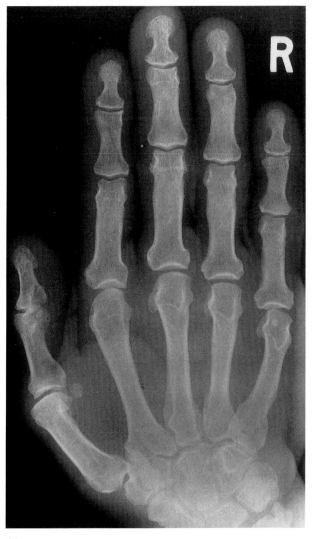

(a)

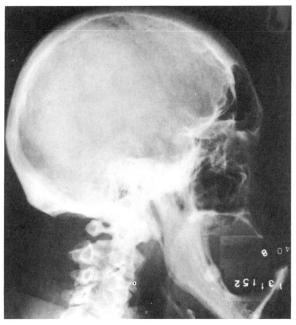

(b)

Fig. 11.44 Acromegaly. (a) The hand is large with prominent tufts to the terminal phalanges. There is widening of metacarpophalangeal joint spaces due to overgrowth of articular cartilage. (b) Note the enlarged pituitary fossa, thickened skull vault, large frontal sinuses and prognathous jaw.

12

Joints

Synovial joints have articular surfaces covered by hyaline cartilage. Cartilage in synovial joints is of the same radiodensity as the soft tissues and, therefore, is not visualised as such; only the space between the adjacent articular cortices can be appreciated (Fig. 12.1). The synovium, synovial fluid and capsule also have the same radiodensity as the surrounding soft tissues and cartilage and, unless outlined by a

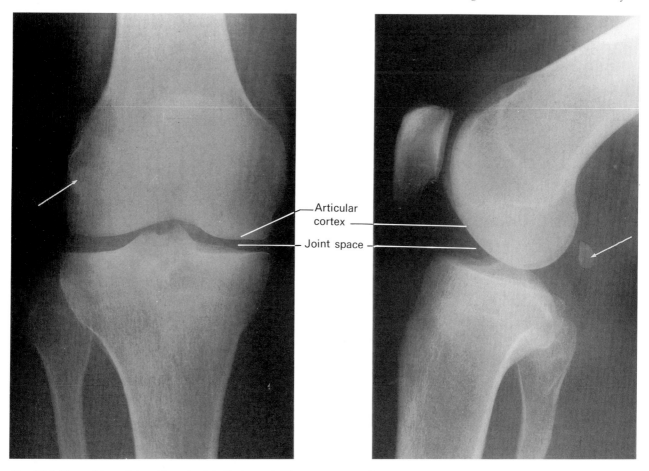

Articular cortex

Joint space

Fig. 12.1 Normal knee joint. Note the fabella (arrow). This is a sesamoid bone in the gastrocnemius. The 'joint space' consists of the articular cartilage and synovial fluid.

plane of fat, cannot be identified as discrete structures. The articular cortex forms a thin, well-defined line which merges smoothly with the remainder of the cortex of the bone.

Techniques

The plain film examination remains the mainstay of imaging joint disease.

Magnetic resonance imaging (MRI) can provide diagnostically useful information in several conditions, notably meniscal and ligamentous tears in the knee, rotator cuff tears of the shoulder and avascular necrosis of the hip.

Arthrography involves injecting contrast medium into the joint space directly and taking plain films or computed tomography (CT) scans. The main use of this technique is to demonstrate meniscal tears of the knee and occasionally rotator cuff tears of the shoulder, but its use is rapidly declining with increasing availability of MRI.

Plain film signs of joint disease

Signs indicating the presence of arthritis

Joint space narrowing

Joint space narrowing is due to destruction of articular cartilage. It occurs in practically all forms of joint disease, except avascular necrosis.

Soft tissue swelling

Swelling of the soft tissues around a joint may be seen in any arthritis accompanied by a joint effusion and whenever periarticular inflammation is present. It is, therefore, a feature of inflammatory, particularly infective, arthritis. The thickened synovium in synovial tumours and haemophilia may give rise to striking soft tissue swelling. Discrete soft tissue swelling around the joints can be seen in gout and rheumatoid arthritis.

Osteoporosis

Osteoporosis of the bones around joints occurs in many painful conditions. Underuse of the bones seems to be an important mechanism, but is not the only factor. Osteoporosis is particularly severe in rheumatoid and tuberculous arthritis.

Signs that point to the cause of the arthritis

Bone erosions

An erosion is an area of destruction of the articular cortex and the adjacent trabecular bone (Fig. 12.2), usually accompanied by destruction of the articular cartilage. Erosions are easily recognised when seen in profile but when viewed *en face*, the appearances can

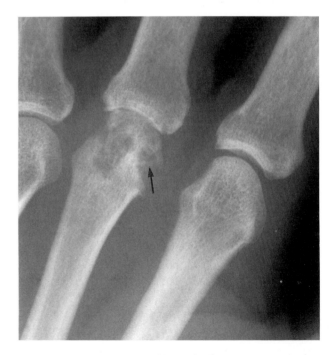

Fig. 12.2 Erosions. Areas of bone destruction are seen affecting the articular cortex of the metacarpophalangeal joint. A typical erosion is arrowed. The joint space is also narrowed.

be confused with a cyst. Oblique views designed to show erosions in profile are often taken.

There are several causes of erosions:

1 Inflammatory overgrowth of the synovium (pannus) which occurs in:
- rheumatoid arthritis, which is by far the commonest cause of an erosive arthropathy
- juvenile rheumatoid arthritis (Still's disease)
- psoriasis
- Reiter's disease
- ankylosing spondylitis
- tuberculosis.

2 Response to the deposition of urate crystals in gout.

3 Destruction due to infection:
- pyogenic arthritis
- tuberculosis.

4 Synovial overgrowth due to repeated haemorrhage in haemophilia and related bleeding disorders.

5 Neoplastic overgrowth of synovium, e.g. synoviosarcoma.

Osteophytes, subchondral sclerosis and cysts

Osteophytes, subchondral sclerosis and cysts are all features of osteoarthritis and neuropathic joints. They are discussed further on page 339. A characteristic increase in the density of subchondral bone is seen in avascular necrosis (see p. 342).

Alteration in the shape of the joint

There are a number of conditions that lead to characteristic alterations in the shape or relationship of the bone ends, e.g. slipped epiphysis, congenital dislocation of the hip, osteochondritis dissecans and avascular necrosis in its later stages.

When dealing with an arthritis it is important to have the following information:

1 *Is more than one joint involved?* Certain diseases typically involve several joints, e.g. rheumatoid arthritis, while others rarely do, e.g. infections and synovial tumours. This information can be helpful since, for example, rheumatoid arthritis and infective arthritis may produce similar changes in individual joints.

2 *Which joints are involved?* Many arthropathies have a predilection for certain joints and spare others. The distribution of joint disease can be very helpful when considering those diseases in which the changes in individual joints appear similar, e.g. various causes of erosion of the articular cortex. The following list highlights certain useful diagnostic features of the distribution of arthritis:
- Rheumatoid arthritis virtually always involves the hands and feet, principally the metacarpo- and metatarsophalangeal joints, the proximal interphalangeal joints and the wrist joints. Psoriatic arthritis usually affects the terminal interphalangeal joints.
- Gout, characteristically, involves the metatarsophalangeal joint of the big toe.
- When osteoarthritis is seen in the hands it almost always involves the terminal interphalangeal joints and often affects the carpometacarpal joint of the thumb. In the feet, it is almost always the first metatarsophalangeal joint that is affected. In the large joints, osteoarthritis is common in the hips and knees but relatively rare in the ankle, shoulders and elbows unless there is some underlying deformity or disease.
- The distribution of neuropathic arthritis depends on the neurological deficit, e.g. diabetes affects the ankles and feet, whereas tabes dorsalis affects the knees, and syringomyelia the shoulders, elbows and hands.

3 *Is a known disease present?* Sometimes an arthritis is part of a known generalised disease, e.g. haemophilia.

Rheumatoid arthritis

Rheumatoid arthritis is a polyarthritis due to inflammatory overgrowth of the synovium, often accompanied by a general systemic disturbance. Any synovial joint may be involved, particularly the wrists and small joints of the hands and feet, with relative sparing of the terminal interphalangeal joints.

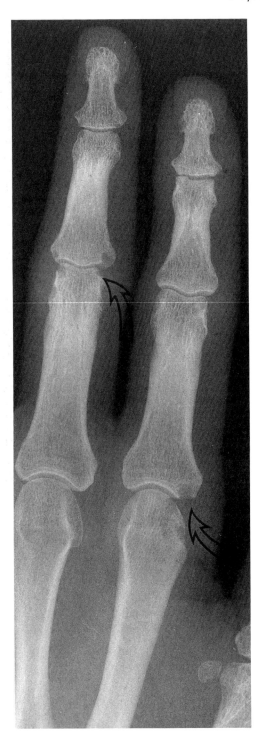

The earliest change is periarticular soft tissue swelling and osteoporosis. This osteoporosis is believed to be due to a combination of synovial hyperaemia and disuse. Destruction of the articular cartilage by pannus leads to joint space narrowing. Further destruction leads to small erosions which occur, initially, at the joint margins (Fig. 12.3). These are often seen first around the metatarso- or metacarpophalangeal joints, proximal interphalangeal joints and on the styloid process of the ulna. Later, extensive erosions may disrupt the joint surfaces. Ulnar deviation is usually present at this stage. With very severe destruction the condition is referred to as arthritis mutilans (Fig. 12.4).

Similar changes are seen in the large joints (Fig. 12.5). In such cases osteoarthritis may be superimposed on the rheumatoid arthritis and may dominate the picture.

With severe disease, there may be subluxation at the atlantoaxial joint due to laxity of the transverse ligament which holds the odontoid peg against the anterior arch of the atlas, so that the distance between it and the front of the odontoid peg becomes greater than 2 mm. Atlantoaxial subluxation may only be demonstrable in a film taken with the neck flexed (Fig. 12.6). Even though it is frequently asymptomatic, there is always the possibility of neurological symptoms due to compression of the spinal cord by the odontoid process. Atlantoaxial instability can be well demonstrated with MRI.

The role of radiology in rheumatoid arthritis

Radiographs assist in the diagnosis of doubtful cases. To this end, the detection of erosions is extremely helpful. A widespread erosive arthropathy is almost diagnostic of rheumatoid arthritis. X-ray films are also useful in assessing the extent of the disease and in observing the response to treatment.

Fig. 12.3 Early rheumatoid arthritis. Small erosions are present in the articular cortex (arrows) and there is soft tissue swelling around the proximal interphalangeal joints.

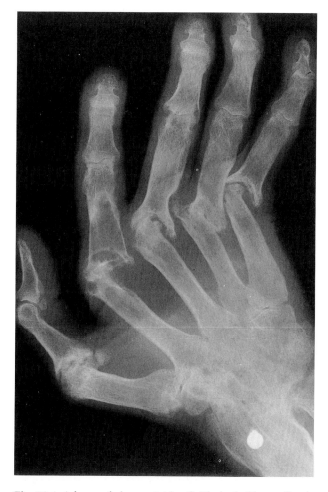

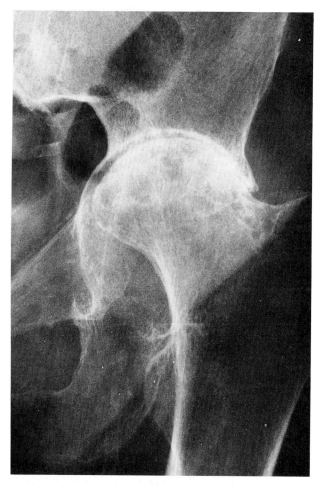

Fig. 12.4 Advanced rheumatoid arthritis (arthritis mutilans). There is extensive destruction of the articular cortex of the metacarpophalangeal joints with ulnar deviation of the fingers. Fusion of the carpal bones and wrist joint has occurred.

Fig. 12.5 Rheumatoid arthritis. Uniform loss of joint space is seen in this hip joint. Sclerosis is also present due to associated osteoarthritis.

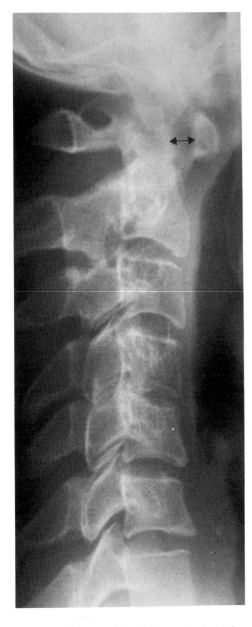

Fig. 12.6 Rheumatoid arthritis—atlantoaxial subluxation. C1 is displaced anteriorly upon C2. The distance between the arch of the atlas and the odontoid peg (arrow) is increased from the normal value of 2 mm to 8 mm. (This is the same patient whose hand is illustrated in Fig. 12.4.)

Other erosive arthropathies

Juvenile rheumatoid arthritis (Still's disease; juvenile chronic polyarthritis) shows many features similar to rheumatoid arthritis but erosions are rarer. The knee, ankle and wrist are the joints most commonly affected. Hyperaemia due to joint inflammation causes epiphyseal enlargement and premature fusion. In *psoriasis*, there is an erosive arthropathy with predominant involvement of the terminal interphalangeal joints (Fig. 12.7). In *Reiter's disease*, few joints are involved and there may be calcaneal erosions with spur formation. *Ankylosing spondylitis* causes an erosive arthritis in synovial joints and the disease always affects the sacroiliac joints.

Gout

In gout, the deposition of urate crystals in the joint and in the adjacent bone gives rise to an arthritis

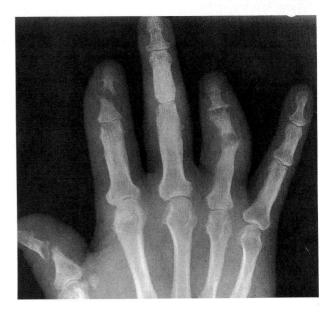

Fig. 12.7 Psoriatic arthropathy. There are extensive erosive changes affecting the interphalangeal joints but sparing the metacarpophalangeal joints.

which most commonly affects the metatarsophalangeal joint of the big toe.

The earliest change is soft tissue swelling. At a later stage, erosions occur which, unlike rheumatoid arthritis, may be at a distance from the articular cortex. These erosions have a well-defined, often sclerotic, edge and frequently have overhanging edges (Fig. 12.8a). They are due to urate deposits in the bone. These deposits may be very large, causing extensive bony destruction. There is usually no osteoporosis.

Localised soft tissue lumps due to collections of sodium urate, known as tophi, may occur in the periarticular tissues (Fig. 12.8b). These swellings can be large; occasionally they show calcification.

Joint infection

Many different bacteria cause infective arthritis but a feature common to them all is that they usually affect only one joint. Infective arthritis can be divided into:
- pyogenic arthritis, *Staphylococcus aureus* being the commonest organism
- tuberculous arthritis.

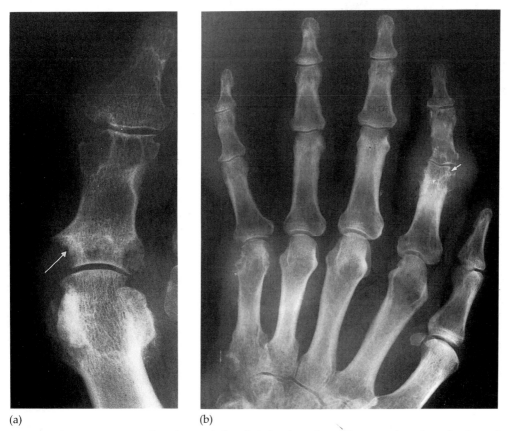

(a) (b)

Fig. 12.8 Gout. (a) Erosion: there is a typical well-defined erosion with an overhanging edge (arrow) at the metatarsophalangeal joint of the big toe. (b) Tophi: these are the large soft tissue swellings. A good example is seen around the proximal interphalangeal joint of the index finger. Several erosions are present (one of these is arrowed).

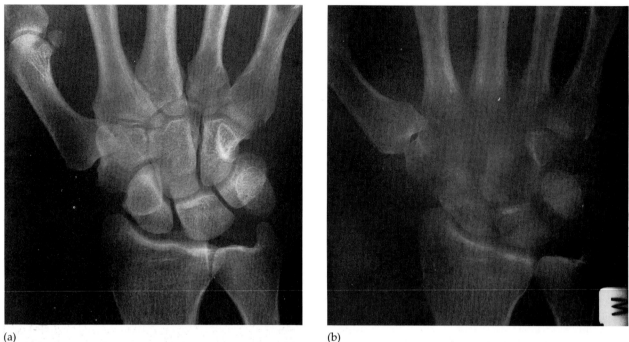

(a)   (b)

Fig. 12.9 Pyogenic arthritis. (a) Initial film of the wrist was normal. (b) Film taken 3 weeks later shows destruction of the carpal bones and bases of the metacarpals.

Synovial biopsy or examination of the joint fluid are necessary in order to identify the infecting organism.

Pyogenic arthritis

In pyogenic arthritis, there is rapid destruction of the articular cartilage followed by destruction of the subchondral bone. A pyogenic arthritis may occasionally be due to spread of osteomyelitis from the metaphysis into the adjacent joint. Soft tissue swelling around the joint may be visible (Fig. 12.9). At a late stage bony ankylosis may obliterate the joint.

Tuberculous arthritis

An early pathological change is the formation of pannus, which explains why a tuberculous arthritis may be radiologically indistinguishable from rheumatoid arthritis. The hip and the knee are the most commonly affected peripheral joints. The features to look for are joint space narrowing and erosions, which may lead to extensive destruction of the articular cortex. A very important sign is a striking osteoporosis, which may be seen before any destructive changes are visible (Fig. 12.10).

At a late stage there may be gross disorganisation of the joint with calcified debris near the joint.

Haemophilia and bleeding disorders

In haemophilia and Christmas disease repeated haemorrhages into the joints result in soft tissue swelling, erosions, and cysts in the subchondral bone. The epiphyses may enlarge and fuse prematurely (Fig. 12.11).

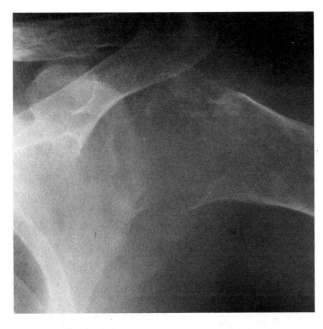

Fig. 12.10 Tuberculous arthritis of the shoulder. Note the striking osteoporosis and erosion of the humeral head.

Osteoarthritis

Osteoarthritis is the commonest form of arthritis. It is due to degenerative changes resulting from wear and tear of the articular cartilage. The hip and the knee are frequently involved but, despite being a weight-bearing joint, the ankle is infrequently affected.

In osteoarthritis, a number of features can usually be seen (Fig. 12.12):

• *Joint space narrowing*. The loss of joint space is maximal in the weight-bearing portion of the joint, e.g. in the hip it is often maximal in the superior part of the joint, whereas in the knee it is the medial compartment that usually narrows the most. Even when the joint space is very narrow it is usually possible to trace out the articular cortex.

• *Osteophytes* are bony spurs, often quite large, which occur at the articular margins.

• *Subchondral sclerosis* usually occurs on both sides of the joint; it is often worse on one side.

• *Subchondral cysts* may be seen beneath the articular

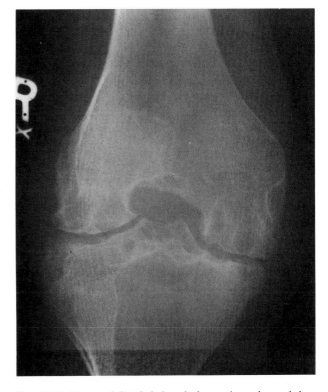

Fig. 12.11 Haemophilia. Subchondral cysts have formed due to repeated haemorrhages into the joint. Note the soft tissue swelling around the joint and the deep intercondylar notch —a characteristic feature of haemophilia.

cortex often in association with subchondral sclerosis. Normally, the cysts are easily distinguished from an erosion as they are beneath the intact cortex and have a sclerotic rim but occasionally, if there is crumbling of the joint surfaces, the differentiation becomes difficult.

• *Loose bodies* are discrete pieces of calcified cartilage or bone lying free within the joint, most frequently seen in the knee. It is important not to call the fabella, a sesamoid bone in the gastrocnemius, a loose body in the knee joint (see Fig. 12.1, p. 331).

Osteoarthritis and rheumatoid arthritis are the two types of arthritis most commonly encountered. They show many distinguishing features which are listed in Table 12.1.

Table 12.1 Comparison of osteoarthritis and rheumatoid arthritis

Osteoarthritis	Rheumatoid arthritis
Joint space narrowing maximal at weight-bearing site	Joint space narrowing uniform
Erosions do not occur but crumbling of the joint surfaces may mimic erosions	Erosions a characteristic feature
Subchondral sclerosis and cysts may be seen	Not a feature but erosions *en face* may mimic cysts
Sclerosis is a prominent feature	Sclerosis not a feature unless there is secondary osteoarthritis
No osteoporosis	Osteoporosis often present

Neuropathic (Charcot) joint

In a neuropathic joint there is an extreme form of degenerative change resulting from the loss of innervation. Typical examples are the shoulder and elbow in syringomyelia and the knee in tabes dorsalis. The joint is completely disorganised with much sclerosis of the surrounding bone. The joint is often subluxed with bone fragments or calcified debris around it (Fig. 12.13).

A different appearance is seen in the feet of diabetics with peripheral neuropathy and in leprosy. In these cases, the predominant feature is resorption of the bone ends. There may also be bone destruction due to infection (Fig. 12.14). Calcification of the arteries in the foot is often present in diabetes.

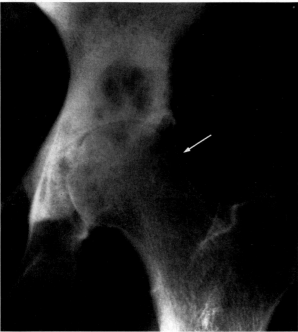

Fig. 12.12 Osteoarthritis of the hip. Note the narrowed superior part of the joint space, subchondral sclerosis and cyst formation and osteophytes (arrow).

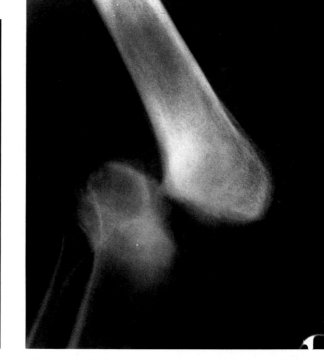

Fig. 12.13 Charcot joint. This knee in a patient with tabes dorsalis is grossly disorganised with sclerosis, calcified debris and bone fragments around the joint.

Chondrocalcinosis

Chondrocalcinosis is a descriptive term for calcification occurring in articular cartilage. In the knee, which is the most frequently affected joint, calcification may occur in the fibrocartilage of the menisci (Fig. 12.15) as well as the articular cartilage. Chondrocalcinosis is usually due to calcium pyrophosphate deposition arthropathy. In a few patients it is secondary to hyper-parathyroidism or haemochromatosis.

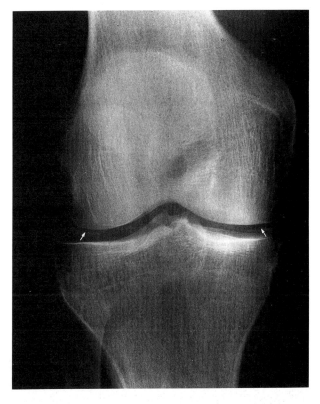

Fig. 12.15 Chondrocalcinosis. Calcification seen in the menisci in the knee (arrows).

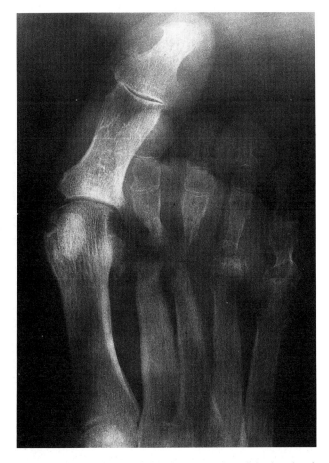

Fig. 12.14 Diabetic foot. There is resorption of the heads of the second and third metatarsals and bases of the proximal phalanges causing disorganisation of the metatarso-phalangeal joints. The patient had a peripheral neuropathy with an anaesthetic foot.

Calcium pyrophosphate deposition disease

In calcium pyrophosphate deposition disease (CPPD), crystals of calcium pyrophosphate are deposited in the joint and are seen as chondrocalcinosis. This may give rise to an arthritis clinically simulating gout, hence the alternative name 'pseudogout'. A severe arthritis resembling degenerative disease may follow, in which subchondral cysts are a prominent feature. Chondrocalcinosis may, however, be an incidental finding.

Synovial sarcoma (synovioma)

This tumour appears as a soft tissue mass adjacent to a joint. Bone destruction on one or both sides of the

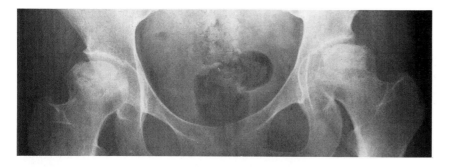

Fig. 12.16 Avascular necrosis. There is fragmentation with some sclerosis of both femoral heads.

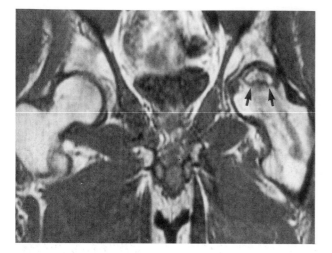

Fig. 12.17 Avascular necrosis of left femoral head (arrows). Coronal MRI scan. A pin tract through the neck of the left femur is also present. The normal appearances are shown in the right femoral head.

joint occurs at a later stage. The soft tissue mass may contain visible calcification.

Avascular necrosis

Avascular or aseptic necrosis occurs most commonly in the intra-articular portions of bones. It is associated with numerous underlying conditions including:
- steroid therapy
- collagen vascular diseases
- radiation therapy
- sickle-cell anaemia

- exposure to high pressure environments, e.g. tunnel workers and deep-sea divers (caisson disease)
- fractures.

There is also a group of conditions, some of which are called osteochondritis, in which no associated cause can be found. These are now regarded as being due to impaired blood supply associated with repeated trauma. Perthe's disease, an avascular necrosis of the femoral head in children, is the most important example.

The radiological features of avascular necrosis are increased density of the subchondral bone with irregularity of the articular contour or even fragmentation of the bone (Fig. 12.16). The cartilage space is preserved until secondary degenerative changes supervene. The diagnosis of avascular necrosis may be made with a radionuclide bone scan or, even better, with MRI (Fig. 12.17) before changes on the x-ray are apparent.

Perthe's disease

The earliest change is increase in density and flattening of the femoral epiphysis which later may progress to collapse and fragmentation. The epiphysis becomes sclerotic due to the combined effect of deposition of new bone on the scaffold of the dead bone (Fig. 12.18). The epiphysis may widen and, in consequence, the femoral neck enlarges and may contain small cysts. The joint space is widened but the acetabulum is not affected.

With healing, the femoral head reforms but may

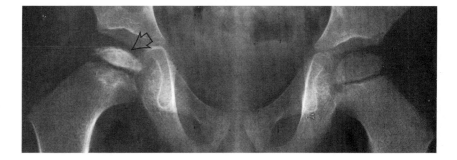

Fig. 12.18 Perthe's disease. The right femoral epiphysis (arrow) in this child is sclerotic and flattened. Compare it with the normal left side.

remain permanently flattened and, therefore, be responsible for osteoarthritis in later life.

Other similar forms of avascular necrosis are: Freiberg's disease, which affects the metatarsal heads; Kohler's disease, which is avascular necrosis of the navicular bone of the foot; Osgood–Schlatter's disease of the tibial tuberosity and Kienböck's disease of lunate bone in the wrist (Fig. 12.19).

Post-traumatic avascular necrosis (Fig. 12.20)

After a fracture, the blood supply may become interrupted and avascular necrosis supervenes. This occurs, particularly, in subcapital fractures of the femoral neck

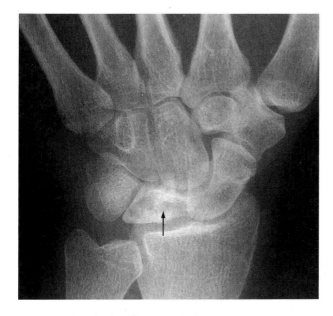

Fig. 12.19 Kienböck's disease. The lunate is flattened and sclerotic (arrow).

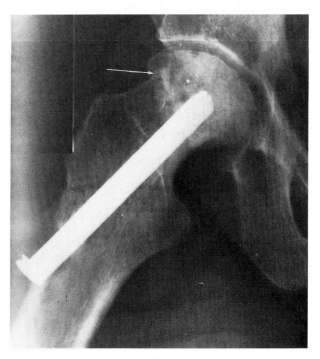

Fig. 12.20 Post-traumatic avascular necrosis. A pin has been inserted because of a subcapital fracture of the femoral neck (arrow) which occurred 10 months before this film was taken. Avascular necrosis has occurred in the head of the femur which has become sclerotic.

and fractures through the waist of the scaphoid. The femoral head and proximal part of the scaphoid become fragmented and dense due to the ischaemia.

Osteochondritis dissecans

Osteochondritis dissecans is thought to be a localised form of avascular necrosis. A small fragment of bone becomes separated from the articular surface of a joint leaving a defect and the bony fragment can often be detected lying free within the joint (Fig. 12.21). It occurs most frequently in the knee and ankle.

Slipped femoral epiphysis

Slipped femoral epiphysis occurs between the ages of 9 and 17 years and may present with pain in the hip or pain referred to the knee. The epiphysis slips posteriorly from its normal position: this is best appreciated on a lateral film of the hip (Fig. 12.22). With a greater degree of slip the condition can be recognised on the frontal view as a downward displacement of the epiphysis.

Congenital dislocation of the hip

Congenital dislocation of the hip can only occasionally be diagnosed by x-ray examination in the neonatal period. Later in life, it becomes easier to diagnose radiologically, but fortunately such cases are now rare, since the condition is usually treated in the neonatal period, the diagnosis having been made clinically. The features to look for are lateral and upper displacement of the head of the femur (Fig. 12.23). Increased slope to the acetabular roof is sometimes present.

Recently ultrasound has replaced x-rays for detecting dislocation or subluxation of the hip in the infant in whom clinical examination is suspicious of an abnormality. Ultrasound allows visualisation of cartilagenous structures which are not seen on x-ray, so the relationship of the cartilagenous femoral head and acetabulum can be determined.

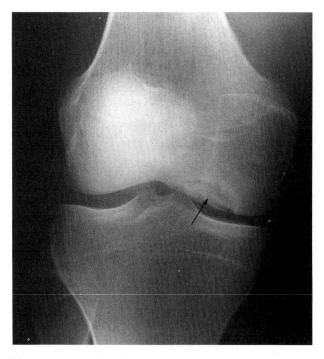

Fig. 12.21 Osteochondritis dissecans. A fragment (arrow) has become separated from the articular cortex of the medial femoral condyle.

Painful hip prosthesis

The two major causes of pain in patients with hip prostheses are infection and loosening. Radionuclide bone scanning permits earlier diagnosis than do plain films. Increased uptake of radionuclide around the prosthesis is seen in both conditions but the pattern differs (Fig. 12.24). A normal scan excludes a significant abnormality.

Osteitis condensans ilii

Osteitis condensans ilii occurs almost exclusively in women who have borne children. The condition is thought to be a stress phenomenon associated with childbearing and is usually asymptomatic. There is a zone of sclerosis on the iliac side of the sacroiliac joints, but the sacroiliac joints themselves are normal (Fig. 12.25).

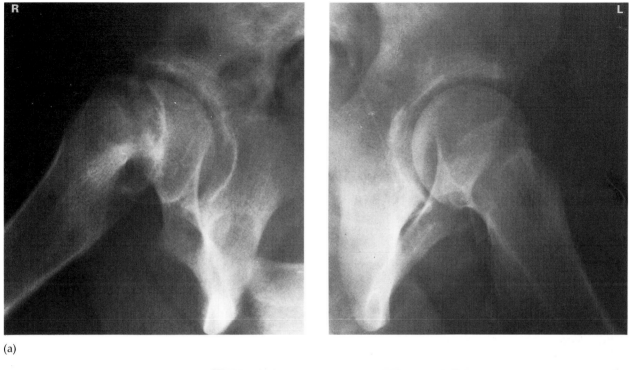

(a)

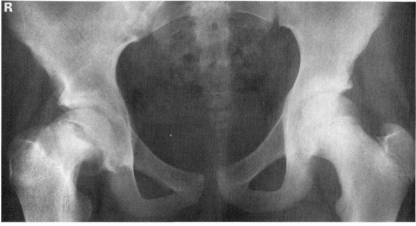

Fig. 12.22 Slipped femoral epiphysis. (a) Lateral view of the hips showing the right femoral epiphysis displaced posteriorly (compare with the normal left side). (b) Frontal view of same patient showing the right femoral epiphysis displaced downwards.

(b)

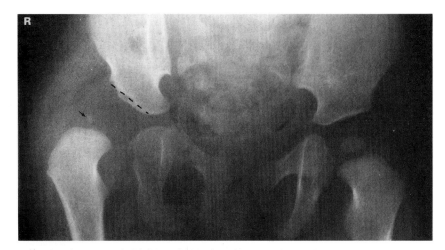

Fig. 12.23 Congenital dislocation of right hip. The right femoral epiphysis (arrow) is smaller than on the normal left side and it does not lie within the acetabulum. Note the sloping roof of the right acetabulum (dotted lines).

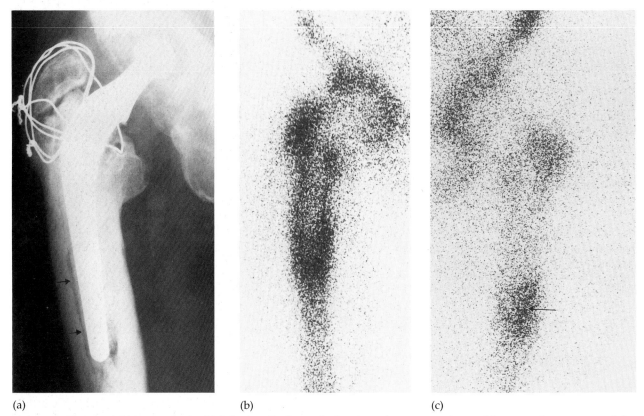

(a) (b) (c)

Fig. 12.24 The painful hip prosthesis. (a) Infection. Radiograph showing a lucent zone (arrows) between the cement and the bone. (b) Bone scan in same patient showing diffuse uptake around the shaft of the prosthesis. (c) Loosening. Radionuclide bone scan showing a localised region of increased uptake around the tip of the prosthesis (arrow).

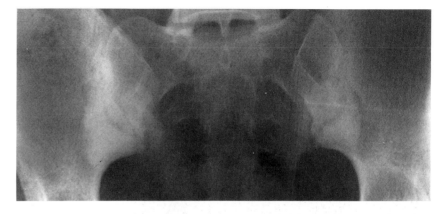

Fig. 12.25 Osteitis condensans ilii. AP view. Sclerosis is seen in both iliac bones just adjacent to the sacroiliac joints. The joints themselves, however, are normal. The patient was a young woman who had borne children.

Scleroderma

In the hands, there may be calcification and atrophy of soft tissues with loss of the tips of the terminal phalanges (Fig. 12.26).

Periarticular and meniscal disorders

Inflammation may occur in the tendons and bursae around a joint, especially the shoulder. The supra-spinatus tendon is particularly affected and on the radiograph there may be amorphous calcification lying directly above the greater tuberosity of the humerus (Fig. 12.27).

Meniscal tears in the knee and rotator cuff tears in the shoulder are frequent clinical problems in which plain films do not reveal the abnormality. MRI is a very good non-invasive method of investigating these conditions.

Magnetic resonance imaging of the knee

The menisci, which are composed of fibrocartilage, are well demonstrated on MRI as they have a different

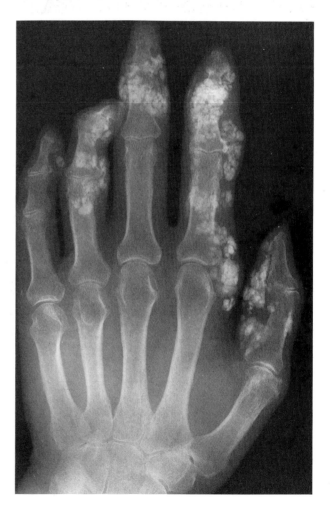

Fig. 12.26 Scleroderma. Extensive soft tissue calcification is present as well as atrophy of soft tissues at the ends of the fingers.

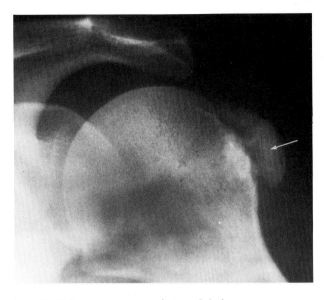

Fig. 12.27 Supraspinatus tendinitis. Calcification is present in the supraspinatus tendon (arrow).

signal intensity from the hyaline cartilage of the adjacent femoral condyle and tibial plateau. A tear can be recognised as a break in the meniscus allowing synovial fluid, which has a different signal intensity, to enter the meniscus (Fig. 12.28). Tears of the cruciate and collateral ligaments may also be recognised at MRI.

Magnetic resonance imaging of the shoulder

The rotator cuff is comprised of the supraspinatus, infraspinatus and teres minor muscles, whose tendons are inserted into the greater tuberosity of the humerus, together with subscapularis, whose tendon is inserted into the lesser tuberosity of the humerus. Tears, which are most frequent in the supraspinatus tendon, can be seen as a break in the tendon with an alteration of signal in the tendon; with tendonitis there is an alteration of signal but the tendon is intact.

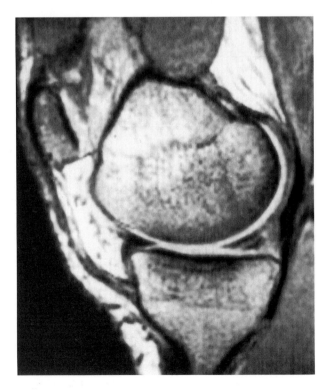

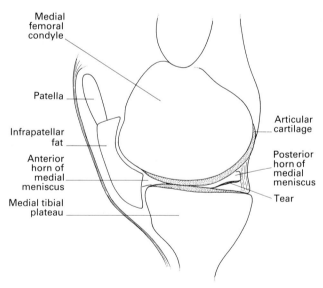

Fig. 12.28 Tear of medial meniscus. Sagittal MRI through the medial part of the knee joint showing a tear in the posterior horn of the medial meniscus. The anterior horn appears normal.

Spine

Plain films and radionuclide bone scans are of great value when diagnosing disorders of the spine. Myelography, computed tomography (CT) and magnetic resonance imaging (MRI) are specialised additional examinations requiring specific indications.

The detailed structure of the vertebrae differs in the cervical, thoracic and lumbar regions, but the general structure is similar. The appearance of a normal vertebra is illustrated in Fig. 13.1. In the lateral projection, the vertebral bodies are approximately rectangular in shape. There may be shallow indentations on the upper and lower surfaces due to protrusion of disc material into the vertebral end plates. These indentations are known as Schmorl's nodes and are of no clinical significance (Fig. 13.2). The appearances of normal vertebrae at CT and MRI are illustrated in Figures 13.3 and 13.4. It should be appreciated that CT and MRI differ from one another in a very important way. At CT, the image is predominantly formed by bone which, being calcified, is shown as high attenuation tissue. The marrow, discs and thecal contents are all of fat or soft tissue density. Bone produces no signal at MRI; the signal responsible for showing the spine on an MR image comes from the bone marrow, thecal contents and discs. Normal bone marrow has a different MRI signal to most soft tissues and, in particular, has a different signal to such pathological tissues as tumour and infection.

Myelography

The spinal cord and spinal nerves are invisible on plain films of the spine, but they may be demonstrated if contrast is introduced into the subarachnoid space by lumbar puncture. Myelography can be performed as a conventional myelogram or as CT myelography. Water-soluble contrast, which is freely miscible with the cerebrospinal fluid and rapidly absorbed from the subarachnoid space, has now replaced oily contrast medium. Myelography is used to examine the lumbar nerve roots in suspected disc protrusions and to elucidate the level and nature of spinal cord compression.

Signs of abnormality

Disc space narrowing

The intervertebral discs are radiolucent on plain radiographs as they are composed of fibrous tissue and cartilage. Normally, the disc spaces are the same height at all levels in the cervical and thoracic spine. In the lumbar spine the disc spaces increase slightly in height going down the spine, except for the disc space at the lumbosacral junction, which is usually narrower than the one above it. CT through the level of the disc itself shows uniform soft tissue density, whereas MRI shows the internal structure of the disc. Disc space narrowing occurs with degenerative disease (Fig. 13.5) and with disc space infection.

Collapse of the vertebral body

A collapsed vertebral body is one which has lost height. Loss of height is most easily appreciated on plain lateral radiographs of the spine, though it is, of course, well demonstrated on sagittal sections with MRI. It is very difficult to assess at CT. If any collapse is present, it is essential to look at the adjacent disc to

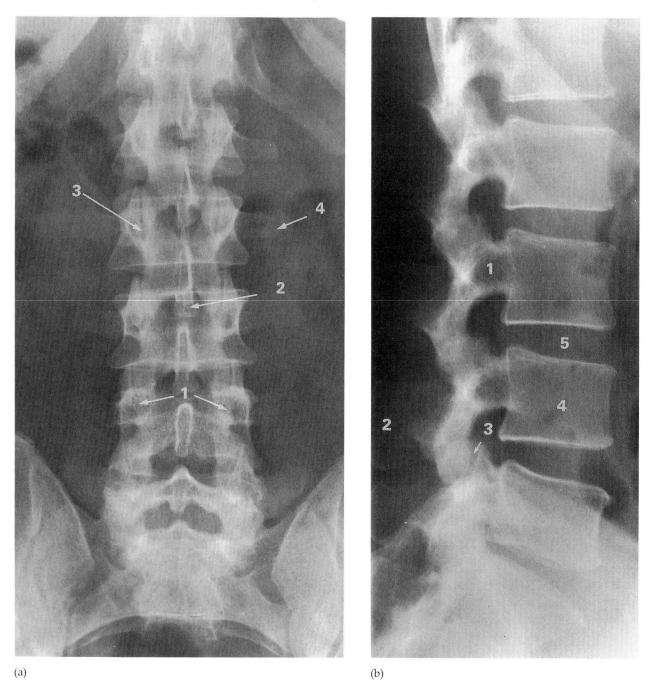

(a)

(b)

Fig. 13.1 Normal lumbar spine. (a) Frontal. **1**, pedicles; **2**, spinous process; **3**, facet joint; **4**, transverse process. (b) Lateral. **1**, pedicles; **2**, spinous process; **3**, facet joint; **4**, vertebral body; **5**, disc space. Note how the height of the disc spaces increases from L1−L5 with the exception of the L5−S1 disc space which is normally narrower than the one above.

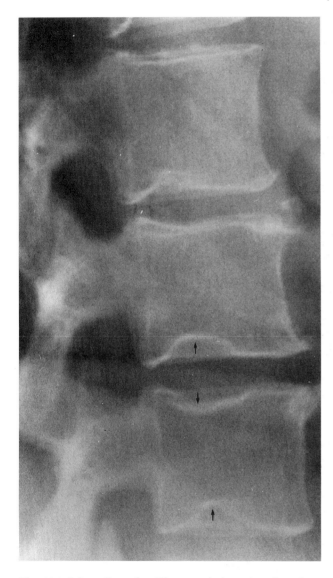

Fig. 13.2 Schmorl's nodes. These are indentations into the end plates of the vertebral bodies (arrows) and are without significance.

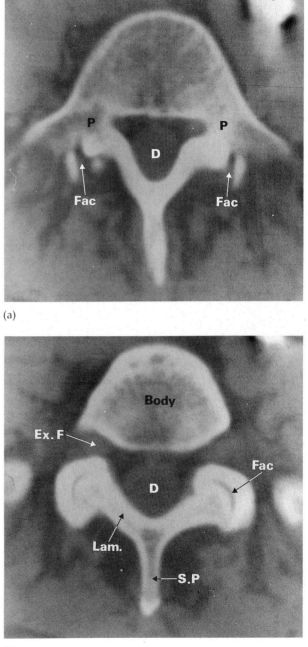

(a)

(b)

Fig. 13.3 CT of lumbar vertebra. (a) Section through pedicles (P). (b) Section through exit foramina (Ex. F). D, dural sac; Fac, facet joint; Lam, lamina; SP, spinous process.

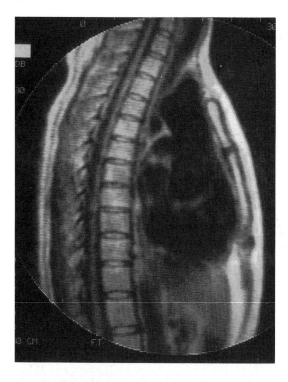

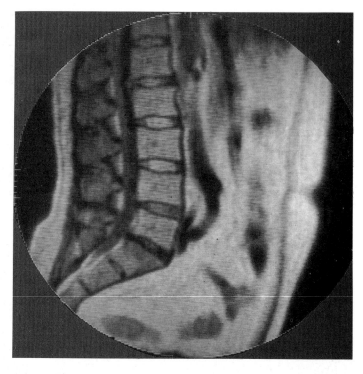

Fig. 13.4 MRI. Sagittal views of the thoracic and lumbar spine. Note how the vertebral bodies and intervertebral discs are very well demonstrated.

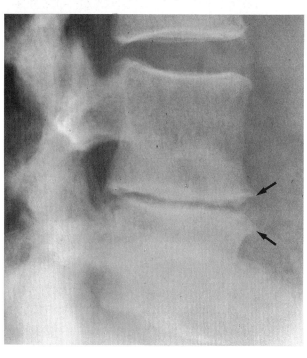

Fig. 13.5 Disc space narrowing. In this case it is due to disc degenerative changes between L3 and L4. Note the osteophytes (arrows) and sclerosis of the adjoining surfaces of the vertebral bodies.

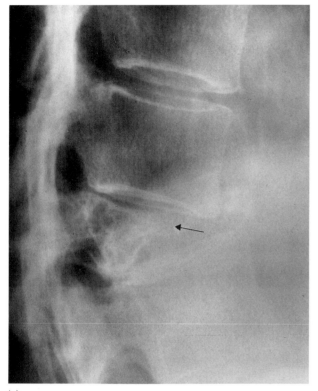

(a)

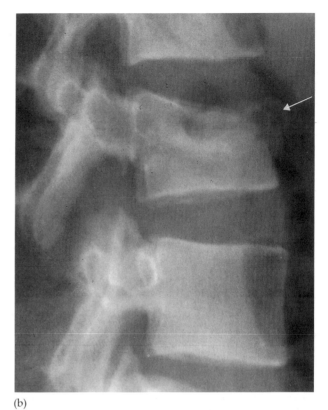

(b)

Fig. 13.6 Collapsed vertebra. (a) Due to a metastasis (arrow). This has caused complete collapse of the vertebral body. The adjacent vertebral discs are unaffected. (b) Traumatic collapse. Note the concave superior surface of the collapsed vertebral body. Some fragments have been extruded anteriorly (arrow).

see if it is narrowed and to check if part of any pedicle is destroyed. The commoner causes of vertebral collapse are listed below together with a synopsis of the signs of importance in differential diagnosis:

• *Metastases and myeloma*. Bone destruction, or replacement of normal marrow signal by tumour in the case of MRI, may be visible. The pedicles are a good place to look for evidence of bone destruction on plain film examination. The disc spaces are usually normal (Fig. 13.6a).

• *Infection*. The adjacent disc space is nearly always narrow or obliterated. There may be bone destruction next to the affected disc but the pedicles are usually intact. MRI will show altered signal within the affected vertebral body and disc.

• *Osteoporosis and osteomalacia*. There is generalised reduction in bone density. The disc spaces are normal or even slightly increased in height and the pedicles are intact. Marrow signal at MRI is normal.

• *Trauma*. A compression fracture is commonly due to forward flexion of the spine, causing the vertebral body to become wedge shaped. The superior surface is usually concave (Fig. 13.6b, c). The discs are normal but may be impacted into the fractured bone. Associated fractures may be seen in the pedicles or neural arch, but otherwise the bone and discs are normal.

• *Eosinophil granuloma*. Complete collapse of one or more vertebral bodies may occur in children or young adults with eosinophil granuloma. The vertebral body is flattened and sometimes referred to as a 'vertebra

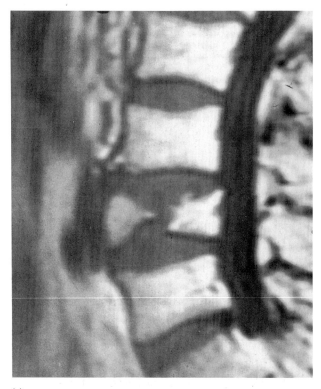

(c)

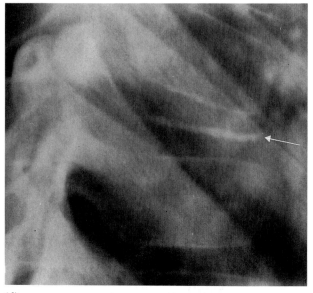

(d)

Fig. 13.6 (Continued) (c) MRI of traumatic collapse. Note how well the fractured vertebral body is shown and that there is no abnormality of the bone marrow of the collapsed vertebra. (d) Collapse due to eosinophil granuloma. In this child the vertebral body is so collapsed that it resembles a thin disc (arrow).

plana' (Fig. 13.6d). The adjacent discs are normal and the pedicles are usually preserved.

The pedicles

On plain films the pedicles are best assessed in the frontal view, except in the cervical spine where oblique views are necessary. They are very well demonstrated on CT scans. Destruction of one or more of the pedicles (Fig. 13.7) is a fairly reliable sign of spinal metastases.

Flattening and widening of the distance between the pedicles occurs with tumours arising within the spinal canal, e.g. neurofibroma or meningioma. Although neurofibromas may be completely intradural, some have a dumb-bell shape with a portion lying outside the spinal canal. In these instances the intervertebral foramen will be enlarged (Fig. 13.8).

The dense vertebra

Sclerosis, which is demonstrated by plain films or CT, may affect just one vertebra or may be part of a generalised process involving many bones. Common causes are:

- *Metastases*, particularly from primary tumours of the prostate or breast (Fig. 13.9).
- *Malignant lymphoma*.
- *Paget's disease*, which may be difficult to distinguish from neoplastic disease. An important diagnostic feature is increase in the size of the vertebra. A coarse trabecular pattern typical of Paget's disease is usually but not invariably present (Fig. 13.10).
- *Haemangioma*, which gives rise to characteristic vertical striations in a vertebra that is normal in size (Fig. 13.11).

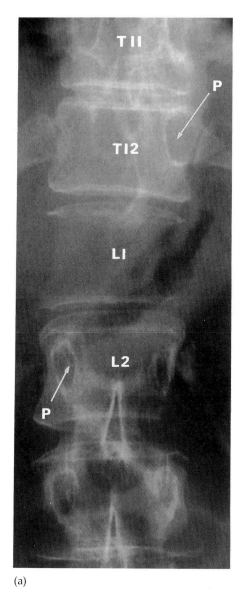

(a)

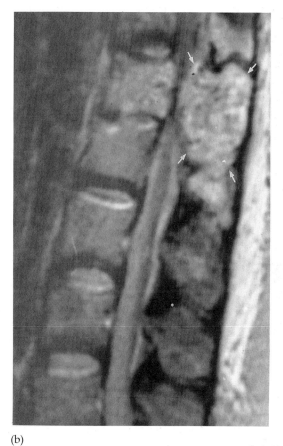

(b)

Fig. 13.7 Destruction of the pedicles due to metastatic renal cell carcinoma. (a) The pedicles of L1 have both been destroyed, as has the right pedicle of T12. Arrows point to representative normal pedicles (P). (b) MRI scan in the same patient showing extensive tumour in the vertebral body and a posterior mass of tumour (arrows) which is compressing the dural sac. (c) CT scan in another patient showing destruction of the left pedicle of a lower thoracic vertebra and the adjacent body, transverse process and medial end of rib.

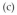

(c)

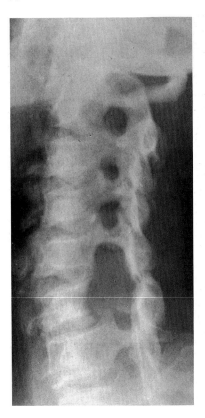

Fig. 13.8 A dumb-bell neurofibroma has enlarged the intervertebral foramina in the cervical spine to cause a large bony defect.

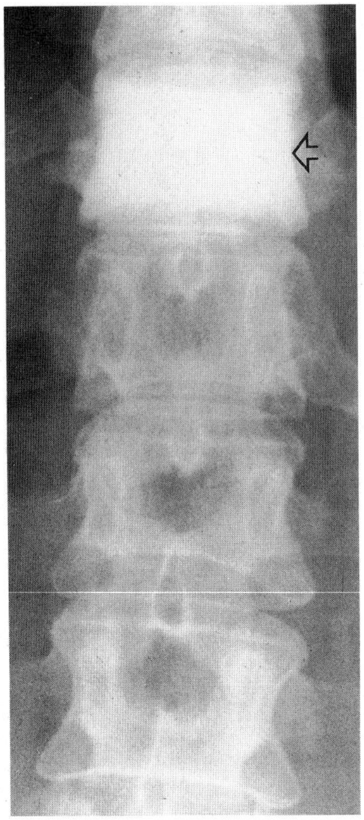

Fig. 13.9 Dense vertebra (arrow) due to metastases from carcinoma of the breast.

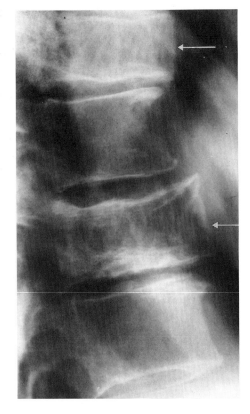

Fig. 13.10 Paget's disease. Note the increased density and coarse trabeculae in the vertebral bodies (arrows). They are also wider than the normal ones.

Lysis within a vertebra

As with sclerosis, lysis may be part of a widespread process or may be confined to one vertebra. The common causes are:
- Metastases, particularly from primary tumours of the lungs or kidneys (Fig. 13.7b).
- Multiple myeloma/plasmacytoma.
- Malignant lymphoma may occasionally give rise to a lytic lesion.
- Infection. Here the lysis usually involves one body or two adjacent bodies and the adjacent disc space is almost invariably narrowed (see below).

Paravertebral shadow

A paravertebral soft tissue shadow may first draw attention to an abnormality in the spine. The easiest place to recognise such swelling on plain radiographs is in the thoracic region where the soft tissue density adjacent to the spine assumes a characteristic fusiform shape (Fig. 13.12). Swellings in the lumbar region have to be very large if they are to displace the psoas outline and be recognisable on plain films. Anterior swelling in the cervical region can be recognised by the forward displacement of the pharyngeal air shadow. Paravertebral soft tissue swelling is readily recognised at all levels with CT and MRI scanning.

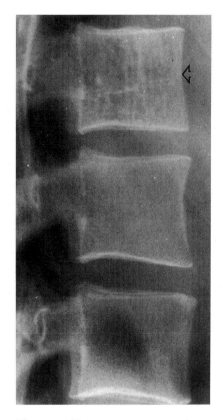

Fig. 13.11 Haemangioma. Vertical striations are present in this normal-sized vertebra (arrow).

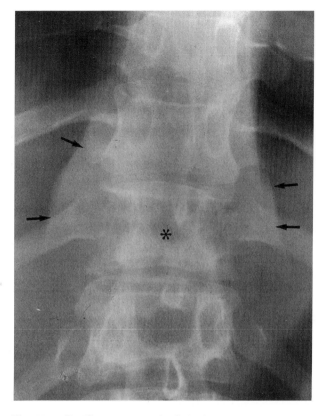

Fig. 13.12 Fusiform paravertebral shadow (arrows) around a thoracic vertebra partially destroyed by Hodgkin's disease (asterisk).

Paravertebral soft tissue swelling occurs with infection, with malignant neoplasms and with haematomas following trauma. Specific diagnostic signs are often present in such cases in the adjacent bones.

Metastases/myeloma

As with the remainder of the skeleton, the important signs of metastases on plain films or CT are areas of lysis or sclerosis, or a mixture of the two (Fig. 13.13). Multiple myeloma, which almost always gives rise to lytic lesions in the vertebral bodies, is frequently in-distinguishable from lytic metastases. A point of difference is that metastases often involve the pedicles as well as the bodies.

Collapse of one or more vertebral bodies may occur with metastases and is a particular feature of myeloma. The collapse may mask the areas of bone destruction in the vertebral body. True destruction of the disc space does not occur with metastases or myeloma.

Radionuclide bone imaging may reveal increased activity around metastatic tumour deposits, because of increased bone turnover, but myeloma lesions may or may not give rise to focal areas of increased activity.

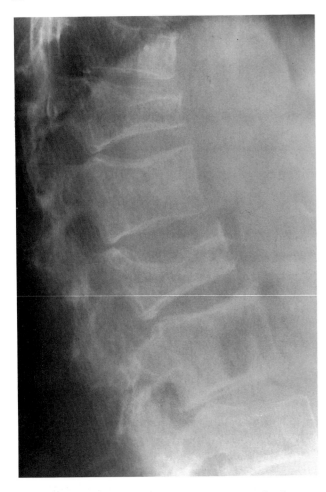

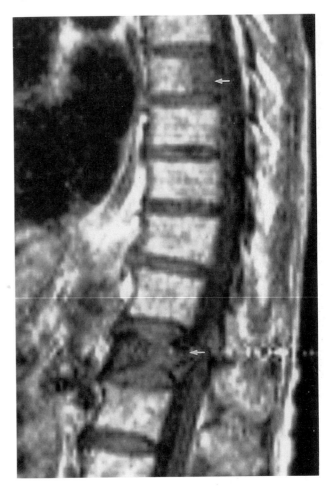

Fig. 13.13 Metastases. Lateral view of the upper lumbar spine. Note the abnormal bony architecture and varying degrees of collapse of several of the vertebral bodies.

Fig. 13.14 Metastases shown by MRI (T_1-weighted scan). The normal marrow signal has been replaced by metastatic tumour (arrows) which shows lower signal.

MRI is the most accurate test for demonstrating metastatic tumour/myeloma. Tumour tissue has significantly different signal characteristics (low signal on T_1-weighted images, high signal on T_2-weighted images) than normal bone marrow (Fig. 13.14), and thus the tumour deposits stand out clearly from the adjacent marrow. The normal bone does not generate any signal and, therefore, does not impair the visibility of the tumour. The use of MRI to detect metastases is limited by its high cost and restricted availability.

Infection

The hallmark of infection is destruction of the intervertebral disc and adjacent vertebral bodies. Early in the course of the disease, there is narrowing of the disc space with erosion of the adjoining surface of the vertebral body. Later, bone destruction may lead to collapse of the vertebral body, resulting in a sharp angulation known as a gibbus (Fig. 13.15). A paravertebral abscess is usually present.

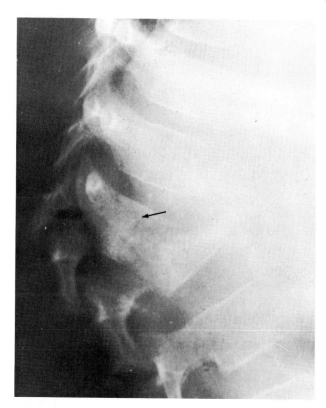

Fig. 13.15 Tuberculosis of the spine. Destruction of the vertebral bodies and the intervening discs has occurred with the formation of a sharp angulation (gibbus). One vertebral body is almost completely destroyed (arrow) and there is destruction of the upper part of the one below it.

Computed tomography shows the bone destruction and paravertebral soft tissue swelling to advantage but is a poor technique for demonstrating disc space narrowing. MRI has the advantage that it can, with one examination, demonstrate the disc space narrowing, altered signal in the adjacent vertebral body and adjacent soft tissue swelling. Needle biopsy/aspiration of the infected disc or adjacent vertebral body under plain film or CT control is a very useful technique to confirm the diagnosis and identify the responsible organism. It should be remembered, however, that positive cultures are rare once antibiotics have been commenced.

The common infecting organisms are tuberculosis and *Staphylococcus aureus*. Though there are some differences in the signs produced by these two infections, there is considerable overlap. The lesion in tuberculosis is usually purely lytic, whereas some sclerosis is often seen in pyogenic infection. Paravertebral abscesses tend to be larger in tuberculosis.

Bony fusion of the vertebral bodies across the obliterated disc spaces occurs with healing. Eventually, tuberculous paravertebral abscesses may calcify.

Spinal trauma

Plain films are the standard investigation for trauma to spine and the following should be looked for:
- Fractures of the vertebral bodies, pedicles, laminae, spinous processes.
- Alignment of fractures and interarticular facets.
- Alignment of the vertebral bodies.

Computed tomography can be very helpful in major trauma, as it will show the extent of any fractures. It is particularly useful for showing fractures of the neural arch and any associated dislocation, because these injuries may result in an unstable spine. CT will also show any bone fragments displaced into the spinal canal—the so-called burst fracture. These fragments may need surgical removal (Fig. 13.16).

When dealing with trauma it can be helpful to divide the spine into the anterior, middle and posterior columns (Fig. 13.17), since spinal stability depends on the integrity of the middle and posterior columns. Fractures confined to the anterior column are stable and these include the commonly seen wedge fractures such as those which occur in osteoporosis.

Degenerative disc disease

Spondylosis results from degeneration of the intervertebral disc. The degenerate disc may herniate into the surrounding tissues and if the herniated disc presses on the spinal cord or spinal nerves, pain and/or neurological deficit may result. Degenerate discs often stimulate the formation of osteophytes, which together with

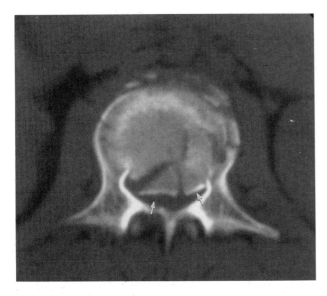

Fig. 13.16 CT scan of fractured vertebral body showing fragments (arrows) displaced backwards into the spinal canal.

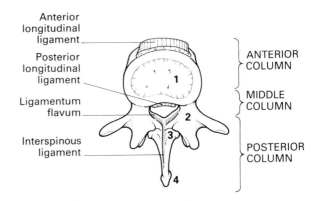

Fig. 13.17 Diagram to show the three columns of the spine. The anterior column includes the anterior longitudinal ligament and anterior two-thirds of the vertebral body. The middle column includes the posterior third of the vertebral body and the posterior longitudinal ligament. The posterior column includes the pedicles, laminae and spinous processes. **1**, vertebral body; **2**, pedicle; **3**, lamina; **4**, spinous process. *Illustration redrawn from Dr T. Jaspan with permission.*

thickening of the soft tissues, may press upon the spinal cord or nerve roots. Osteoarthritic changes in the apophyseal joints may exacerbate this problem. Spondylosis occurs maximally in the lower cervical and lower lumbar regions.

Plain radiographs in spondylosis

In most cases in which spondylosis is seen, the patient is asymptomatic. When neurological symptoms or signs are present, radiographs of the spine have limited clinical value, as there is little correlation between the symptoms, the signs and the radiological changes. Even when there is disc protrusion producing neurological signs, plain films of the spine may be normal. Usually, the major purpose of requesting radiographs of the spine is to exclude other diseases that may be present.

The signs of spondylosis on plain films (Fig. 13.18) are:
- Disc space narrowing.
- Osteophyte formation and sclerosis, which fre-

quently occur on the adjoining surfaces of the vertebral bodies. Osteophytes on the posterior surface of the vertebral bodies narrow the spinal canal and may encroach on the exit foramina through which the spinal nerves travel. In the cervical spine osteophytic encroachment of the exit foramina is best shown on oblique views.

Myelography for disc herniation (prolapse)

The common sites for disc herniation are the lumbar and cervical regions.

Lumbar disc herniation. In a normal myelogram (a lumbar myelogram is sometimes called a radiculogram) the contrast medium fills the nerve root sheaths and the nerve roots can be seen surrounded by contrast medium. Herniated discs may compress any portion of the thecal sac, but most symptomatic disc herniations occur posterolaterally. Provided the disc herniation does not lie too laterally, the disc will compress one of the spinal nerves in its nerve root sheath. This

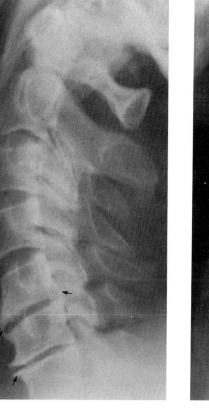

(a)

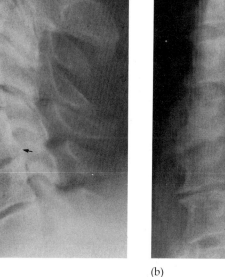

(b)

Fig. 13.18 Cervical spondylosis. (a) Lateral view. The C5–C6 and C6–C7 disc spaces are narrowed and there are osteophytes on the anterior and posterior aspects of these vertebral bodies (arrows). (b) Oblique view. The intervertebral foramina have been drawn in. The osteophytes (arrows) are narrowing the foramina.

is recognised as narrowing or absence of filling of the nerve root sheath on myelography (Fig. 13.19).

Cervical disc herniation. Herniation of a cervical disc may press on a nerve root sheath, as in the lumbar region, or may compress the spinal cord, often at multiple levels. Cervical spondylosis is accompanied by hypertrophy of the adjacent spinal ligaments which also contribute to the compression. At myelography there may be multiple transverse indentations of the thecal sac and obliteration of nerve root sheaths.

Computed tomography of disc herniation

The CT diagnosis of disc herniation needs high resolution images. High resolution scanning requires many

thin sections to be taken, so spinal CT is limited to imaging only those portions of the spine likely to show disc herniation of clinical importance.

The boundaries of the normal spinal canal are formed by vertebral bodies, pedicles, laminae and intervertebral facets to form an approximately triangular shape, interrupted by the exit foramina which are seen as gaps between the pedicles (Fig. 13.20). The vertebral bodies are recognised as bone by their cancellous structure and by the surrounding dense cortical bone, which is deficient only where the cortex is perforated by the posteriorly located vertebral veins. The disc is of lower density than bone and of uniform opacity. The nucleus pulposus cannot be separately distinguished from the surrounding annulus fibrosis at CT. The contents of the dural sac without contrast

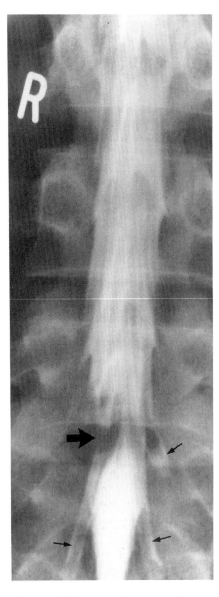

are all of the same density, therefore swelling of the intrathecal nerves and of the spinal cord are not recognisable. The nerve root sheaths are seen as circular dots adjacent to the dural sac surrounded by fat within the spinal canal. The posterior margin of the disc is outlined by fat and it is displacement of this fat by a tissue of higher attenuation that allows one to recognise disc herniation.

Disc herniations are directly visualised as small focal projections from the disc (Fig. 13.21). They are usually directed posterolaterally to one or other side of the midline. They point toward the neural exit foramen and therefore compress the adjacent root sheath or nerve root, which may become swollen. It should be appreciated that more than a third of demonstrably herniated discs are asymptomatic, so the criterion for surgery must be clear-cut evidence of compression of the clinically affected nerve root. CT is particularly useful for postoperative cases and for the rare disc herniations that are situated lateral to the root sheaths, because it shows the herniation itself, not just the compressive effects on the subarachnoid space, as does myelography. CT has largely superseded myelography for diagnosing disc herniation but in turn MRI is now replacing CT.

Magnetic resonance imaging of disc herniation

Magnetic resonance imaging is very sensitive for showing the altered signal in the nucleus pulposis that occurs with disc degeneration, but this is of limited value since the presence of degeneration bears little

Fig. 13.19 Disc protrusion on myelogram. Contrast is in the subarachnoid space below the termination of the spinal cord. Note the filling of the nerve root sheaths (arrows). There is a large disc protrusion (large arrow).

Fig. 13.20 (Upper part of facing page) CT scan of normal lumbar disc. Note the normal shape of the disc with no protrusions into the spinal canal or exit foramina. Ao, aorta; IVC, inferior vena cava.

Fig. 13.21 (Lower part of facing page) Disc herniation. CT scan. There is a large posterior herniation, maximal on the left and centrally. The thecal sac (very difficult to see at these settings) is pushed backward. IVC, inferior vena cava.

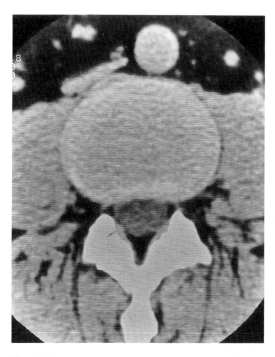

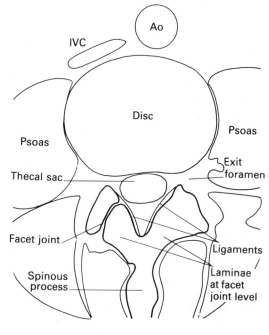

Fig. 13.20

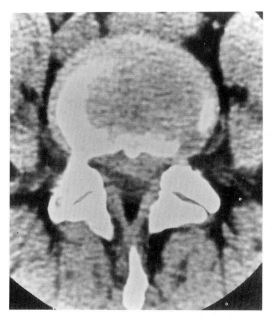

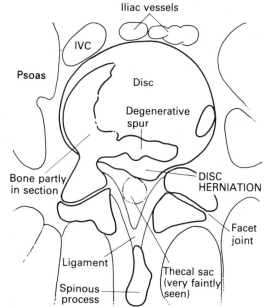

Fig. 13.21

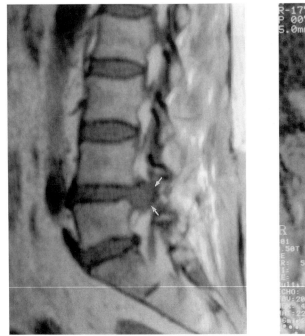

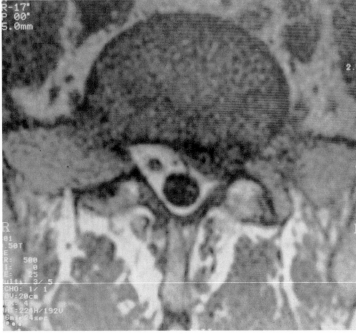

(a)

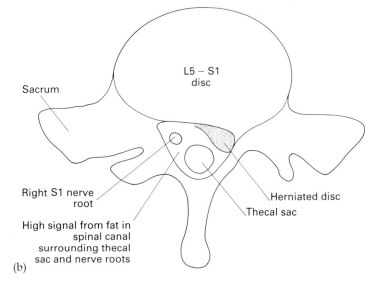

(b)

Fig. 13.22 Disc herniation. MRI scans. (a) Sagittal
T_1-weighted scan showing a large posterior
herniation of the L4—5 disc (arrows). (b) Axial
T_1-weighted scan of an L5-S1 disc showing a
disc herniation compressing the adjacent nerve
root. The opposite equivalent nerve root can be
clearly seen.

relationship to the presence of symptoms. The main value of MRI is that it can demonstrate herniation of disc material into the spinal canal or exit foramina better than CT or myelography (Fig. 13.22). The principles of diagnosis are similar to those described above for the diagnosis of disc herniation by CT.

Magnetic resonance imaging is now being increasingly used in patients who continue to have symptoms following surgery for back pain. Postoperative scarring can be distinguished from disc herniation with a high degree of accuracy, particularly if contrast enhanced images are obtained following intravenous gadolinium.

Spinal stenosis

A narrow spinal canal may give rise to cord or nerve root compression especially when spondylotic changes supervene. Symptomatic spinal stenosis is encountered in the cervical and lumbar regions.

In the cervical region the anteroposterior diameter of the spinal canal can be easily measured on the lateral radiograph. It is more difficult to assess the dimension of the lumbar spinal canal on conventional films, but stenosis can be suspected if the interpedicular distance is small and the depth of the pedicles is reduced.

Computed tomography or MRI are ideal methods of demonstrating the size and shape of the spinal canal and so diagnosing spinal stenosis. They will also show disc protrusions and any bony or soft tissue encroachment upon the narrowed spinal canal.

Myelography can be used to visualise the narrowed spinal canal. In some cases, there is complete obstruction of the contrast column due to the associated spondylotic changes.

Spondylolisthesis

The term spondylolisthesis refers to forward slip of one vertebral body on the one below it, a condition which occurs most frequently at the lumbosacral junction and between the fourth and fifth lumbar vertebrae. It is usually the result of a defect between the superior and inferior articular facets (the pars interarticularis). The defect in the pars interarticularis is thought to be a stress fracture. It can usually be identified on the lateral projection but may sometimes be better seen on oblique films (Fig. 13.23). Minor degrees of slip can also occur without a break in the pars interarticularis, if there is degenerative disc disease with osteoarthritis in the apophyseal joints.

Spondylolysis is the term given to a defect in the pars interarticularis without a forward slip of one vertebral body on the other.

Defects in the pars interarticulares are readily identified with CT, but the plain film examination usually suffices.

Spina bifida

Spina bifida is a result of incomplete closure of the vertebral canal, usually in the lumbosacral region, which may be associated with an abnormality affecting the spinal cord. In severe cases presenting at birth there may be protrusion of the spinal cord (meningomyelocele) or its membranes (meningocele) from the spinal canal. In these cases the laminae of several vertebrae will be absent and the distance between the pedicles will be increased. Complex malformations of the vertebral bodies and the contents of the spinal canal (spinal dysraphism) may also be present. In such cases, CT/MRI can provide useful information. Antenatal diagnosis by ultrasound is now possible (see p. 277).

Frequently, the patient has no externally visible abnormality and no neurological defect, but failure of bony fusion of the two laminae is seen radiologically. This may occur at any level but is common in the lumbosacral region, and in these cases it is without significance (Fig. 13.24).

Ankylosing spondylitis

Ankylosing spondylitis affects principally the sacroiliac joints and the spine, although occasionally other

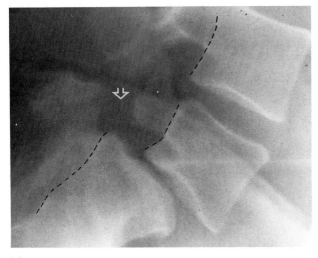

(a)

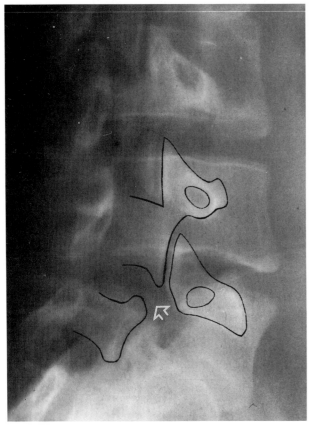

(b)

joints may be involved as well. Both sacroiliac joints are invariably affected by the time spinal involvement has occurred. The earliest radiological change is fuzziness of the joint margins, followed by frank erosions (Fig. 13.25a). Eventually, the process leads to obliteration of the joint space.

In the spine the spinal ligaments ossify, forming vertically oriented bony bridges between the vertebral bodies. The posterior apophyseal and the costotransverse joints become fused. In advanced cases the whole spine is rigidly fused and becomes a solid block of bone. From its plain radiographic appearance this is known as a 'bamboo spine' (Fig. 13.25b).

Spinal cord compression

A conventional or CT myelogram (see Fig. 13.27) is performed in most cases of spinal cord compression, but examining the plain films and CT scans without myelographic contrast medium is also important, because in some instances the cause will be visible and the injection of a contrast agent can be avoided. Although the level of compression will be correctly

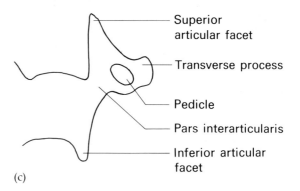

(c)

Fig. 13.23 Spondylolisthesis. (a) Lateral view. There is forward slip of L5 upon S1. The dotted lines which mark the posterior aspects of the vertebral bodies should form a smooth curve. The defect in the pars interarticularis is arrowed. (b) Oblique view showing the defect in the pars interarticularis (arrow). On the oblique view a shape resembling the front end of a 'scottie dog' can be recognised. (c) The 'scottie dog'. A defect in the pars interarticularis is seen as a break in the dog's neck.

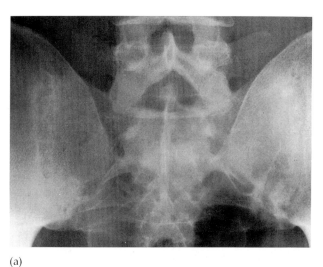

(a)

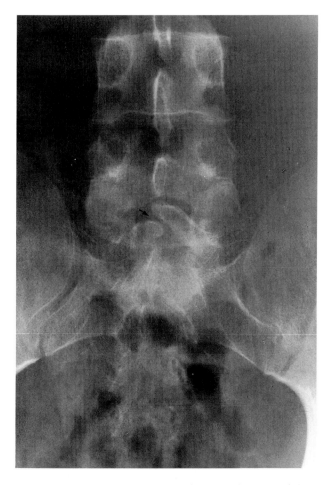

Fig. 13.24 Failure of bony fusion of the two laminae of the first part of the sacrum (arrow) is a common finding without significance.

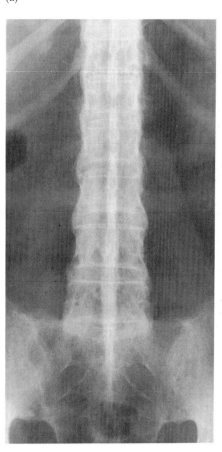

Fig. 13.25 Ankylosing spondylitis. (a) The sacroiliac joints have an irregular fuzzy outline. (b) With advanced disease the whole spine becomes fused (bamboo spine). Note that the sacroiliac joints are also fused.

(b)

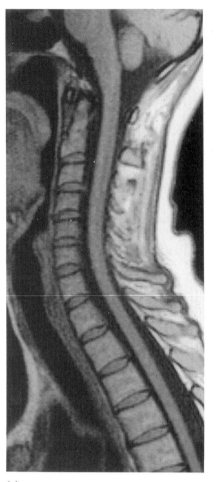

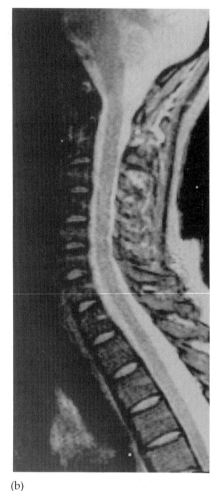

(a)

(b)

Fig. 13.26 MRI of normal spinal cord and thecal sac. Sagittal sections. (a) T_1-weighted image. (b) T_2-weighted image. The spinal cord and the surrounding cerebrospinal fluid can be clearly seen on both images. Note also how well the vertebral bodies and discs are demonstrated.

predicted by clinical examination, a myelogram will also demonstrate the exact site, and often the nature and extent, of the abnormality; information that is important should surgery be necessary.

Magnetic resonance imaging is an excellent test to demonstrate the cause of spinal cord compression, since it shows the spine, extradural tissues, subarachnoid space and intrathecal contents with one non-invasive examination (Fig. 13.26).

The causes of compression of the spinal cord are usually divided according to the site of origin of the responsible space-occupying lesion:

1 Extradural lesions, e.g. metastases (Fig. 13.27), spinal tuberculosis, cervical disc herniation and the bone and soft tissue reactions that accompany cervical spondylosis. It is worth remembering here that lumbar disc herniations are too low to compress the spinal cord, which does not extend below L1.

2 Intradural but extramedullary lesions, i.e. within the dura but not within the spinal cord, e.g. neurofibroma (Fig. 13.28) and meningioma.

3 Intramedullary lesions, i.e. within the spinal cord, e.g. spinal cord tumour or haemorrhage into the spinal cord (Fig. 13.29).

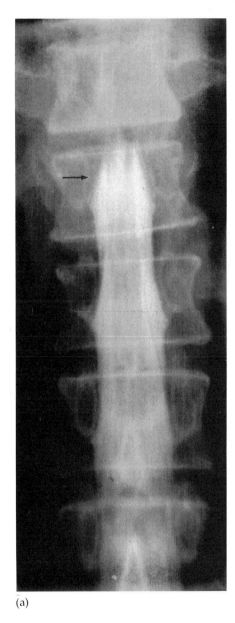

(a)

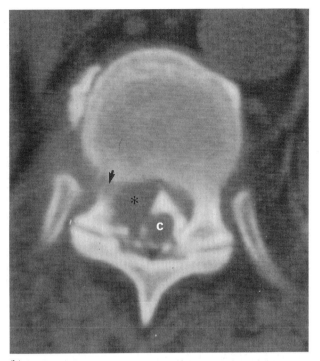

(b)

Fig. 13.27 Spinal cord compression. (a) Myelogram. Contrast has been injected into the subarachnoid space. This film has been taken with the patient lying head downwards and the flow of contrast is arrested in the lower thoracic region due to an extradural block (arrow) caused by metastatic deposits from a carcinoma of the bronchus. (b) CT myelogram, in the same patient, at the level of the block, showing extradural tumour (∗) displacing the opacified subarachnoid space to the left and destroying the right pedicle at this level (arrow). C, spinal cord.

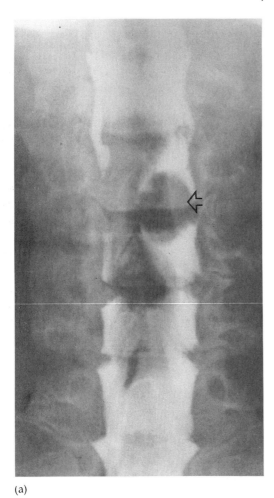

(a)

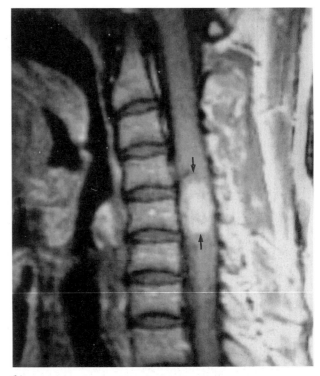

(b)

Fig. 13.28 Intradural neurofibroma. (a) Myelogram showing a filling defect in the contrast column (arrow) in the cervical region. (b) MRI of a similar lesion. The high signal intensity tumour (arrows) on a contrast-enhanced scan was shown to be outside the spinal cord but inside the spinal canal on the axial sections.

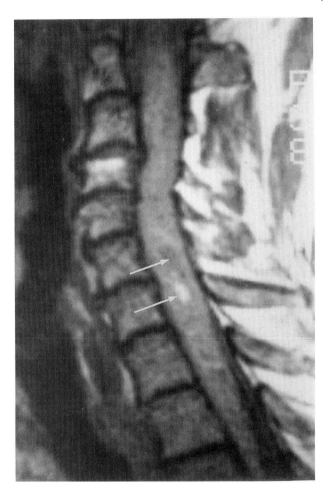

Intrinsic disorders of the spinal cord

Prior to the introduction of CT and MRI, the only disorders of the spinal cord that could be imaged were those that produced deformity of the outline of the cord at myelography, such as tumours and syringomyelia. Computed tomography scanning added comparatively little. Magnetic resonance imaging is rapidly becoming the modality of choice for imaging the spinal cord. Conditions which expand the cord, such as tumours, syringomyelia and hydromyelia, and some haematomas, are readily diagnosed by a combination of altered signal within the cord and expansion of its outline (Fig. 13.29). It is also possible to diagnose some conditions which do not give rise to space-occupying lesions, such as plaques of demyelination in multiple sclerosis and small areas of haemorrhage, because the signal from these pathological processes is very different to that of the adjacent normal nerve tissue.

Fig. 13.29 MRI scan showing haematoma within the spinal cord. The small area of mixed high signal (lower arrow) and low signal (upper arrow) is due to a spontaneous haemorrhage.

14

Bone Trauma

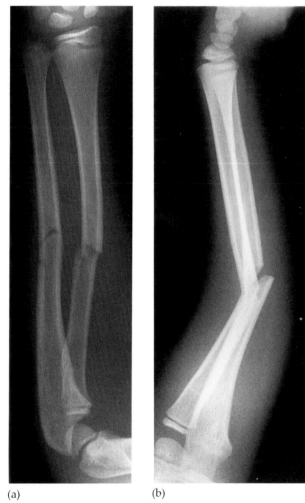

(a)　　　　　(b)

Fig. 14.1 Fracture of forearm showing the value of two views. (a) The fractures of the radius and ulna show little displacement on the frontal projection. (b) The lateral view, however, shows a marked angulation.

Plain radiographs

Plain radiography in bone trauma is invaluable in order to:

- Diagnose the presence of a fracture or dislocation.
- Determine whether the underlying bone is normal or whether the fracture has occurred through abnormal bone (pathological fracture).
- Show the position of bone ends before and after treatment of a fracture.
- Assess healing and complications of fractures.

The latter two subjects and details of individual fractures will not be discussed as they are best dealt with in textbooks of orthopaedics. Head injury is discussed on page 411.

In any case of trauma it is essential to take at least two views, preferably at right angles to one another. Sometimes a fracture or dislocation will be seen on only one view and so may be missed unless two views are taken. Similarly, the position of a fracture should never be assessed from a single film (Fig. 14.1).

Some injuries are likely to produce fractures in more than one site. With tibial fractures, for example, the fibula is frequently also broken but the fractures may be a considerable distance apart. Certain bones, e.g. the pelvis and mandible, often fracture in two sites, only one producing severe symptoms. In these situations all likely fracture sites should be included on the films.

Fracture

Frequently, a fracture is very obvious but in some cases the changes are more subtle. Fractures may be

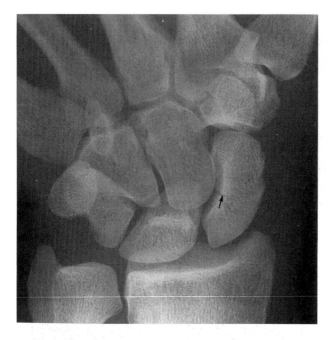

Fig. 14.2 Fracture of the scaphoid appearing as a lucent line (arrow).

recognised or suspected by the following signs:

- *Fracture line*. The fracture usually appears as a lucent line. This may be very thin and easily overlooked (Fig. 14.2). Occasionally, the fracture appears as a dense line due to overlap of the fragments (Fig. 14.3).
- *A step in the cortex* may be the only evidence of a fracture (Fig. 14.4).
- *Interruption of bony trabeculae* is of use in impacted fractures where there is no visible lucent line. This is, however, a difficult sign to evaluate (Fig. 14.5).
- *Bulging or buckling of the cortex* is a particularly important sign in children, where fractures are frequently of the greenstick type (Fig. 14.6).
- *Soft tissue swelling* may be a valuable guide to the presence of an underlying fracture.
- *A joint effusion* may become visible following trauma. In the elbow, where an effusion often indicates a fracture, fat pads lie adjacent to the joint capsule and if there is an effusion they will be displaced away

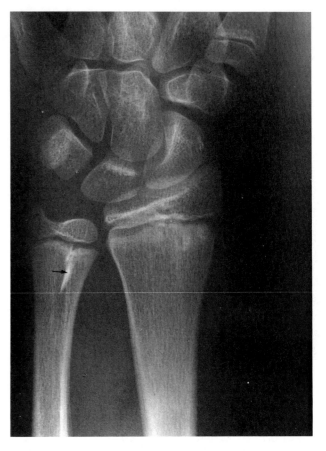

Fig. 14.3 Fracture of the ulna appearing as a sclerotic line (arrow).

from the shaft of the humerus on the lateral view (Fig. 14.7).

Dislocation

The joint surfaces no longer maintain their normal relationship to each other. An associated fracture should be carefully looked for.

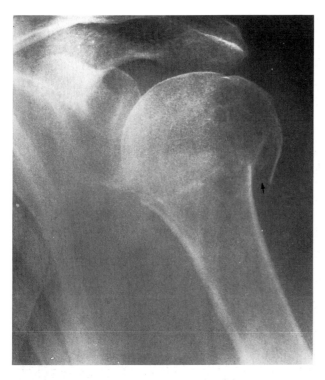

Fig. 14.4 Fracture of neck of humerus appearing as a step in the cortex (arrow).

Further plain film views

Injuries may sometimes be invisible even with two views taken at right angles to each other. If the radiographic findings are equivocal, or if there is clinical suspicion of bony injury with normal radiographs, then further films should be taken as follows:

• *Different projections*, e.g. oblique views (Fig. 14.8).

• *Stress films*. A film taken with a joint under stress may show that it is unstable, due to ligamentous damage. Stress films are helpful in ankle injuries when forced inversion and eversion may show movement of the talus.

• *Flexion and extension views*. In the cervical spine, injury may cause alteration in the alignment of the posterior borders of the vertebral bodies. This is usually much more obvious on a film taken with the neck flexed (Fig. 14.9). In the conscious patient pain

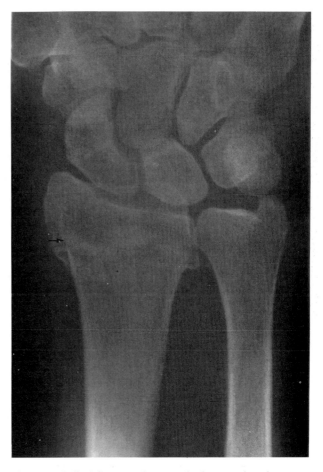

Fig. 14.5 Colles' fracture showing the bony trabeculae are interrupted across the fracture site (arrow). There is also a step in the cortex.

will prevent damage to the spinal cord from instability of the cervical spine, providing the movement is carried out by the patient himself. Flexion and extension views should not be carried out on the unconscious patient.

• *X-ray the other side*. Comparing with the normal side can be useful in the problem case, particularly if expert help is not available. This applies largely in children where epiphyseal lines and unusual patterns of ossification may simulate a fracture.

• *Delayed films*. If films are taken about 2 weeks after

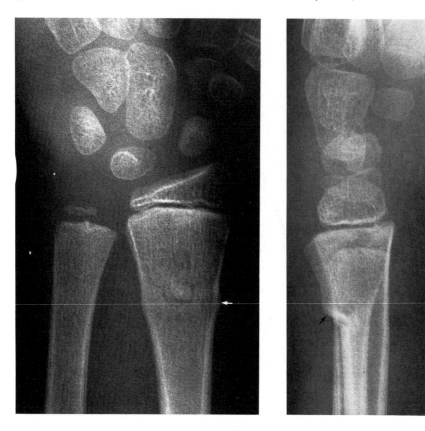

Fig. 14.6 Greenstick fracture of lower end of radius in a child. There is buckling of the cortex (arrows).

injury, resorption of the bone at the fracture site may then reveal the fracture line. This is particularly useful in detecting scaphoid fractures which may be invisible immediately after the injury (Fig. 14.10).

Although plain films suffice in almost all patients who have undergone trauma, in certain incidences other imaging modalities are employed.

Radionuclide bone scanning in bone trauma

Radionuclide bone scans show increased activity at injured sites within 2−3 days (Fig. 14.11a). Increased activity persists for as long as the fractures are healing, often lasting several months. Multiple fractures occasionally give a picture resembling metastases (Fig. 14.11b), but usually the distribution suggests injury (Fig. 14.11c).

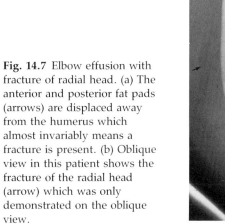

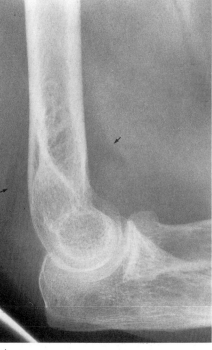

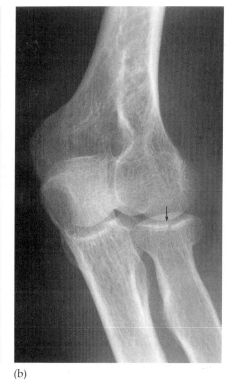

Fig. 14.7 Elbow effusion with fracture of radial head. (a) The anterior and posterior fat pads (arrows) are displaced away from the humerus which almost invariably means a fracture is present. (b) Oblique view in this patient shows the fracture of the radial head (arrow) which was only demonstrated on the oblique view.

(a)

(b)

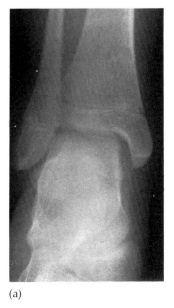

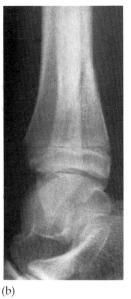

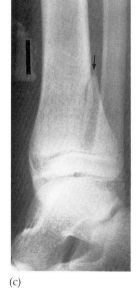

Fig. 14.8 Oblique view to demonstrate a fracture. (a) and (b) AP and lateral views in this child's ankle do not show an obvious fracture. (c) Oblique view clearly demonstrates the fracture (arrow).

(a)

(b)

(c)

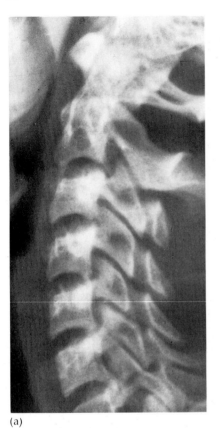

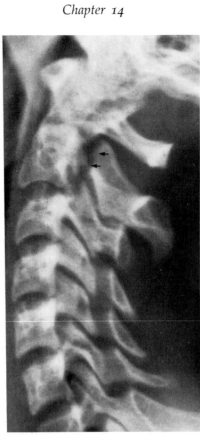

(a)   (b)

Fig. 14.9 Flexion and extension views to demonstrate a fracture. (a) Extension view of cervical spine does not reveal a fracture. (b) Flexion view clearly shows the fracture of the arch of C2 (arrows).

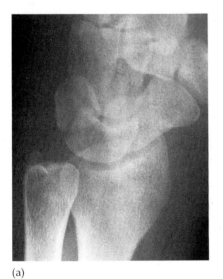

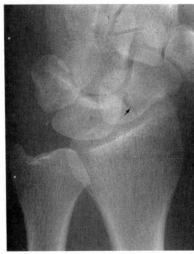

(a)   (b)

Fig. 14.10 Delayed films to demonstrate a fracture. (a) Films taken immediately after injury do not show a fracture. (b) Films taken 2 weeks after injury show a fracture through the scaphoid (arrow).

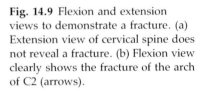

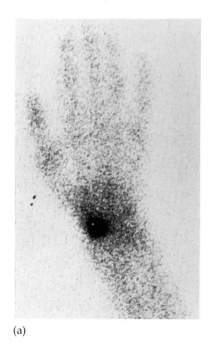

(a)

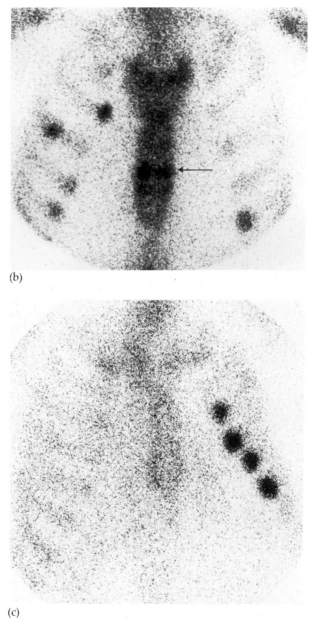

(b)

(c)

Fig. 14.11 Radionuclide bone scans in trauma. (a) Fracture of scaphoid. There is increased activity in the scaphoid in this patient who suffered continuing pain after trauma to the wrist. In spite of normal x-rays the bone scan indicates there is a fracture which was not visible on the radiographs. (b) Multiple fractures following steering wheel injury to the chest. The increased activity due to the many fractures could easily be mistaken for metastases. (The arrow points to a sternal fracture.) (c) Fractures in the anterior ends of four adjacent ribs. Here, the distribution of increased activity is diagnostic of injury; metastases would be more randomly distributed.

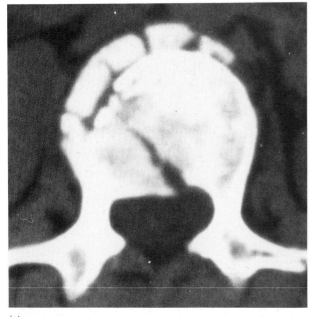
(a)

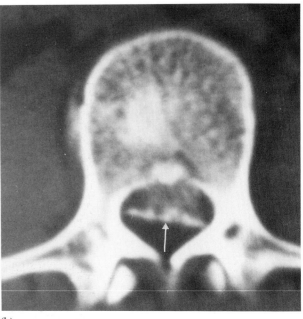
(b)

Fig. 14.12 CT scanning in fractures of the lumbar spine. (a) A comminuted fracture of a vertebral body with slight backward displacement of one half. (b) A large bone fragment (arrow) displaced into the spinal canal.

Computed tomography in bone trauma

The major advantages of computed tomography (CT) over plain films are:
- Better assessment of fractures in bones of complex shape, such as the spine and pelvis. The plan view and the multiplicity of sections are major advantages here. In the spine, fractures of the pedicles, laminae and articular facets as well as fragments displaced into the spinal canal are particularly well seen (Fig. 14.12). In fractures of the pelvis, especially those around the hip joints, CT shows the relationship of the fractures to the joint as well as loose fragments within the joint (Fig. 14.13). Fractures and their displacement, as well as bone fragments in pelvic fractures may be better appreciated by three-dimensional reconstruction of the CT image.
- Better assessment of the extent of soft tissue damage and haematomas and of internal visceral injuries.
- In general, less manipulation of the patient is re-

quired, so that the examination of the severely injured individual is more comfortable and often safer. With modern equipment the examination is often quicker, an important factor in patients with serious internal injuries.

Magnetic resonance imaging in bone trauma

Though useful in demonstrating injury to soft tissues such as muscles, tendons and ligaments, magnetic resonance imaging (MRI) plays no part in the diagnosis of the bone injury itself.

Stress fracture

Stress fractures are due to repeated, often minor, trauma. They occur in athletes, particularly in the tibia and fibula. Another example is the so-called march fracture occurring in the shafts of the metatarsals. Initially, despite the presence of pain, a radiograph

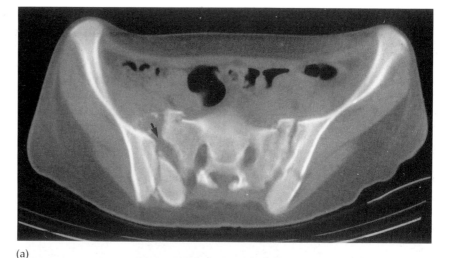

(a)

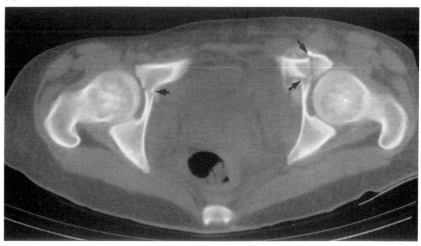

(b)

Fig. 14.13 Fracture of the pelvis. (a) A section through the sacrum shows fractures of the sacrum and iliac bones. There is separation of the right sacroiliac joint (arrow). (b) A lower section shows fractures through the acetabula (arrows). The fractures and their displacement were much better demonstrated with CT than with radiographs of the pelvis.

will show no evidence of a fracture but if a further film is taken after 10–14 days a periosteal reaction may draw attention to the fracture site, where a thin crack may be visible (Fig. 14.14).

Radionuclide bone scanning can be helpful in distinguishing stress fractures from other causes of pain, since a stress fracture will appear as an area of increased uptake before any changes are visible on the radiographs (Fig. 14.15).

Pathological fractures

A pathological fracture is one that occurs through abnormal bone. Pathological fractures may be the presenting feature of both primary and secondary bone tumours (Fig. 14.16). Often, the causative lesion is obvious. Sometimes, particularly in ribs, metastases responsible for fractures are ill defined and difficult to see. In such cases the diagnosis rests on recognising the irregularity of the margins of the fracture. If there is doubt about the diagnosis it is

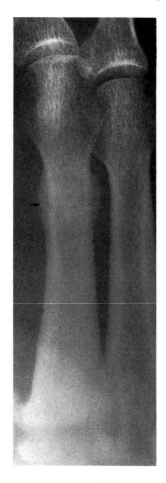

Fig. 14.14 March fracture. This film was taken 2 weeks after the onset of pain. It shows a periosteal reaction (arrow) around the metatarsal shaft although a fracture cannot be seen.

helpful to look elsewhere in the skeleton for other metastases.

Pathological fractures may also occur in osteoporosis and osteomalacia, but the underlying condition may be difficult to diagnose.

Transverse fractures occur through abnormal bone, particularly in Paget's disease. In these instances the Paget's disease is always obvious (Fig. 11.37, p. 324).

Non-accidental injury (battered baby syndrome)

It is essential that everyone looking at radiographs should be fully aware of this condition, as the radiological findings may suggest the diagnosis in otherwise unsuspected cases. If child abuse is suspected the whole skeleton including the skull should be x-rayed, as clinically unsuspected injuries may be detected.

Certain patterns suggest that the injury is not accidental (Fig. 14.17):
- *Multiplicity of fractures* is an important sign, particularly if the fractures are of different ages, because the injuries often take place on separate occasions. Some fractures appear recent, while others show periosteal reaction indicating healing (see also Fig. 11.2a, p. 298).
- *Metaphyseal fractures* frequently appear as small chips from the metaphyses of the long bones. They most probably result from twisting and pulling the limbs of a struggling baby.
- *Metaphyseal sclerosis* is probably due to repeated injury and repair.
- *Epiphyseal separation* is frequently associated with a metaphyseal fracture.
- *Periosteal reactions*. Haemorrhage under the periosteum occurs easily in children. The elevated periosteum lays down new bone which may be so extensive that it envelopes the shaft.

Radionuclide bone scanning is sometimes used to show multiple bone and joint injuries in the non-accidental injury. Such injuries appear as areas of increased uptake and detailed radiographs of these sites can be taken at presentation and again during the follow-up period if the initial radiographs show no abnormality.

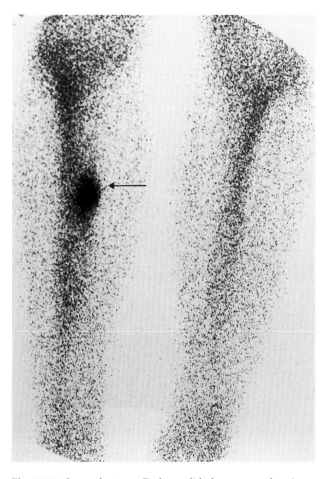

Fig. 14.15 Stress fracture. Radionuclide bone scan showing increased uptake in the tibia (arrow) of this athlete with pain in the leg. The radiographs at the time of the scan were normal.

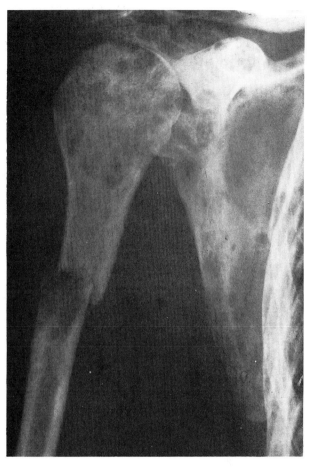

Fig. 14.16 Pathological fracture of the humerus. There are widespread lytic metastases from a carcinoma of the breast.

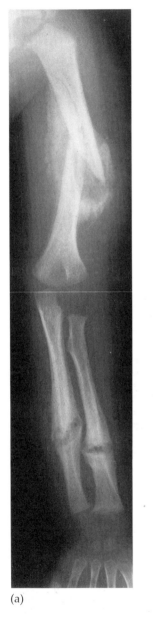

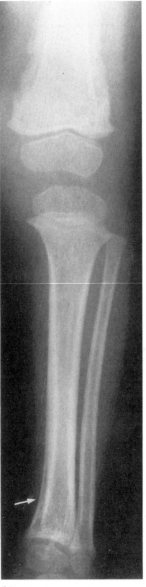

(a)

(b)

(c)

Fig. 14.17 Non-accidental injury. (a) Multiplicity of
fractures. There is a recent fracture of the humerus with
florid callus formation. The fractures of the radius and ulna
are of longer duration and show healing with organised
callus. (b) Periosteal reaction along the shaft of the tibia
(arrow) due to previous trauma with haemorrhage under the
periosteum. There has been recent trauma to the lower end
of the femur with marked periosteal reactions.
(c) Metaphyseal fractures (arrows) and sclerosis around the
knee.

15

Skull and Brain

The newer imaging modalities have had a greater impact on the diagnosis of diseases of the central nervous system than on any other body system. Computed tomography (CT) and magnetic resonance imaging (MRI) have become the standard investigations for most disorders of the brain. Plain films are still the initial investigation for disorders of the bones of the skull—particularly fractures, but otherwise have limited uses. Radionuclide imaging has been almost entirely replaced by CT and MRI. Arteriography, pre-viously a mainstay for many serious disorders, is now limited to demonstrating arterial stenoses, aneurysms and some arteriovenous malformations.

Plain skull films

Normal

The standard views of the normal skull and pituitary fossa are shown in Figure 15.1a–e.

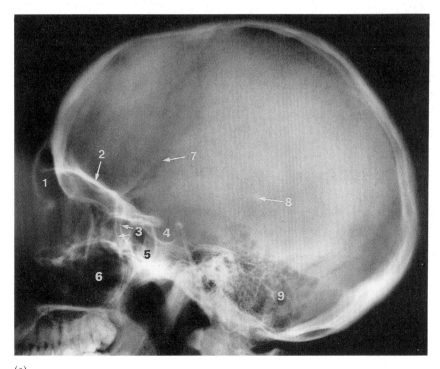

(a)

Fig. 15.1 Standard view of the skull (diagrams show the position in which the films are taken). (a) Lateral view: **1**, frontal sinus; **2**, roof of right and left orbits superimposed; **3**, anterior border of middle cranial fossa; **4**, pituitary fossa; **5**, sphenoid sinus; **6**, maxillary antrum; **7**, vascular groove; **8**, pineal; **9**, mastoid air cells.

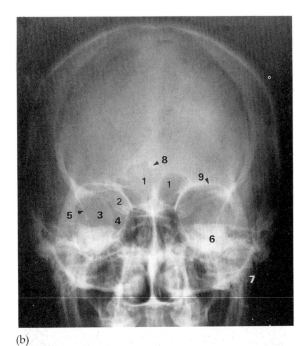

(b)

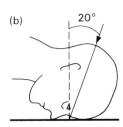

(b)

Fig. 15.1 (Continued) (b) Posteroanterior view: **1**, frontal sinuses; **2**, lesser wing of sphenoid; **3**, greater wing of sphenoid; **4**, superior orbital fissure; **5**, wall of middle cranial fossa; **6**, petrous bone; **7**, mastoid air cells; **8**, pineal; **9**, superior orbital margin.

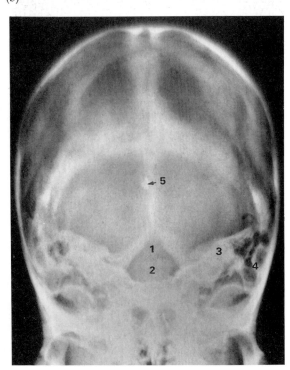

(c)

(c)

Fig. 15.1 (Continued) (c) Towne's view: **1**, foramen magnum; **2**, dorsum sellae of pituitary fossa; **3**, petrous bone; **4**, mastoid air cells; **5**, pineal.

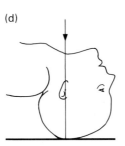

(d)

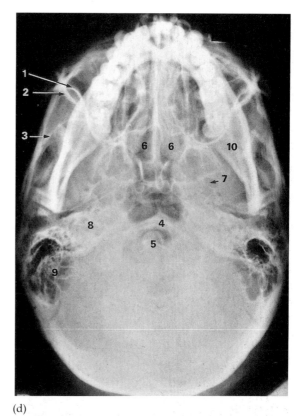

(d)

Fig. 15.1 (Continued) (d) Base or submentovertical view:
1, lateral border of maxillary sinus; **2**, lateral border of orbit;
3, anterior border of middle cranial fossa; **4**, anterior arch of
atlas; **5**, odontoid peg; **6**, sphenoid sinus; **7**, foramen ovale;
8, petrous bone; **9**, mastoid air cells; **10**, mandible.

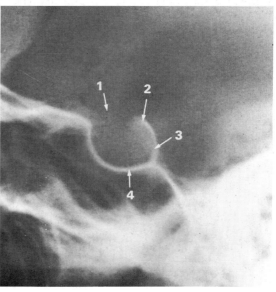

(e)

Fig. 15.1 (Continued) (e) Normal pituitary fossa: **1**, anterior
clinoid process; **2**, posterior clinoid process; **3**, dorsum
sellae; **4**, floor. The white line forming the floor and the
dorsum sellae is known as the lamina dura.

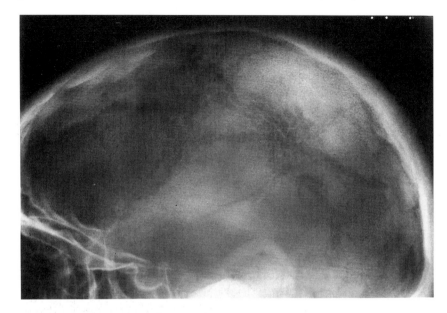

Fig. 15.2 Vascular markings. In this normal skull the vascular markings are very prominent. Note how they form a star-shaped translucency in the parietal region.

The bones of the normal vault have an inner and outer table of compact bone with spongy bone (diploë) between them; the sutures remain visible even when fused and should not be mistaken for fractures. A normal but inconstant suture—the metopic suture, is sometimes seen dividing the frontal bone. Blood vessels cause impressions on the bones of the vault, resulting in linear or star-shaped translucencies (Fig. 15.2) and small lucencies are often seen normally in the inner table near the vertex due to normal arachnoid granulations; they may be difficult to distinguish from small lytic lesions.

The position of a *calcified pineal gland* is the only method of identifying the midline on plain films. The incidence of calcification of the pineal increases with age; it is rarely calcified in children but is seen in about 60% of plain films in adults. The density of the external occipital protuberance on the Towne's view can easily be mistaken for the pineal, so a calcified pineal should never be diagnosed unless it can be seen on the lateral view.

Abnormal plain films

A good method of reviewing plain skull films is to look first for intracranial calcification, then to examine the pituitary fossa and, lastly, to review the bones of the vault and base for areas of lysis or sclerosis and for fractures.

The important plain film signs of intracranial disease are calcification and signs of raised intracranial pressure. Pituitary tumours can be recognised by enlargement of the pituitary fossa.

Intracranial calcifications on plain films

Most intracranial calcification is normal and of no significance to the patient. These calcifications can usually be readily identified from their site (Fig. 15.3). It is, however, very important to recognise those few occasions where the calcification is pathological. The major causes of focal areas of calcification are primary tumours (Fig. 15.4), notably meningioma and glioma, arteriovenous malformation, large aneurysms and old abscesses. Computed tomography or MRI is almost invariably required, either to make the diagnosis

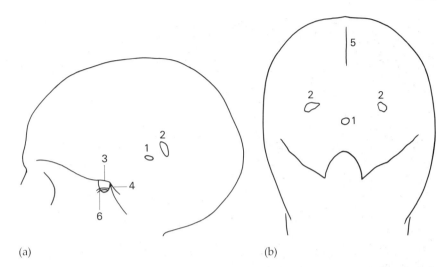

Fig. 15.3 Innocent calcification. (a) Lateral view. (b) Towne's view: **1**, pineal; **2**, choroid plexus, the calcification may be asymmetrical and only one side may calcify; **3**, interclinoid ligament; **4**, petroclinoid ligament; **5**, falx, best seen on frontal projection; **6**, atheromatous calcification in carotid artery.

(a)

(b)

or to show the shape and extent of the underlying abnormality.

Tuberose sclerosis, congenital toxoplasmosis and cytomegalic virus infection may cause multiple small discrete calcifications within the brain.

Raised intracranial pressure

Plain film abnormalities are only seen in prolonged cases of raised intracranial pressure. In children under eight, the sutures are widened (Fig. 15.5) whereas in older children and adults there is erosion of the lamina dura of the dorsum sellae, i.e. it becomes ill defined (Fig. 15.6). This may be very hard to evaluate, particularly in older people.

Enlargement of the pituitary fossa

Tumours of the pituitary are the commonest cause of enlargement or 'ballooning' of the pituitary fossa (Fig. 15.7). With prolactin secreting adenomas the rest of the skull will be normal, but in patients with growth hormone secreting adenomas there may additionally be changes of acromegaly (see p. 329). ACTH secreting tumours responsible for Cushing's disease are usually too small to enlarge the pituitary fossa.

A craniopharyngioma is the common suprasellar

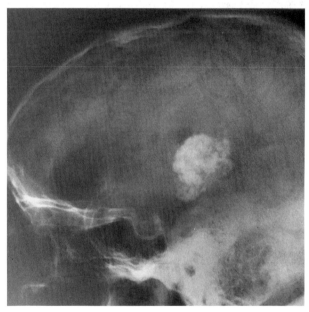

Fig. 15.4 Calcification in a glioma.

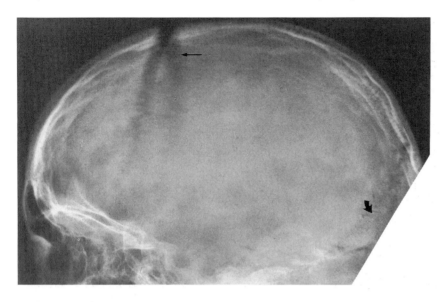

Fig. 15.5 Raised intracranial pressure in a child. The sutures become widened affecting the coronal suture first (straight arrow). Compare this widened suture with the normal lambdoid suture (curved arrow).

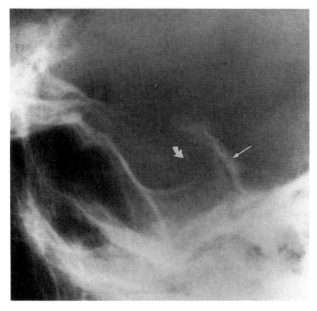

Fig. 15.6 Raised intracranial pressure in an adult. The dorsum sellae of the pituitary fossa (curved arrow) has lost its sharp outline and appears indistinct. The petroclinoid ligament is calcified (arrow).

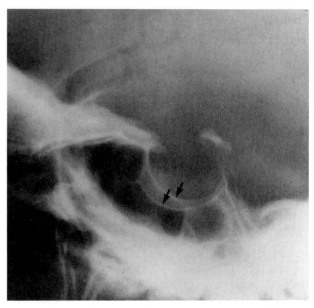

Fig. 15.7 Enlargement of the pituitary fossa with a sloping floor. The floor appears as a double line on the lateral view (arrows).

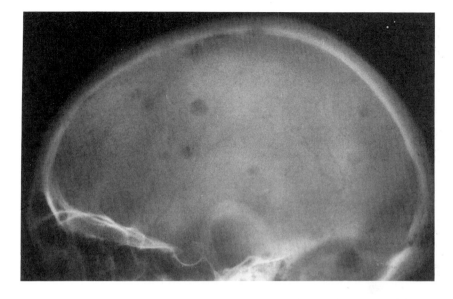

Fig. 15.8 Myeloma. Several well-defined lytic lesions of various sizes are seen in all areas of the skull vault.

tumour in children. It may flatten or enlarge the pituitary fossa and commonly calcifies.

Bone lysis

Areas of bone lysis usually indicate metastasis or myeloma (Fig. 15.8). Large areas of bone destruction are seen in histiocytosis X, giving the appearance known as 'geographical skull' (Fig. 15.9), and in osteoporosis circumscripta, which is a form of Paget's disease.

Bone sclerosis

The commonest cause of bone sclerosis is hyperostosis frontalis interna: a condition of no clinical significance, in which there is irregular thickening of the inner table of the skull in the frontal regions sparing the midline (Fig. 15.10).

Localised sclerosis, sometimes mixed with lytic areas, may be caused by a meningioma (Fig. 15.11), metastasis or fibrous dysplasia. An osteoma causes a well-defined density which may arise from the outer table of the skull. Osteomas occur particularly in the frontal sinuses.

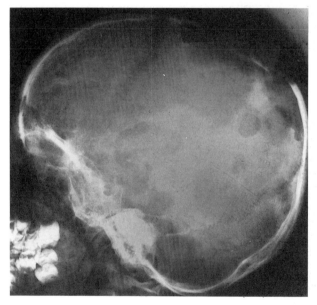

Fig. 15.9 Histiocytosis X. In this child's skull vault there are large irregularly shaped lytic areas. This appearance is known as a geographical skull.

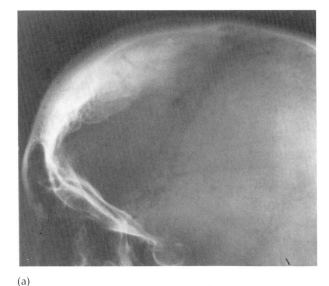

(a)

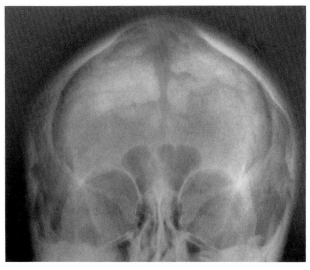

(b)

Fig. 15.10 Hyperostosis frontalis interna. (a) Lateral view showing sclerosis in the frontal region near the vertex. (b) The frontal view shows the characteristic sparing of the midline.

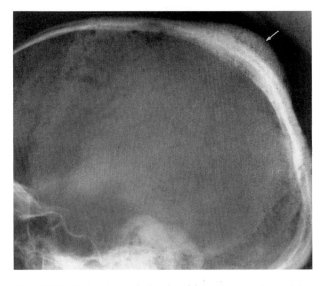

Fig. 15.11 Meningioma. A localised hyperostosis (arrow) is seen on the parietal bone.

Paget's disease (Fig. 15.12) is the commonest cause of generalised sclerosis in the United Kingdom, but is much less common in the United States. It may take the form of multiple patchy areas of increased density. A striking feature is thickening of the skull vault. Recognition of this thickening is important in distinguishing Paget's disease from sclerotic metastases. Basilar invagination may also be seen due to softening of the bone. In basilar invagination the odontoid peg encroaches on the foramen magnum and may press on the brain stem, giving rise to clinical symptoms and signs.

Skull fractures

Skull fractures are discussed on page 411 together with the other plain film signs of head injury.

Computed tomography and MRI

In most neurological disorders, the plain films are either normal or the abnormalities are too non-specific for the diagnosis to be made. Computed tomography

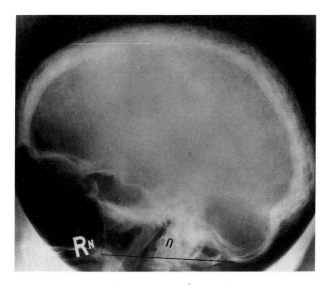

Fig. 15.12 Paget's disease. There is generalised sclerosis with marked thickening of the bone. Basilar invagination is present which can be detected by drawing a line from the back of the hard palate to lowermost part of the occiput. The tip of the odontoid peg should not be more than 6 mm above this line. In this case it is 18 mm.

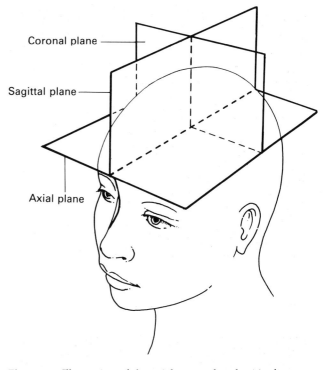

Fig. 15.13 Illustration of the axial, coronal and sagittal planes.

and MRI give vastly more information and one or other investigation is indicated in practically all patients with intracranial disease.

Computed tomography of the brain

A routine examination of the brain involves making nine or ten axial sections. The axial plane is the routine projection but it is sometimes possible to obtain direct coronal scans, or alternatively computer reconstructions can, in selected circumstances, be made from the axial sections which then provide images in the coronal or sagittal planes (Fig. 15.13). The window settings are selected for the brain, but may be altered to show the bones.

Contrast enhancement for CT

An intravenous injection of contrast medium is often given because an abnormality not seen on pre-contrast scans may be rendered visible following contrast enhancement. Occasionally, this is due to the contrast accumulating in larger blood spaces, but more commonly it is due to breakdown of the blood−brain barrier allowing contrast to enter the lesion. Such breakdown occurs mainly with neoplasm, ischaemia and inflammation.

The use of contrast enhancement varies in different centres. It tends not to be used in patients who are known to have a very recent cerebral haemorrhage or infarct, because it has been shown that contrast medium has an injurious effect on acutely ischaemic brain.

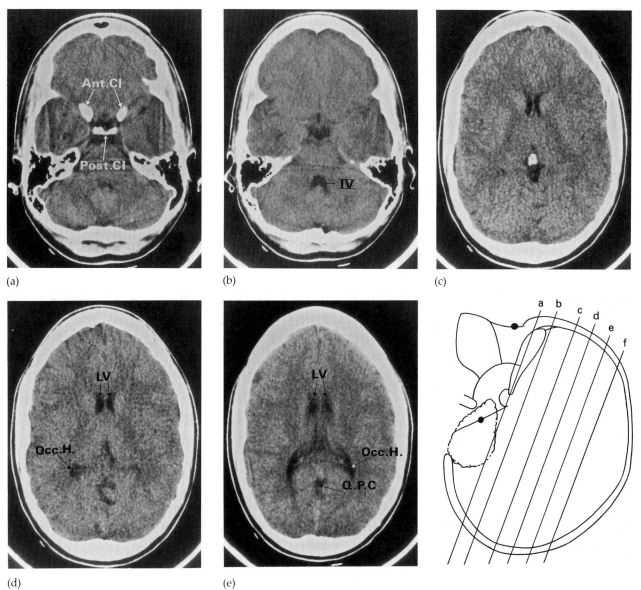

(a)   (b)   (c)

(d)   (e)

Fig. 15.14 Normal head CT. The images on the page opposite are representative sections from a post-contrast series. Those on this page are the pre-contrast images from the same patient. The levels at which the sections were taken are indicated in the diagram.

a.c.a	anterior cerebral artery	LV	lateral ventricle	Post. Cl	posterior clinoid process
Ant. Cl	anterior clinoid process	Occ. H	occipital horns	PS	pituitary stalk
CP	choroid plexus	P	pineal gland	Q.P.C.	quadrigeminal plate cistern
Fa	falx cerebri	Pe	petrous bone	III	third ventricle
m.c.a.	middle cerebral artery	p.c.a.	posterior cerebral artery	IV	fourth ventricle

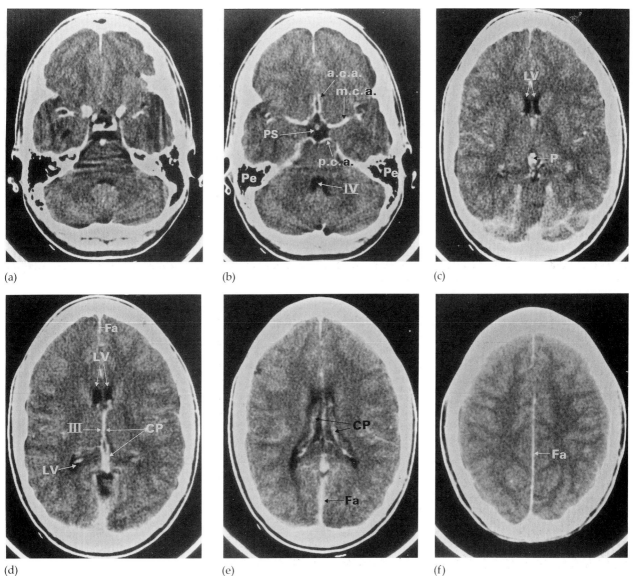

Fig. 15.14 (Continued)

Normal head CT

A normal CT scan of the head is illustrated in Fig. 15.14. The cerebrospinal fluid (CSF) is seen as water density within the ventricular system and subarachnoid space, and is clearly different in density to the normal brain substance. With modern scanners and the use of intravenous contrast enhancement, it is possible to distinguish the white and grey matter of the brain. The larger arteries at the base of the brain as well as the venous sinuses can be recognised when opacified by contrast medium. The falx appears denser than the brain. The supratentorial regions are usually well shown, but details of the posterior fossa may be

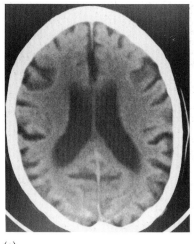

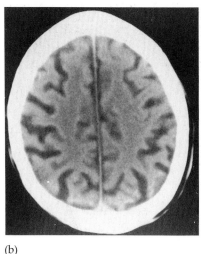

(a)   (b)

Fig. 15.15 Cerebral atrophy. CT scan. The ventricles are dilated due to atrophy of the brain substance and the cortical sulci are widened. (a) Section through bodies of lateral ventricles. (b) Section above level of lateral ventricles (the midline linear density is the falx).

obscured by artefacts from the overlying temporal and occipital bones.

Abnormal head CT

The cardinal signs of an abnormality on a CT scan are:
- abnormal tissue density
- mass effect
- enlargement of the ventricles.

Abnormal tissue density

Abnormal tissue may be of higher or lower density than the normal surrounding brain. High density is seen with recent haemorrhage (see Fig. 15.25, p. 406), calcified lesions (see Fig. 15.20a, p. 401) and areas of contrast enhancement (see Fig. 15.19, p. 400). Low density is usually due to neoplasms or infarcts, or is due to oedema, which commonly surrounds neoplasms, infarcts, haemorrhages and areas of inflammation. Oedema characteristically shows finger-like projections and does not enhance with intravenous contrast medium (see Fig. 15.18, p. 399). As a rule it is not possible to diagnose the nature of a mass based on attenuation values alone; an exception being lipoma which, because it contains fat, has a value of approximately − 100 Hounsfield units.

Mass effect

The lateral ventricles should be examined to see if they are displaced or compressed. Shift of midline structures, such as the septum pellucidum (the thin membrane separating the lateral ventricles), the third ventricle, or the pineal, is a common finding with masses. Ventricular dilatation will occur if the mass obstructs the flow of CSF. Specific diagnoses are suggested by combining the clinical features with information about multiplicity, size, shape, position and density of the lesion, all of which are known with great accuracy from CT.

Enlargement of ventricles

There are two basic mechanisms which cause the cerebral ventricles to enlarge:
1 Obstruction to the CSF pathway — either within the ventricular system (non-communicating hydrocephalus) or over the surface of the brain (communicating hydrocephalus).
2 Secondary to atrophy of brain tissue (Fig. 15.15).

CT scanning can provide an accurate picture of the size of the various ventricles, cerebral sulci and subarachnoid cisterns. With this information it may be possible to predict the nature of the hydrocephalus.

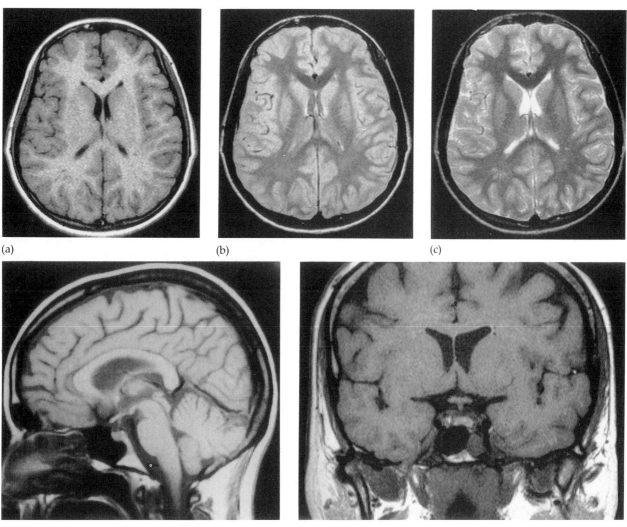

(a)   (b)   (c)

(d)   (e)

Fig. 15.16 Normal brain MRI. The top row of images are axial sections at the level of the lateral ventricles. (a) T_1-weighted image. (b) Balanced image. (c) T_2-weighted image. The bottom two images are (d) midline sagittal section (T_1-weighted) and (e) coronal section through level of frontal horns (T_1-weighted).

Magnetic resonance imaging of the brain

The routine techniques used for magnetic resonance imaging vary from centre to centre. Axial, coronal and sagittal projections are all considered standard (Fig. 15.16) and two of these are usually chosen for a routine examination. This multiplanar capability is particularly useful for assessing the extent of pituitary tumours and for visualising structures in the posterior fossa and craniovertebral junction. A variety of signal sequences are used to create the images: usually T_1-weighted, T_2-weighted and balanced (proton density) images.

No signal is produced from bone, so there is no

bone artefact, which means that the posterior fossa structures are more clearly demonstrated than with CT. It is possible to recognise flowing blood and, therefore, the larger arteries and veins stand out clearly without the need for contrast medium. The characteristics of grey and white matter are different, and both are clearly different from the CSF in the ventricular system and subarachnoid space. Therefore, the anatomy of the brain can be exquisitely displayed.

Contrast enhancement for MRI

The natural differences in signal intensity are sufficiently great that the need for artificial contrast agents is much less with MRI than it is with CT. As discussed on page 12, an MRI contrast agent must have magnetic properties. The first agent introduced for intravenous administration was gadolinium DTPA. Like the intravenous iodinated agents used for computed tomography, gadolinium is excluded from the normal brain substance by the blood–brain barrier (it does, however, accumulate in the pituitary gland). Breakdown of the blood–brain barrier due to tumours, abscess and infarcts means that gadolinium will accumulate within these pathological processes. The tissues containing the gadolinium show very high signal intensity (i.e. appear white) on T_1-weighted images (see Fig. 15.22, p. 403).

The disadvantages of MRI compared to CT are the inability to show calcification, lack of bone detail and the relative expense of the technique, and the difficulty of monitoring seriously ill patients whilst lying within the scanner.

Abnormal MRI of the brain

The range of abnormalities that can be shown by MRI is very great. The principles of diagnosis are the same as with CT, in that the basic signs are a change in signal intensity and evidence of mass effect. The difference is that the range of signal intensities is more various and usually more obvious at MRI than with CT. Fat, subacute and chronic haemorrhage, oedema,

CSF and flowing blood all have characteristic signal intensities. Thus it is more often possible to make a specific diagnosis of an intracranial disorder with MRI than with CT. Nevertheless, many mass lesions such as the various cerebral neoplasms and infections can appear similar to one another in all respects. A note-

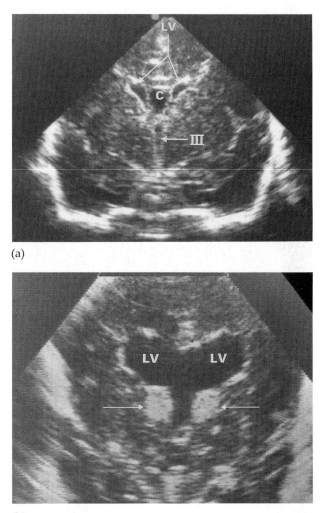

(a)

(b)

Fig. 15.17 Neurosonography. (a) Normal coronal section taken through the anterior fontanelle in a neonate. C, cavum septum pellucidum; LV, lateral ventricle; III, third ventricle. (b) Coronal section showing bilateral subependymal haemorrhages (arrows). The lateral ventricles are dilated.

worthy feature of MRI is its ability to demonstrate plaques of demyelination in multiple sclerosis (see Fig. 15.32, p. 411) and abnormal blood vessels such as arteriovenous malformations (see Fig. 15.29, p. 409).

Neurosonography (Fig. 15.17)

With ultrasound it is simple to scan the heads of neonates and young babies to obtain images of the ventricular system and the adjacent brain. Scanning is best done through an open fontanelle where there is no bone to impede the transmission of ultrasound. Little discomfort is caused to the baby and the procedure is readily carried out even on ill babies in

intensive care units. Neurosonography has proved particularly useful in detecting intracerebral haemorrhage and the ventricular dilatation that may follow. It has also been used to demonstrate the presence and cause of other forms of hydrocephalus and congenital abnormalities of the brain.

Brain tumours

Glioma

At CT (Fig. 15.18), a glioma typically appears as a solitary, irregular mass surrounded by oedema. Compression or displacement of the ventricles can usually

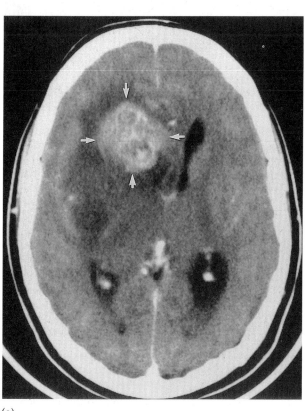

(a)

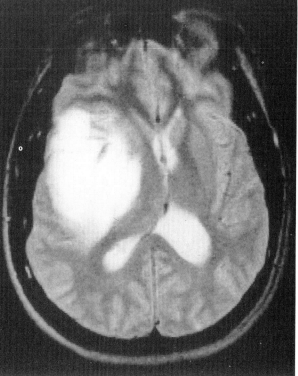

(b)

Fig. 15.18 Glioma. (a) CT scan, post i.v. contrast, showing round mass (arrows) with contrast enhancement and surrounding oedema. Note the compression and displacement of the adjacent lateral ventricles. (b) MRI scan (T_2-weighted) in another patient, showing a large, high-intensity rounded lesion with displacement of the adjacent ventricular system.

be demonstrated. The CT attenuation values of the tumour itself are usually low, but may be high or mixed. Gliomas may calcify; some, particularly the low grade tumours, may be very densely calcified and even visible on plain film (see Fig. 15.4). Most gliomas show partial enhancement with intravenous contrast medium (Fig. 15.18); sometimes only the outer portion enhances, giving the so-called 'ring enhancement' pattern.

AT MRI, the signs are basically the same as for CT. The essential features are a mass, often with adjacent oedema. The mass may show a variety of signal intensities. In general, the tumour is lower in signal intensity than the normal brain on the T_1-weighted images and higher in signal intensity on the T_2-weighted images (Fig. 15.18b). Calcification, though sometimes recognisable as absence of signal, is less evident that it is with CT. The enhancement pattern with gadolinium is similar to the pattern of contrast enhancement at CT.

Brain metastases (Fig. 15.19)

Metastases in the brain may be of high or low density at CT. They usually show contrast enhancement and are often surrounded by substantial oedema. The MRI features are essentially similar. Metastases are typically multiple. A solitary metastasis is indistinguishable from a glioma with either technique.

Meningioma

Meningiomas arise from the vault, falx or tentorium in characteristic sites, the commonest being the para-sagittal region, over the cerebral convexities and the sphenoid ridges. On an unenhanced CT scan, a meningioma is slightly denser than the brain due to calcium in the lesion (Fig. 15.20a). Following intravenous contrast injection the tumour shows marked enhancement (Fig. 15.20b). Sclerosis and thickening of the adjacent bone may also be seen (Fig. 15.11, p. 392).

The multiplanar imaging capability of MRI gives the radiologist the ability to predict the site of origin of the tumour with greater confidence than is usually

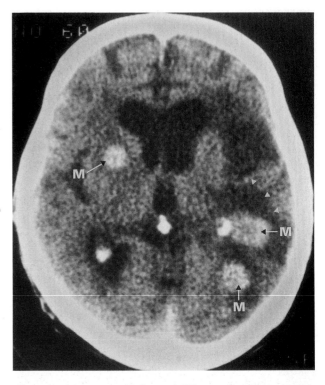

Fig. 15.19 Metastases. Enhanced CT scan showing several rounded areas of increased density (M) surrounded by oedema. The arrow heads indicate the edge of the oedema around one of the larger lesions. The remaining very dense areas are due to the choroid plexus and pineal.

possible with CT (Fig. 15.21). Once it can be ascertained that the tumour is pressing in from outside the brain, the diagnosis of meningioma becomes highly likely.

Acoustic neuroma

Neurofibromas of the acoustic nerve arise in the internal auditory canal or immediately adjacent to the internal auditory meatus in the cerebello-pontine angle. When large, they can be recognised at CT or MRI. When small, they may only be identifiable with MRI. Contrast enhancement improves their visibility with either technique (Fig. 15.22).

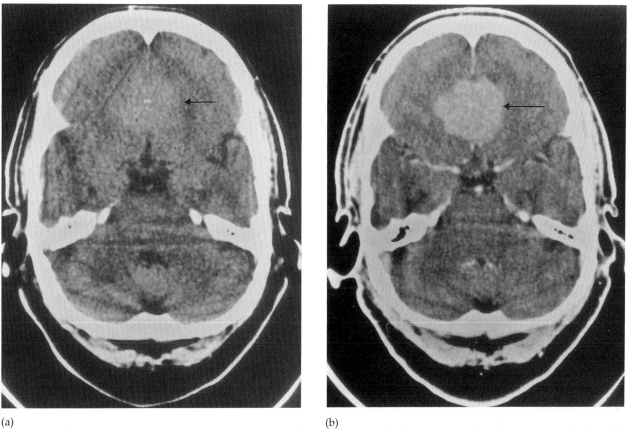

(a)   (b)

Fig. 15.20 Meningioma. (a) Pre-contrast image showing that the density of the meningioma (arrow) is slightly greater than the brain substance due to fine calcification in the tumour. (b) Enhanced CT scan showing a large midline tumour (arrow) beneath the frontal lobes. Note the marked contrast enhancement.

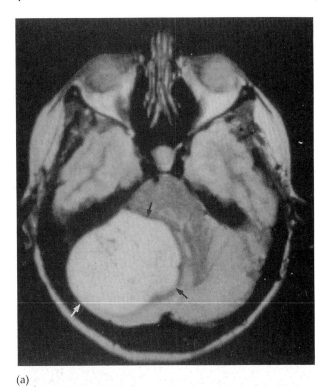

(a)

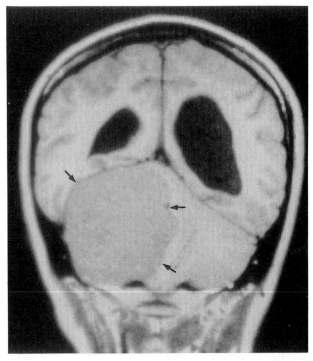

(b)

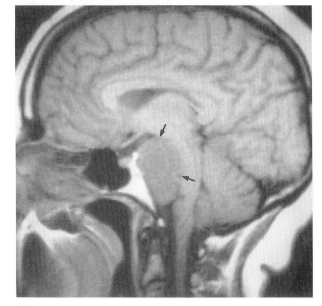

(c)

Fig. 15.21 Meningioma, illustrating the advantages of the multiplanar imaging capability of MRI in a patient with a large meningioma in the posterior fossa (arrows). (a) T_2-weighted axial section. (b) T_1-weighted coronal section. (c) Meningioma (arrows) of the clivus, in a different patient, pressing on the pons (T_1-weighted midline sagittal section).

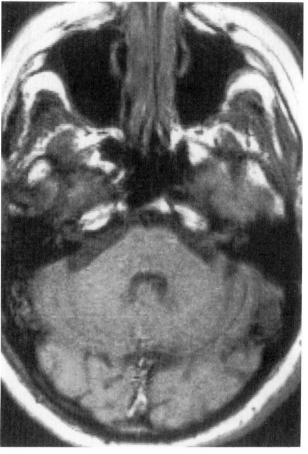 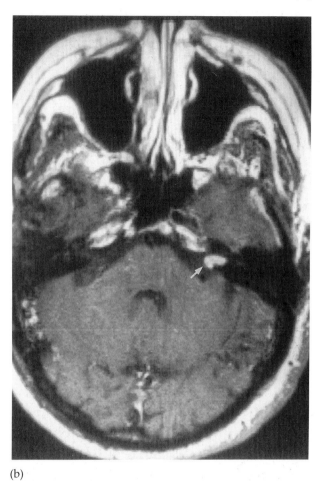

(a)   (b)

Fig. 15.22 Acoustic neuroma, illustrating the use of contrast enhancement at MRI. (a) Pre-contrast MRI scan. The acoustic neuroma is virtually invisible. (b) Post gadolinium enhancement. The small acoustic neuroma (arrow) in the left internal auditory canal is clearly demonstrated.

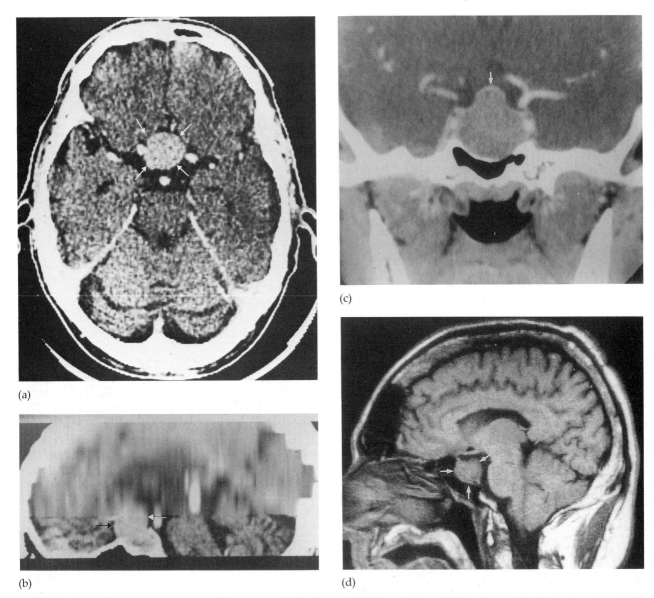

Fig. 15.23 Pituitary tumour. (a) CT scan after contrast shows a mass in the pituitary fossa which enhances vividly (arrows). (b) Sagittal reconstruction indicates the extent of the tumour (arrows). Note that the image reconstructed from thin sections provides adequate detail, whereas that in the upper part of the picture reconstructed from the standard 1 cm thick sections is uninterpretable. (c) Direct coronal image. Post-contrast CT scan in another patient, showing a large tumour expanding the pituitary fossa and projecting superiorly (arrow). (d) MRI scan, in yet another patient, showing a similar tumour (arrows).

Pituitary tumours

To perform CT of the pituitary region entails making thin sections through the pituitary fossa and suprasellar region in the axial and/or coronal plane (Fig. 15.23). Computed tomography not only confirms the enlarged sella but can also demonstrate the pituitary tumour directly, together with any suprasellar extension which may be pressing on the optic chiasm. A large pituitary adenoma may enhance vividly following intravenous contrast administration. Similar appearances, however, may be seen with a large aneurysm, a meningioma and a craniopharyngioma.

Magnetic resonance imaging is particularly suitable for demonstrating the presence and extent of a pituitary tumour (Fig. 15.24). The combined sagittal and coronal imaging planes are ideal, showing very small tumours, smaller than can be seen with CT. Gadolinium en-hancement is particularly useful in finding small, so-called microadenomas of the pituitary. The upward extent of a pituitary tumour, particularly its relationship to the optic chiasm and optic nerves, can be readily demonstrated with MR imaging.

Cerebral infarction and haemorrhage

Acute cerebral infarction and haemorrhage are often clinically similar. Computed tomography can help distinguish between these two entities, because acute intracerebral haemorrhage gives rise to a specific appearance, namely high density due to the haematoma itself (Fig. 15.25). The high density area may be surrounded by a lower density region due to oedema. Depending on the site and amount of bleeding, blood may also be identified in the subarachnoid space and within the ventricles. An acute infarct, on the other

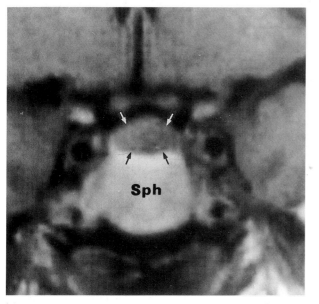

(a)

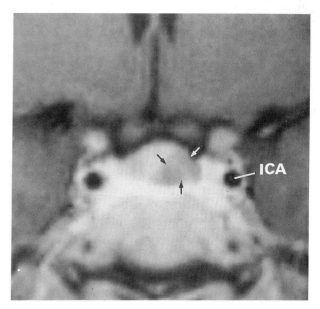

(b)

Fig. 15.24 Very small pituitary adenoma (microadenoma) demonstrated by MRI using gadolinium enhancement. (a) T$_1$-weighted pre-contrast image, which shows slight enlargement of the pituitary. The arrows point to the pituitary. (b) Post-contrast image on which the normal portion of the gland enhances whereas the adenoma (arrows) does not enhance. ICA, internal carotid artery; Sph, sphenoid sinus.

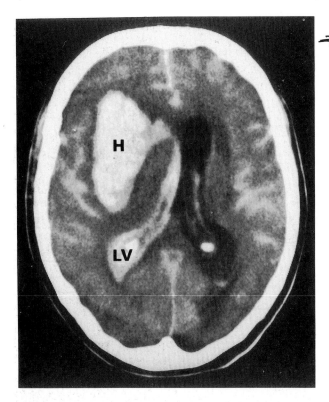

Fig. 15.25 Intracerebral haemorrhage. CT scan showing the haematoma as a high density area (H). Blood is also seen in the displaced lateral ventricle (LV) and in the sub-arachnoid spaces over the cerebral hemispheres. The patient had suffered head trauma.

hand, does not produce any recognisable CT abnormality for the first 24 hours. Interestingly, MRI is not as useful as CT in the first 24 hours following an acute stroke. Even though MRI can demonstrate altered signal from both infarction and haemorrhage, the appearances in the two conditions are indistinguishable from one another using MRI at this early stage.

In the ensuing few days after the onset of stroke, the changes of intracerebral haemorrhage at MRI become more specific. A subacute or chronic haemorrhage develops a specific signal pattern due to breakdown products of haemoglobin, which have a paramagnetic effect that profoundly alters the MR signal in a highly characteristic way (Fig. 15.26). The appearances of intracerebral haemorrhage at CT also change with time. The initial high density of the haemorrhage itself lessens over a week or two, eventually leaving a low density area indistinguishable from an infarct.

Subacute and chronic infarction are recognisable at both CT and MRI. The changes are essentially those of oedema conforming in shape to a known arterial distribution (Fig. 15.27), gradually resolving and sometimes leaving a recognisably atrophic area and/or persistent scar.

Subarachnoid haemorrhage is usually due to a ruptured aneurysm. Only the largest aneurysms are directly visualised at CT, even with intravenous contrast enhancement (Fig. 15.28). Computed tomography is nevertheless the best initial investigation as it may localise the site of bleeding, so that arteriography of the appropriate vessels can be performed. If multiple aneurysms are found at arteriography, the information from CT may indicate which aneurysm has bled. Magnetic resonance imaging can also demonstrate the presence of aneurysms. It will show smaller aneurysms than can be demonstrated with CT, but MRI is not as sensitive as arteriography in this regard. Like CT, MRI may show haematoma adjacent to a ruptured aneurysm.

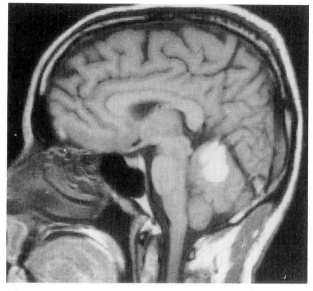

(a)

Fig. 15.26 Cerebral haemorrhage on MRI. (a) A 7-day-old haemorrhage into the superior portion of the cerebellum is clearly shown as a high signal intensity collection on a T_1-weighted image. (b) A chronic haemorrhage in the right cerebral hemisphere shows the complex mixture of high and low signal typical of old haemorrhage.

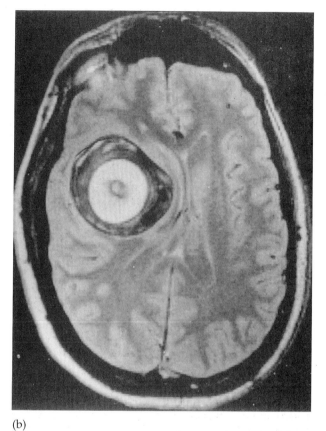

(b)

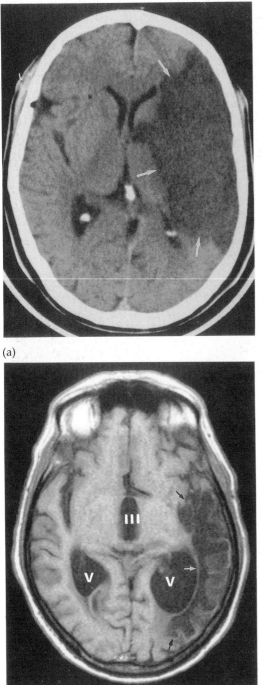

(a)

(b)

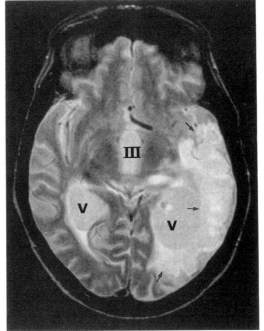

(c)

Fig. 15.27 Cerebral infarction. (a) Unenhanced CT scan showing low density region of left cerebral hemisphere conforming to the distribution of the middle cerebral artery (arrows). (b) and (c) MRI scans of another patient with a large middle cerebral artery territory infarct. The infarcted area (arrows) shows low signal intensity on the T_1-weighted image (b) and high signal intensity on the T_2-weighted image (c). The lateral ventricles (V) and the third ventricle (III) are dilated in this patient.

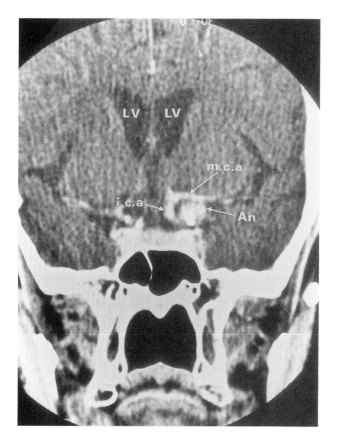

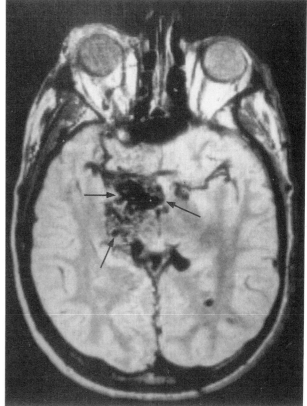

Fig. 15.28 Aneurysm (An) of the left internal carotid artery. This image, unlike most of the other CT scans in this chapter, is a direct coronal scan. LV, lateral ventricle; i.c.a., internal carotid artery; m.c.a., middle cerebral artery.

Fig. 15.29 Large arteriovenous malformation lying deep within the right cerebral hemisphere shown by MRI. The signal void from the fast-flowing blood in the vascular malformation (arrows) and its feeding and draining blood vessels are well demonstrated without the need for contrast medium.

An *arteriovenous malformation* may present with haemorrhage. Computed tomography can demonstrate the abnormal vessels in the region of the haemorrhage, particularly with contrast enhancement. MRI is particularly suitable for demonstrating arteriovenous malformations, because the signal from fast-flowing blood is so very different to that of stationary tissues (Fig. 15.29). It has become the best method of investigation to confirm or exclude this particular diagnosis. As with aneurysms, angiography is then needed to define the vascular anatomy for those cases where surgery is contemplated (Fig. 15.30).

Infection

Inflamed tissue within the brain can be identified as increased contrast enhancement on CT. If abscess formation has occurred, the pus in the centre is of low density. Abscesses, therefore, typically show a 'ring enhancement' pattern (Fig. 15.31). The features at MRI are essentially similar.

Herpes encephalitis may give a near diagnostic appearance of enhancing areas at CT, or altered signal intensity on MR scanning in the temporal lobes.

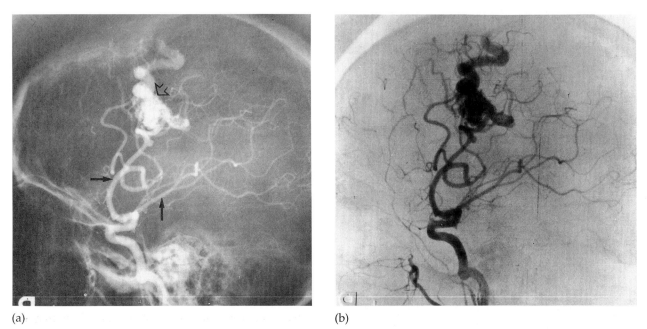

(a)   (b)

Fig. 15.30 Arteriovenous malformation. (a) Carotid angiogram showing a collection of large abnormal vessels (large arrow) supplied by the middle cerebral artery (horizontal arrow). On this injection the posterior cerebral artery (vertical arrow) but not the anterior cerebral artery has filled. (b) Subtraction. With this technique the shadowing due to the bones has almost been eliminated so that the contrast-filled vessels stand out more clearly.

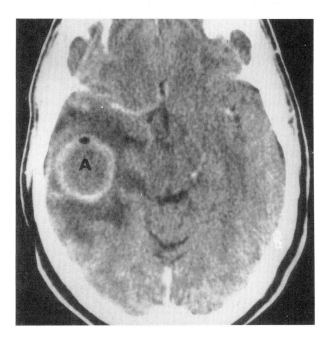

Fig. 15.31 Cerebral abscess in temporal lobe. Post-contrast CT scan showing a spherical mass with central low density and marked ring enhancement from the edge of the abscess (A). A small bubble of gas is seen at the top of the abscess.

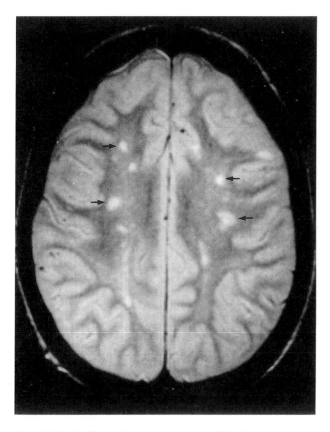

Fig. 15.32 Multiple sclerosis shown by MRI. The high signal intensity plaques of demyelination are well shown on this mildly T_2-weighted image. (The arrows point to representative plaques.)

Multiple sclerosis (Fig. 15.32)

Prior to the introduction of MRI, there was no clinically useful imaging examination for diagnosing multiple sclerosis (MS). It is possible to see severe long-standing MS plaques on contrast-enhanced CT, but it is too insensitive a test to be of clinical use. Magnetic resonance imaging, however, can demonstrate plaques at a time when the diagnosis of MS is not yet certain and can also be used to follow the progress of the disease.

Head injury

Fractures

Most fractures of the skull are still diagnosed on plain films. Fractures appear as linear translucencies, which can be difficult to distinguish from normal vascular markings and sutures. The following analysis may be helpful (Fig. 15.33):

• Fractures sometimes appear more translucent than vascular markings because they traverse the full thickness of the bone.

• Fractures may branch abruptly.

• Fractures have straight or jagged edges, and it is usually possible to see how these edges fit together. Conversely, venous channels have undulating irregular edges which cannot be fitted together.

• Arterial grooves have parallel sides and are, therefore, more easily mistaken for fractures, but they occur in known anatomical sites.

• Sutures also occur in recognised anatomical positions and show definite regular interdigitations. Widening of one suture has the same significance as a fracture.

A depressed fracture often has a different appearance. It appears dense rather than lucent because the fragments overlap. A tangential view is required to show the inward depression. Such a fracture may require surgery in order to elevate it (Fig. 15.34).

An extradural haematoma should be carefully considered if a fracture crosses the groove for the middle meningeal artery.

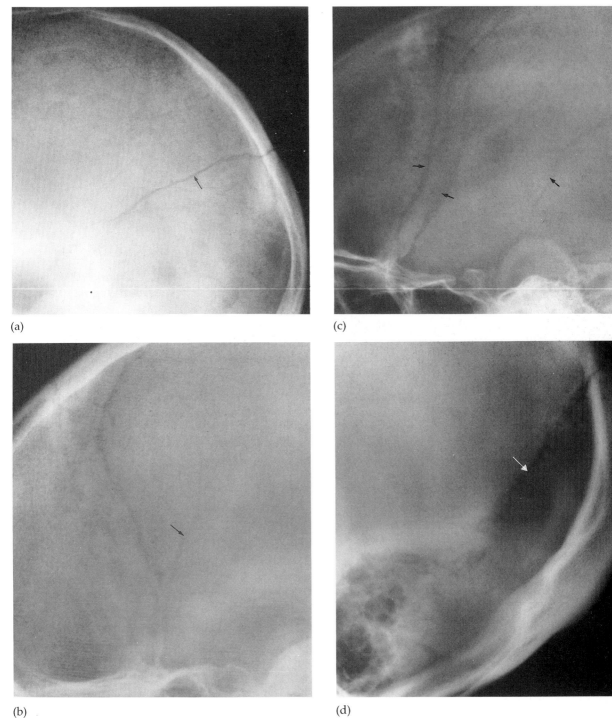

(a)

(b)

(c)

(d)

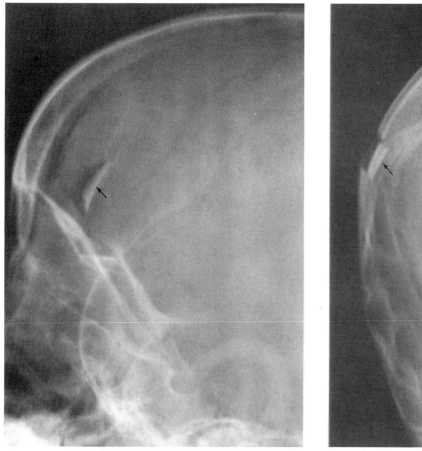
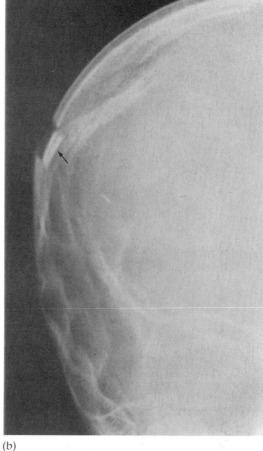

(a)   (b)

Fig. 15.34 Depressed fracture. (a) The fracture is seen as a curvilinear density (arrow) due to the overlapping fragments. (b) In a tangential view (another patient) the fragment can be seen to be depressed inwards (arrow).

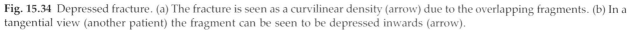

Fig. 15.33 (facing page) Linear markings in the skull vault. (a) Fracture line with straight edges (arrows). (b) Arterial groove for middle meningeal artery (arrow) — line with straight edges occupying a recognised site. (c) Venous channels: wider, more undulating grooves (arrows) — the more posterior groove ends in a venous star. (d) Suture. These show regular interdigitations (arrow).

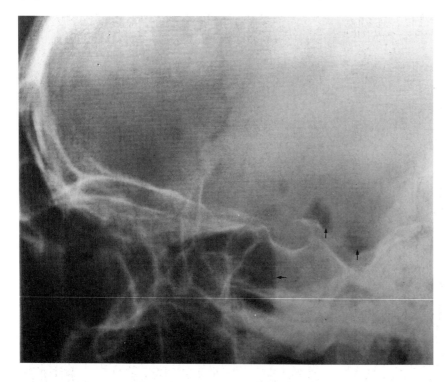

Fig. 15.35 Head injury. Horizontal ray lateral film showing a fluid level in the sphenoid sinus (horizontal arrow) and air in the subarachnoid space (arrows). Although a fracture cannot be identified, these findings indicate that there has been severe skull trauma with a fracture of the skull base and a tear of the dura.

The value of plain films following head injury

Although a fracture is a valuable sign of a head injury, the appearance of a fracture often bears little correlation to the underlying brain damage, and severe brain damage and subdural haematomas can occur in patients with normal skull films.

Plain film signs which indicate significant head injuries are:

1 Shift of the pineal from the midline. This is an important sign as it often indicates an extradural or subdural haematoma. Swelling of one hemisphere due to contusion of the brain can also cause pineal displacement.

2 Fluid levels in the sinuses, or air in the subarachnoid space or ventricles, indicate a fracture with a tear of the dura (Fig. 15.35). Antibiotic treatment is often advocated with this type of injury to prevent meningitis. As with the detection of all fluid levels, it is necessary to take the lateral film with a horizontal ray.

Computed tomography in head injuries

Computed tomography should be carried out in all patients who have had a significant head injury, particularly if there is deterioration in the patient's conscious level or worsening of neurological deficit. (MRI can be used instead, but is rarely necessary.) Computed tomography is initially performed without intravenous contrast administration. Selected cases are then given contrast. Computed tomography scans can distinguish between extracerebral and intracerebral lesions and can separate those patients with compressing haematomas who require immediate surgery from those in whom craniotomy might be of no benefit or might even be harmful.

Extracerebral lesions

Haematomas have a high density for about 2 weeks following the injury (Fig. 15.36a) but after 3–4 weeks

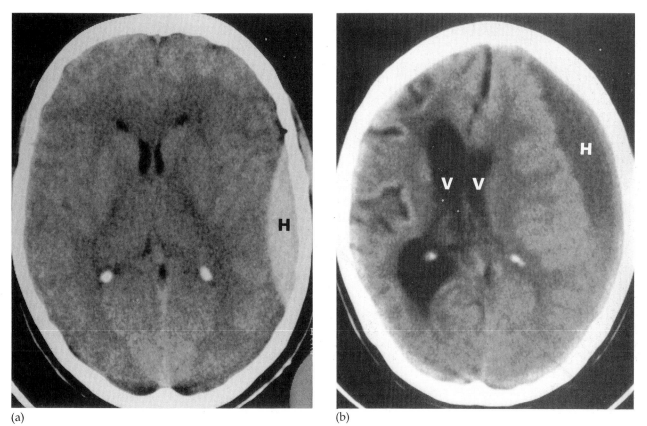

Fig. 15.36 Extracerebral haematoma. (a) CT scan showing a high density lentiform area typical of an acute extradural haematoma (H). (b) CT scan in another patient taken a month after injury showing a subdural haematoma (H) as a low density area. Note the substantial ventricular displacement. V, ventricles.

the density decreases to become lower than that of the brain (Fig. 15.36b). In the intervening period, they pass through a phase of being isodense with the brain and so are invisible on CT scans taken without contrast. Nevertheless, they should be suspected if there is midline or ventricular displacement. The displacement may not be obvious if the haematomas are bilateral.

Extradural haematoma is seen as a lens-shaped, smoothly demarcated high density area situated over the surface of the hemisphere associated with a skull fracture.

Subdural haematoma is similarly shaped and also situated over the surface of the cerebral hemisphere. A fracture somewhere in the skull may or may not be present.

Fractures of the skull base or vault. Fractures of the skull base and through the paranasal sinuses may be difficult or impossible to identify with plain films and should be carefully looked for on CT. Special settings, known as bone windows, may be needed to see subtle fractures.

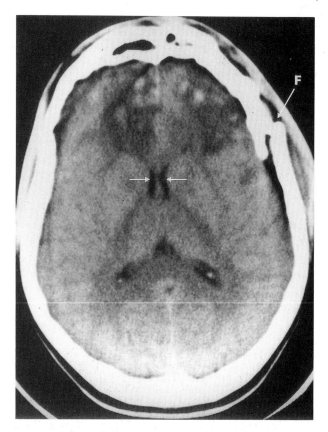

Intracerebral lesions

Oedema. With oedema the whole brain may show swelling with homogeneous low density and compression of the ventricles (Fig. 15.37).

Contusion shows as patchy areas of low density associated with swelling of the brain, causing displacement of the ventricles.

Haematomas are seen as areas of high density which may be multifocal. There may be mass effect causing displacement of the ventricles.

Occasionally a severe head injury can exist with no abnormal CT scan features.

Fig. 15.37 CT scan showing several bilateral frontal lobe contusions. The widespread ill-defined low density is due to oedema: the small high density areas are focal haemorrhages. The lateral ventricles are compressed and therefore small (horizontal arrows). A depressed fracture (F) is also demonstrated.

16

Sinuses, Orbits and Neck

Sinuses

On plain radiographs the normal sinuses are translucent because they contain air. Because of the contrast afforded by the air, plain films still have an important role in sinus disease. It so happens that on an occipitomental view the maxillary antra are approximately the same translucency as the orbits. The frontal sinuses are often asymmetrical and part or all of them may be absent. The mucosa lining the normal sinus is too thin to be visualised.

Thickened mucosa can be recognised on plain films providing there is some air in the sinus (Figs 16.1 and 16.2), by noting the soft tissue density between the air in the sinus and the bony wall. The mucosal thickening may be smooth in outline or it may be polypoid. Polyps may be sufficiently large to extend into the nasopharynx.

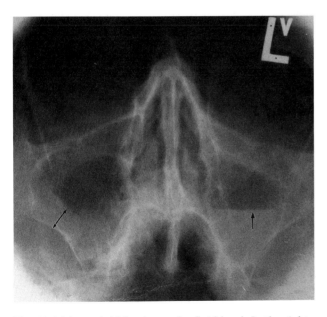

Fig. 16.1 Mucosal thickening and a fluid level. In the right antrum, thickening of the mucosa (arrows) results in the sinus no longer having a thin outline. The horizontal line in the left antrum on this erect film (arrow) indicates a fluid level which remains horizontal even when the patient's head is tilted.

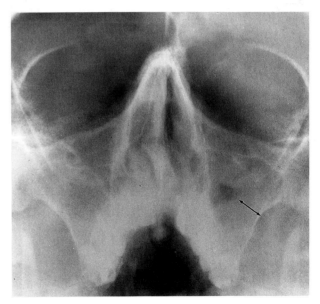

Fig. 16.2 Opaque antrum and mucosal thickening. The right antrum is completely opaque and it appears denser than the orbit. There is gross mucosal thickening in the left antrum (arrow) with only a small amount of air left in the antrum.

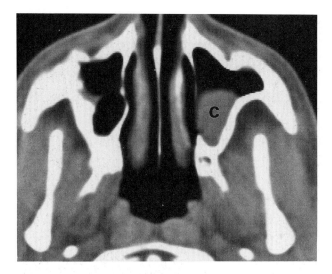

Fig. 16.3 CT scan of maxillary antra. Note the excellent demonstration of the bony margins and how easy it is to see the soft tissue swelling in this case a retention cyst (C). The sinuses are otherwise normal.

Allergy and infection both cause mucosal thickening and it is impossible to say radiologically which condition is responsible.

Fluid in the sinuses is recognised by the presence of a fluid level. With the patient erect, a fluid level appears as a horizontal line across the sinus which remains horizontal even when the patient's head is tilted (Fig. 16.1). Fluid levels are seen with infection in the sinus and also with trauma, when a fracture allows blood or CSF to collect in the sinus.

Both computed tomography (CT) and magnetic resonance imaging (MRI) provide an excellent view of the sinuses (Fig. 16.3). The bony walls are clearly displayed and any mucosal thickening can be readily detected.

The opaque sinus

The sinus becomes opaque when all the air is replaced and it then appears as dense or denser than the adjacent orbit (Fig. 16.2).

The causes of an opaque sinus are:
• *Infection or allergy*. The air in the sinus is replaced

by fluid, or a grossly thickened mucosa, or a combination of the two.
• *Mucocele*. Mucoceles are obstructed sinuses. Secretions accumulate and the sinus becomes expanded. A frontal sinus mucocele may erode the roof of the orbit and cause exophthalmos. Computed tomography clearly shows the size and extent of a mucocele.
• *Carcinoma of the sinus or nasal cavity*. In all opaque sinuses, particularly the antra, special attention should be paid on both plain films and CT to the bony margins, because if these are destroyed, the diagnosis of carcinoma becomes almost certain (Fig. 16.4). Computed tomography is superb at visualising bone destruction, but its greatest value is in demonstrating tumour invasion, by showing the extent of any soft tissue mass which may extend beyond the sinus cavity. The same features can also be seen with MRI. CT and MRI have an important role in treatment planning and in assessing the response to radiotherapy.

Nasopharynx

The adenoids are normally seen on the lateral film in children as a bulge projecting into the nasopharyngeal air passage (Fig. 16.5). Computed tomography and MRI give excellent visualisation of the nasopharynx and can demonstrate the presence of tumour together with any spread into the skull base (Fig. 16.6).

Orbits

Computed tomography and MRI clearly demonstrate the anatomy of the orbits. Imaging is indicated in all patients with exophthalmos since it is possible to distinguish between masses arising within the orbit, masses arising outside the orbit and thyroid eye disease. With an intraorbital mass its relationship to the optic nerve can be determined.

The main causes of intraorbital masses include various tumours, including tumours of the optic nerve (Fig. 16.7), vascular malformations and granulomas. The most common orbital masses originating outside the orbit are tumours or mucoceles of the frontal or

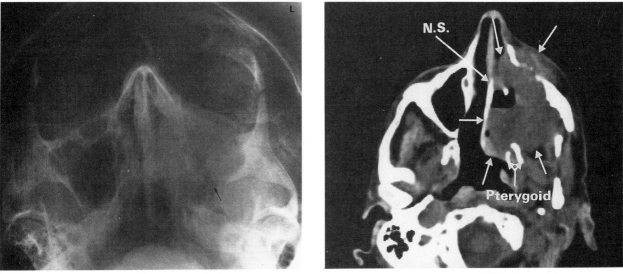

(a)   (b)

Fig. 16.4 (a) Carcinoma of the antrum. The left antrum is opaque and there is extensive destruction of its walls (arrow). Compare with the normal right antrum. (b) CT scan in another patient showing a large mass arising from the antrum destroying its bony walls extending into the adjacent soft tissues and obliterating the nasal cavity. The arrows point to the extent of the tumour. The opposite antrum and pterygoid plates are normal. N.S., nasal septum.

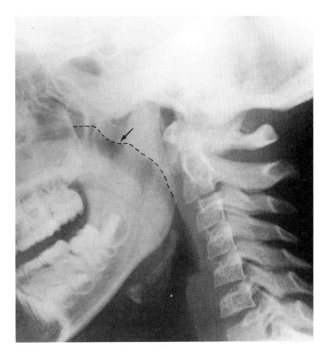

Fig. 16.5 Normal lateral view of postnasal space in a child. The posterior boundary of nasopharyngeal air passage has been marked with dotted lines and there is an impression into it (arrow) caused by the adenoids.

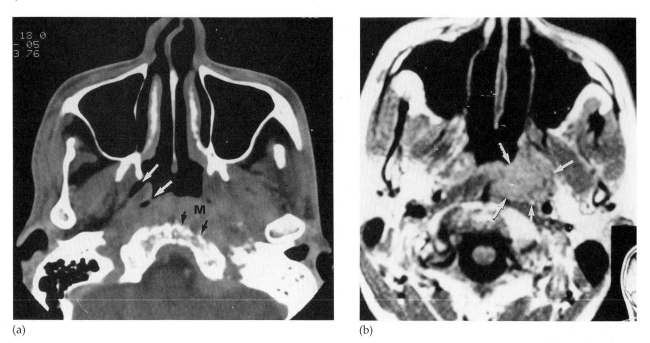

(a)   (b)

Fig. 16.6 Nasopharyngeal carcinoma. (a) CT scan showing a mass (M) in the nasopharynx on the left extending into the soft tissues of the postnasal space and eroding the skull base (black arrows). Note how the tumour obliterates the fossa of Rosenmuller and eustacian recess which are shown on the normal right side (white arrows). (b) MRI scan in another patient clearly showing the extent of the tumour (arrows).

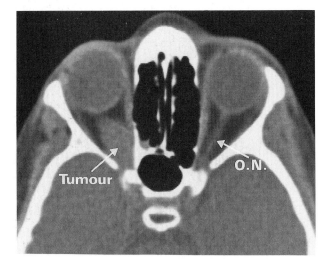

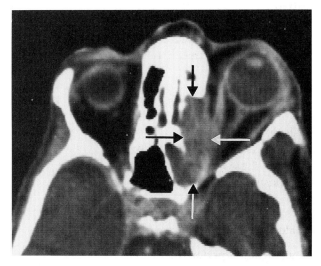

Fig. 16.7 Optic nerve glioma. CT scan showing a soft tissue mass arising from the optic nerve. The opposite orbit demonstrates the normal anatomy. O.N., optic nerve.

Fig. 16.8 Carcinoma of the ethmoid sinus invading the orbit and causing proptosis. The tumour is arrowed.

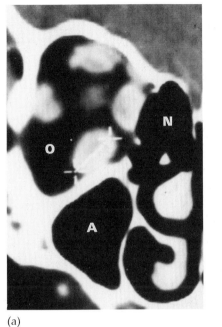

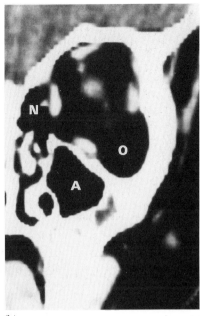

(a) (b)

Fig. 16.9 Thyroid eye disease. (a)
Coronal scan through the orbit
showing enlargement of the
oculomotor muscles; one of them is
shown by crosses. (b) Coronal scan
showing normal eye muscles for
comparison. The ill-defined central
density is the optic nerve; the other
oval densities are the eye muscles.
A, antrum; N, nasal cavity; O, orbit.

ethmoid sinuses (Fig. 16.8), and a meningioma arising
from the sphenoid ridge.

In thyroid eye disease, there is enlargement of the
extraocular muscles (Fig. 16.9) which is frequently
bilateral and may affect one, several, or all the eye
muscles. There is also infiltration of the fat behind the
eye which adds to the exophthalmos.

Salivary glands

Calculi, which occur most commonly in the submandibular duct or gland, normally contain calcium
and can therefore be seen on plain films. In order to
demonstrate the duct system sialography is necessary.

Sialography

A sialogram is performed by injecting contrast into the
ducts of the salivary glands. Only the submandibular
and parotid glands have ducts which can be cannulated
(Fig. 16.10). Stones and strictures in the ducts can be

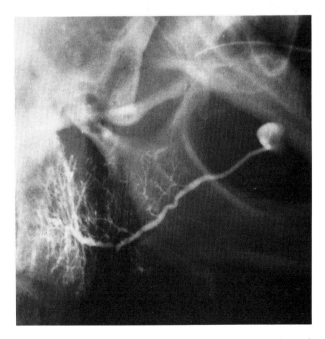

Fig. 16.10 Normal parotid sialogram. Note the long duct of
even calibre and the fine branching of the ducts within the
gland.

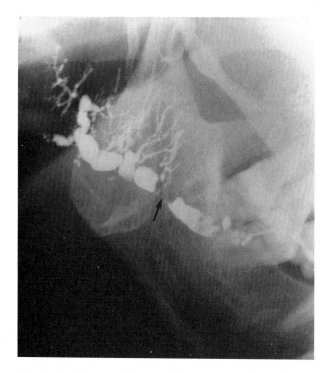

Fig. 16.11 Sialectasis. There is dilatation of the ducts due to a stone (arrow) in the main parotid duct.

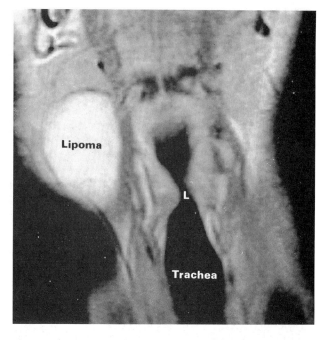

Fig. 16.12 Lipoma in the neck. Coronal MRI scan of a patient presenting with a lump in the neck. The signal characteristics of the mass indicate that it contained fat. Note how the larynx (L) has also been demonstrated.

identified. There may be dilatation of small ducts, which is known as *sialectasis*, and this may occur with obstruction to the main duct (Fig. 16.11) but may also be seen without obvious obstruction. Tumours of the salivary gland may cause stretching and displacement of the ducts within the gland.

Computed tomography is performed occasionally in patients with masses in or adjacent to a salivary gland to answer a specific question in clinically selected cases.

Neck

Computed tomography and MRI can be carried out to investigate a mass in the neck, to stage a primary tumour arising in the neck and to determine the presence and extent of enlarged cervical lymph nodes.

For CT, intravenous contrast enhancement is usually necessary as this opacifies the many vessels which might otherwise be mistaken for small lymph nodes. The thyroid gland, which is situated on either side of the trachea, normally enhances quite markedly after intravenous contrast administration. Unless the mass is cystic, e.g. a branchial cleft cyst or cystic hygroma, it may be difficult to determine its nature although the size, shape and position may help in this regard. Masses in the neck are also shown well with MRI (Fig. 16.12).

Computed tomography can demonstrate enlarged lymph nodes in the neck that are too small to palpate or in sites not amenable to clinical examination. Enlarged nodes may be due to lymphoma, metastases (Fig. 16.13) or infection but their appearance on CT is similar irrespective of the cause.

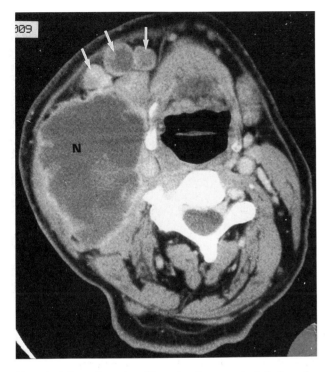

Fig. 16.13 Lymph nodes. There is a huge metastatic lymph node (N) and several small nodes (arrows) in the neck from a carcinoma of the floor of the mouth.

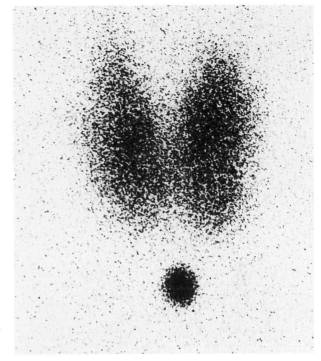

Fig. 16.14 Normal thyroid. ^{123}I radionuclide scan. The intense activity below the thyroid is a marker indicating the position of the suprasternal notch.

Larynx

The larynx is best examined with MRI because of its excellent demonstration of soft tissues and its ability to produce images in the coronal plane. Alternatively, CT can be employed. Direct inspection by laryngoscopy reveals a great deal of information about the larynx, particularly in regard to the vocal cords. However, imaging can provide additional information regarding the spread of tumours outside the larynx, particularly into the subglottic space which cannot be inspected directly.

Thyroid imaging

The thyroid may be imaged by ultrasound or alternatively with nuclear medicine techniques by giving an intravenous injection of technetium-99m-pertechnetate or iodine-123 (Fig. 16.14). It is rarely necessary to use CT to examine the thyroid.

Thyroid imaging is useful in the patient with a suspected thyroid nodule, to help determine its nature. Most solitary nodules do not take up radionuclide and are referred to as 'cold' nodules. A 'cold' nodule can be due to a cyst, an adenoma or a carcinoma (Fig. 16.15). Ultrasound will show whether the mass is cystic or solid (Fig. 16.16). As a solid mass could be an adenoma or carcinoma, biopsy or surgical excision is often performed. Sometimes a nodule is functioning or 'hot' and takes up the radionuclide; such nodules are invariably benign adenomas (Fig. 16.17).

With multinodular goitre, ultrasound or CT shows an enlarged gland with several nodules, often of varying size. The radionuclide scan shows an enlarged

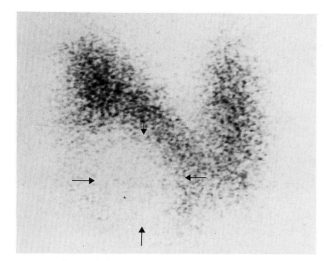

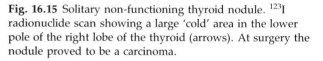

Fig. 16.15 Solitary non-functioning thyroid nodule. ^{123}I radionuclide scan showing a large 'cold' area in the lower pole of the right lobe of the thyroid (arrows). At surgery the nodule proved to be a carcinoma.

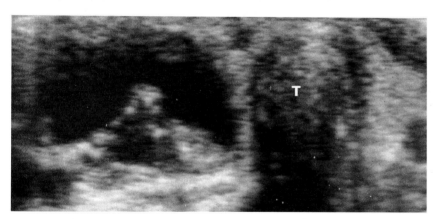

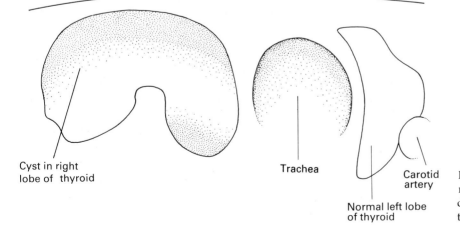

Cyst in right
lobe of thyroid

Trachea

Normal left lobe
of thyroid

Carotid
artery

Fig. 16.16 Ultrasound of a thyroid nodule showing a complex-shaped degenerative cyst in the right lobe of the thyroid. T, trachea.

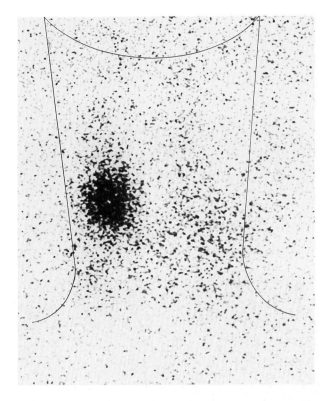

Fig. 16.17 Solitary functioning thyroid nodule. [123]I radionuclide scan showing intense uptake in the functioning adenoma. The remainder of the gland shows substantially reduced activity because of suppression of TSH production. As these nodules function independently of pituitary control they are known as autonomous nodules. The outlines of the neck and jaw have been drawn in.

thyroid gland with several cold areas. The risk of malignancy is no higher in this condition than it is in the general population.

Thyroid masses may extend into the mediastinum and thyroid imaging using ^{123}I is the best method of detecting whether such a mass is due to thyroid tissue.

Iodine-131 has limited uses because of high radiation dose to the thyroid. It has, however, an important role in the management of thyroid cancer. Most thyroid cancers present as 'cold' nodules. Imaging for metastatic spread at this stage is of no avail as the tumours do not take up sufficient radionuclide. However, after the normal thyroid tissue has been ablated by surgery or by a therapeutic dose of ^{131}I, thyroid stimulating hormone (TSH) levels rise and stimulate any functioning metastatic or recurrent tumour, thus allowing them to be identified by radionuclide imaging.

Parathyroid imaging

The usual cause of primary hyperparathyroidism is a parathyroid adenoma, which may be detected on ultrasound as a mass lying behind the thyroid. A parathyroid adenoma will take up thallium-201 when injected intravenously. The thyroid, which overlies the parathyroids, also accumulates thallium but if the thyroid is imaged using ^{99m}Tc, the thallium and technetium images can be subtracted electronically from one another so that the uptake of thallium in the thyroid is removed and the resulting image is that of the parathyroids. The normal parathyroid glands are too small to be visualised, but even a small adenoma can be detected (Fig. 16.18). Localisation of a parathyroid adenoma prior to surgery for hyperparathyroidism is important because about 10% of adenomas occur in an ectopic position, often in the mediastinum.

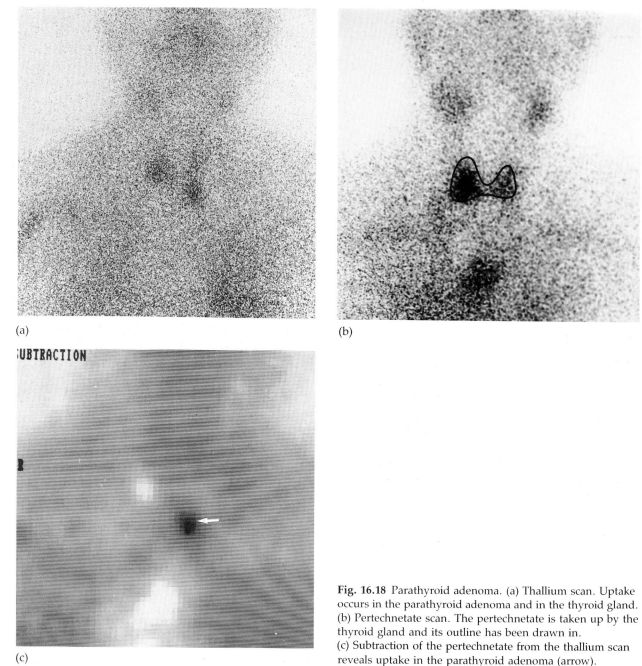

(a)

(b)

SUBTRACTION

(c)

Fig. 16.18 Parathyroid adenoma. (a) Thallium scan. Uptake occurs in the parathyroid adenoma and in the thyroid gland. (b) Pertechnetate scan. The pertechnetate is taken up by the thyroid gland and its outline has been drawn in. (c) Subtraction of the pertechnetate from the thallium scan reveals uptake in the parathyroid adenoma (arrow).

17

Angiography and Interventional Radiology

Angiography

An angiogram is an x-ray examination in which the blood vessels are opacified by an iodine-containing contrast medium. The low-osmolar agents are used in order to avoid the pain and complications encountered with high-osmolar materials. Angiograms are broadly divided into arteriograms and venograms, depending on the vessels injected.

Arteriography

Although it is possible to inject the contrast medium directly through a needle, almost all arteriograms are done via a catheter. The most widely used method of catheterising a blood vessel is the 'Seldinger technique' illustrated in Figure 17.1. At the end of the procedure, the catheter is pulled out. A few minutes compression of the puncture site with the fingers is enough to stop the bleeding in most patients. The advantages of the Seldinger technique are that it is easy and quick to do, that the hole in the artery is no bigger than the catheter and that catheters of any length may be used.

The punctured artery may occasionally become blocked, or alternatively it may be difficult to stop the bleeding once the catheter has been withdrawn. Either complication may require surgical intervention.

The major indications for arteriography are to demonstrate:
• Disorders of the blood vessels, particularly occlusions, stenoses, thrombi, aneurysm formation and vascular malformations (Fig. 17.2).
• Arterial anatomy before surgery. This is only necessary where such information will influence a subsequent surgical procedure.
• Some tumours, by showing abnormal areas of vascularity. This indication has now been largely replaced by the newer imaging modalities.

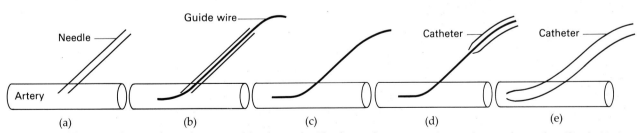

Fig. 17.1 Seldinger technique for catheterising blood vessels. The femoral artery or vein are the usual vessels utilised. (a) A needle is inserted through the skin into the blood vessel. (b) A guidewire is passed through the needle into the lumen of the vessel. (c) The needle is withdrawn, leaving the guidewire in the lumen of the vessel. (d) A catheter is threaded over the guidewire and passed into the lumen of the vessel. (e) The guidewire is withdrawn, leaving the catheter in position in the lumen of the vessel.

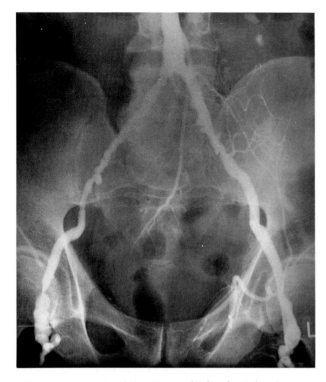

Fig. 17.2 Arteriogram showing multiple atheromatous stenoses in the iliac and femoral arteries bilaterally. The internal iliac arteries are occluded at their origins on both sides. The normal anatomy is shown in Figure 17.8a.

Venography (phlebography)

Thrombi in the deep veins of the legs or in the iliac veins can be demonstrated by leg and pelvic phlebography. A large volume of contrast medium is injected into a small vein close to the toes. The contrast is forced into the deep venous system of the calf by means of tourniquets or by performing the examination with the patient semi-erect. Provided enough contrast is used, it is possible to demonstrate the pelvic veins and the inferior vena cava as well as the leg veins. Thrombi may cause a complete blockage or they may be seen as filling defects in the opacified veins (Fig. 17.3).

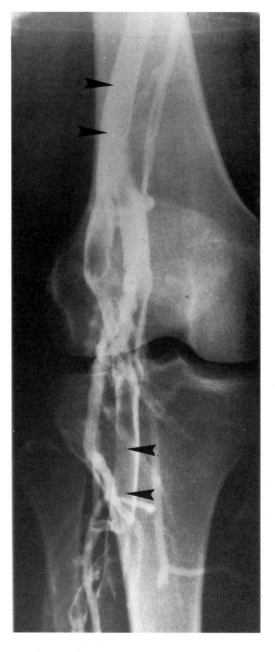

Fig. 17.3 Leg venogram showing deep vein thrombosis. The lower arrows point to the filling defect of the thrombus in the popliteal vein. Compare with the uniform opacity of the normal vein higher up (upper arrows).

Ultrasound techniques in arterial and venous disorders

Ultrasound allows examination of arteries and veins in a completely non-invasive manner. As the examination is carried out with both conventional ultrasound and Doppler imaging, the term 'duplex sonography' is sometimes employed.

Ultrasound of the venous system is an alternative to venography for the detection of venous thrombosis. With a venous thrombosis, intraluminal echogenic material is visible and the veins lose their normal compressibility; thrombus-free veins should be compressible by direct pressure using the ultrasound transducer. Colour Doppler scanning shows that there is a lack of spontaneous flow in the affected veins.

Ultrasound can readily visualise the iliac, common femoral and popliteal veins. A disadvantage with ultrasound is that it is unreliable for examining the calf veins and the femoral vein within the adductor canal. The calf veins, however, are a frequent site for deep vein thrombosis and it is hoped that with the use of colour Doppler it will be eventually possible to examine these veins satisfactorily.

Ultrasound of the arterial system has been used extensively in examining the carotid arteries in patients with suspected cerebral ischaemia. Ultrasound techniques may also be used to visualise the aorta, iliac, femoral and renal arteries, but as yet they are not suitable for arteries below the knee.

The common, internal and external carotid arteries can be readily visualised in the neck. The location or size of any atheromatous plaques and the severity of any luminal narrowing can be determined. With colour Doppler imaging a stenosis in the artery can be visualised and an occlusion will show as an absence of flow (see Plate 2c). Because a stenosis disrupts the normal flow pattern, analysis of the flow velocity waveform can give further information regarding the degree of stenosis.

Subtraction films

It is possible to photographically subtract the shadows that are present on the plain film from the films taken after the contrast has been injected for the angiogram. The result is a film containing details of the opacified structures only (see Fig. 15.30, p. 410).

Digital subtraction angiography

The same principles of subtraction are employed in digital subtraction angiography (DSA), also known as digital vascular imaging (DVI), except that the images are digitised and stored in a computer (Fig. 17.4). It is then possible to subtract electronically the plain image from the equivalent one containing the contrast, leaving only the contrast-filled vessels visible. Digital subtraction angiography is used mainly as an adjunct to conventional arteriography which is done in the usual way, but with the advantage that much smaller catheters can be used and much less contrast medium given (Fig. 17.5). Digital subtraction angiography can produce images of the aorta and its branches from an intravenous injection (Fig. 17.4), but such arteriograms are often degraded for various technical reasons and their use is limited.

Interventional radiology

The radiologist is now involved in carrying out various percutaneous techniques under imaging control. These include dilating stenoses, occluding vessels, draining abscesses and other fluid collections, and obtaining biopsy samples. These procedures greatly assist and may modify surgery, or even replace it altogether. They are carried out with the help of a variety of imaging modalities, notably fluoroscopy, angiography, ultrasound or computed tomography, and are usually performed under local anaesthesia, causing only relatively minor discomfort to the patient. Only the basic principles of the interventional techniques in widespread use will be described here.

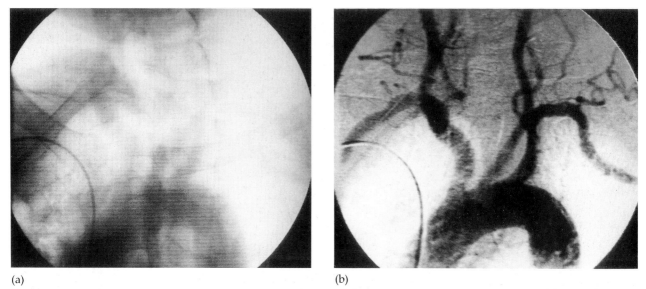

(a)   (b)

Fig. 17.4 Digital subtraction angiography. (a) Unprocessed image following intravenous contrast injection. The vessels can scarcely be discerned. (b) Same image, the only difference being electronic subtraction of bone and soft tissues, leaving the aorta and its branches clearly visible.

Angioplasty

Arterial stenoses and even occlusions may be traversed with a guidewire. A balloon catheter can be passed through the abnormal site, which has been previously determined by arteriography (Fig. 17.6). The stenosis is then dilated by inflating the balloon (Fig. 17.7). This percutaneous technique, which usually uses the femoral artery as an access route, has been widely employed in peripheral vascular disease and gives results as good as bypass surgery, particularly for iliac and superficial femoral artery disease. However, it can only be used in selected patients. Short stenoses are the ideal lesions to treat with angioplasty. Occlusions are less successful and if the occlusion is very long, angioplasty may not be an appropriate treatment. Angioplasty has also been effective in renal artery stenosis, in patients with renal vascular hypertension and in patients with coronary artery stenosis.

Therapeutic embolisation

Arteries can be occluded by introducing a variety of materials through a catheter selectively placed in the vessel. Metal coils covered with thrombogenic filaments, gelatin foam, or even special cyanoacrylate glues that solidify in contact with blood, have all been used for therapeutic embolisation. These techniques have been used primarily to control bleeding. Once arteriography has demonstrated the bleeding site, the offending vessel can then be embolised. Arterial embolisation is also of use in patients with tumours, e.g. renal cell carcinoma, to reduce tumour vascularity prior to surgery, or with inoperable tumours, to treat intractable pain and bleeding (Fig. 17.8). Vascular occlusion has also been successfully used in treating arteriovenous malformations in various organs, most notably the brain and the lungs.

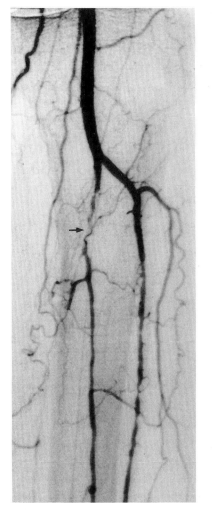

Fig. 17.5 Digital subtraction angiogram (DSA) using an intra-arterial injection of contrast medium. Note that the bones and soft tissues are barely visible. The angiogram shows the left popliteal artery and its branches with severe atheromatous stenosis of the proximal posterior tibial artery (arrow).

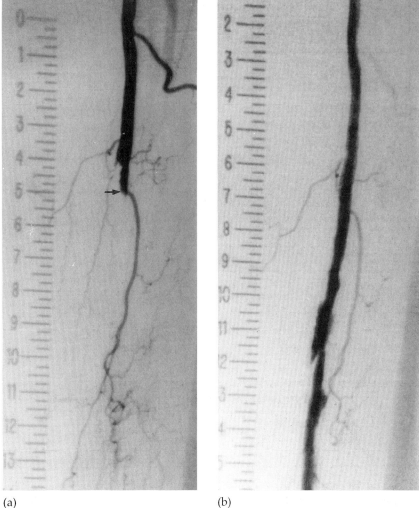

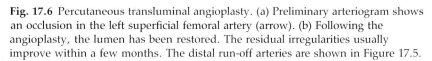

(a)   (b)

Fig. 17.6 Percutaneous transluminal angioplasty. (a) Preliminary arteriogram shows an occlusion in the left superficial femoral artery (arrow). (b) Following the angioplasty, the lumen has been restored. The residual irregularities usually improve within a few months. The distal run-off arteries are shown in Figure 17.5.

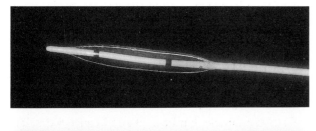

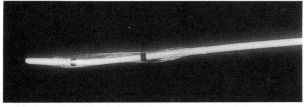

Fig. 17.7 Percutaneous angioplasty balloon catheters. The bottom image shows the catheter prior to inflating the balloon. The top image shows the catheter with the balloon distended as it would be if it were inside the artery.

Vascular catheterisation for infusion purposes

Arterial catheters can be accurately placed for infusion of cytotoxic agents directly into malignant tumours and for the infusion of fibrinolytic agents to dissolve fresh clots from the vascular system.

Percutaneous needle biopsy

Needle biopsy techniques are particularly useful for the non-operative confirmation of suspected malignancy. Under fluoroscopic, ultrasound or computed tomographic guidance (Fig. 17.9), a needle is passed to the desired site and a small amount of tissue is removed. Most intrathoracic or intra-abdominal sites can be sampled. With a fine aspiration needle (20–22 gauge), material can be obtained for cytology. This needle can pass through blood vessels, vascular

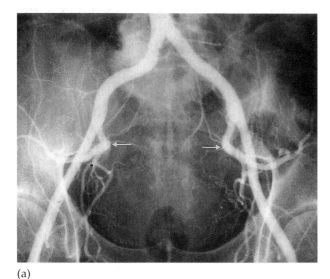

(a)

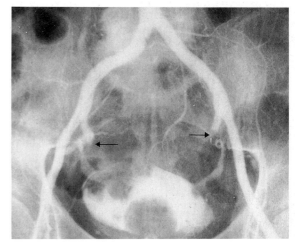

(b)

Fig. 17.8 Therapeutic embolisation. (a) Arteriogram prior to embolisation showing patent internal iliac arteries (arrows) in a patient with uncontrollable bleeding from a large bladder tumour. (b) Following embolisation, both iliac arteries are occluded. The arrows point to the level of occlusion.

masses, loops of bowel and solid organs with only minimal risk of infection or bleeding. Apart from a small pneumothorax with intrathoracic biopsy, complications are extremely rare. To obtain material for histological study a larger needle (14–18 gauge for soft tissues, 10–13 gauge for bone) is used. The larger needles require specific approaches to avoid damage to intervening structures and require stricter indications than fine needle aspiration.

Percutaneous drainage of abscesses and other fluid collections

Specially designed drainage catheters can be introduced percutaneously into abscesses or other fluid collections. The catheters vary in diameter from 8–14 French depending on the nature of the fluid to be drained. The larger catheters may have a double lumen

to assist with irrigation of an abscess cavity. They are introduced under the control of whichever imaging modality is most convenient; the essential feature is that the operator must know exactly where the abscess is and must know that the route chosen for the catheter will be safe (Fig. 17.10). Ultrasound, CT and fluoroscopy are the usual methods.

Once the catheter has been placed in an abscess, it is usually necessary to allow the pus to drain for several days. Irrigation of the tube and the abscess cavity is often essential for continued effective drainage. Thus, the placement of the tube is only the first step in successful percutaneous abscess drainage.

The technique is suitable for most abdominal abscesses, though the success with some forms of abscess is considerably greater than with others. For example, percutaneous drainage is usually successful for liver and intraperitoneal abscesses (Fig. 17.11), but much

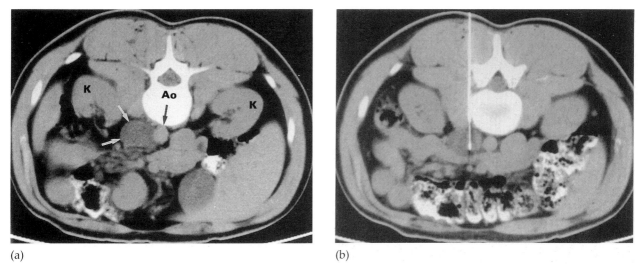

(a) (b)

Fig. 17.9 Needle biopsy of an enlarged para-aortic lymph node under CT control with the patient prone. (a) An enlarged lymph node (arrow) is seen to the left of the abdominal aorta (Ao) at the level of the kidneys (K). (b) The tip of an 18-gauge cutting needle has been placed in the enlarged lymph node. The tissue obtained confirmed that the lesion was a metastasis from a germ cell tumour of the testis.

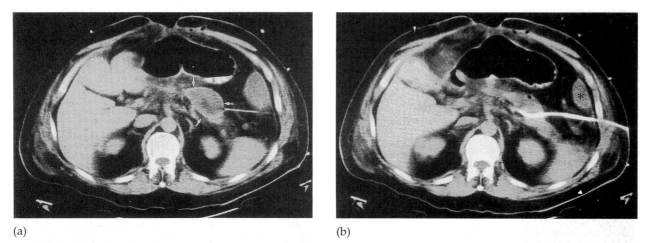

(a)   (b)

Fig. 17.10 Pancreatic abscess drainage. (a) CT scan showing abscess (arrows) in the body of the pancreas and a fine needle introduced from the left flank, avoiding the spleen, kidney and colon. (b) The needle has been exchanged for a 12 French drainage catheter and the abscess is now smaller. Another abscess is also present (∗).

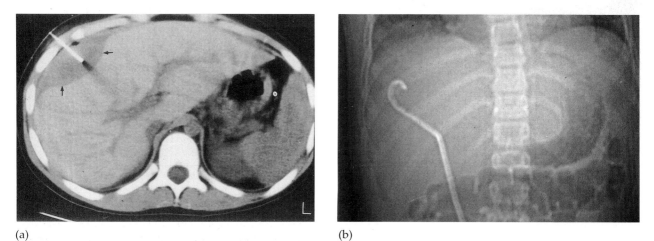

(a)   (b)

Fig. 17.11 Subphrenic abscess in a 14-year-old boy following acute appendicitis and appendicectomy. (a) An 18-gauge needle has been placed into the subphrenic abscess (arrows) anterior to the liver. A guidewire was passed through this needle and the needle was exchanged for a drainage catheter. (b) Film to show the position of the drainage catheter.

less satisfactory for pancreatic abscesses (Fig. 17.10), particularly if they follow pancreatitis and are multiple or multiloculated.

Drainage of the biliary system

The last decade has seen an explosion of techniques designed to drain an obstructed biliary system. The methods used can be broadly divided into those in which the drainage tube is introduced endoscopically and those in which it is introduced percutaneously.

The two most common causes of bile duct obstruction are tumours, notably carcinoma of the pancreas or cholangiocarcinoma, and stones in the common bile

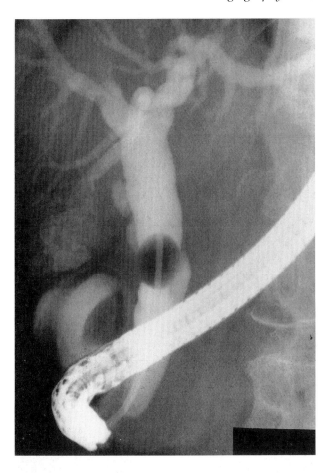

Fig. 17.12 Endoscopic removal of stones in the common bile duct (CBD). A balloon catheter has been passed into the CBD after endoscopic intubation of the papilla of Vater. The stones were then pulled out of the CBD. A sphincterotomy was performed.

duct. If the obstruction is due to stones, then endoscopic removal of all the stones and sphincterotomy of the papilla of Vater is a frequently chosen option (Fig. 17.12).

The results of surgery for curative treatment of malignant bile duct obstruction are usually most disappointing. Non-operative stenting and drainage procedures for patients in whom curative surgery is impossible have, therefore, become far more frequent in recent years. Patients may live for a considerable

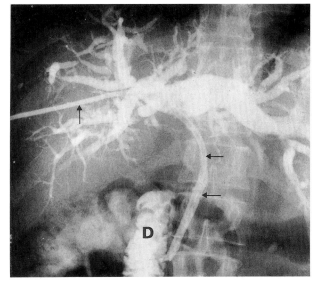

Fig. 17.13 Percutaneous placement of a stent (horizontal arrows) to bypass an obstruction in the common hepatic duct, so that bile drains into the duodenum (D). The vertical arrow points to a catheter that was used to push the stent through the common bile duct.

time with biliary stents in place, particularly if the responsible tumour is slow-growing, as is the case with many cholangiocarcinomas. The stents can be placed over guidewires that have been introduced percutaneously following needle puncture of a dilated bile duct within the liver (Fig. 17.13). The guidewire can be manipulated through the tumour and into the duodenum via the common bile duct. The stent is then passed over the guidewire to effect long-term internal drainage. Alternatively, a stent can be passed retrogradely via endoscopic cannulation of the papilla of Vater, up the common bile duct and through the tumour, so that bile from the obstructed biliary tree drains into the duodenum.

Drainage of the urinary system

Internal drainage of the urinary system using double-J stents placed into an obstructed pelvicalyceal system with the distal end of the catheter in the bladder has become standard practice. These stents are usually placed via a cystoscope, the catheters being passed into the ureteric orifice under direct vision. Alternatively, the double-J stents for long-term internal drainage catheters may be introduced percutaneously via the loin under ultrasound and fluoroscopic control. Short-term drainage (24–48 hours) can be achieved by simply puncturing an obstructed kidney under ultra-sound or fluoroscopic control, passing the guidewire through the needle and exchanging the needle for a small catheter in order to establish temporary external drainage. This procedure, known as percutaneous nephrostomy, is used almost exclusively to establish drainage in such emergency situations as acute obstruction following extracorporeal shock-wave lithotripsy or to drain an acute pyonephrosis.

Appendix

CT Anatomy of Abdomen

The normal appearances of the abdomen and pelvis of an adult male are shown in this appendix. The levels of the sections chosen are illustrated in the two diagrams. Each section is 10 mm thick. Gastrografin was given orally twice: 15 minutes and 1.5 hours before-

hand. Intravenous contrast was injected during the examination.

Other images from this particular patient were used to illustrate the normal retroperitoneum (Fig. 10.8a, p. 289), and the normal bladder (Fig. 7.9d, p. 230)

Ao   Aorta
D   Diaphragm
Du   Duodenum
D III   Third part of duodenum
GB   Gall bladder
IVC   Inferior vena cava
K   Kidney
Ps   Psoas muscle
PV   Portal vein
SMA   Superior mesenteric artery
SMV   Superior mesenteric vein
Sp   Spine
SV   Splenic vein

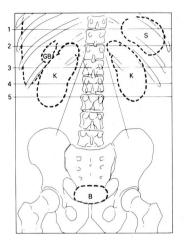

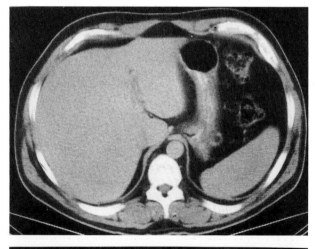

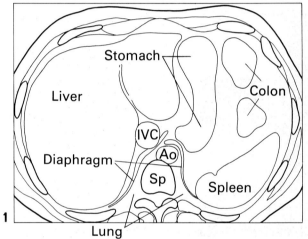

1

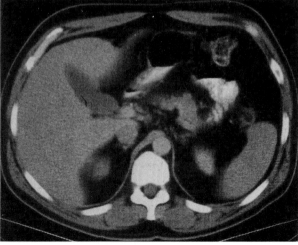

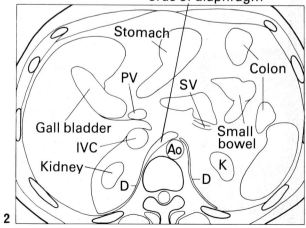

2

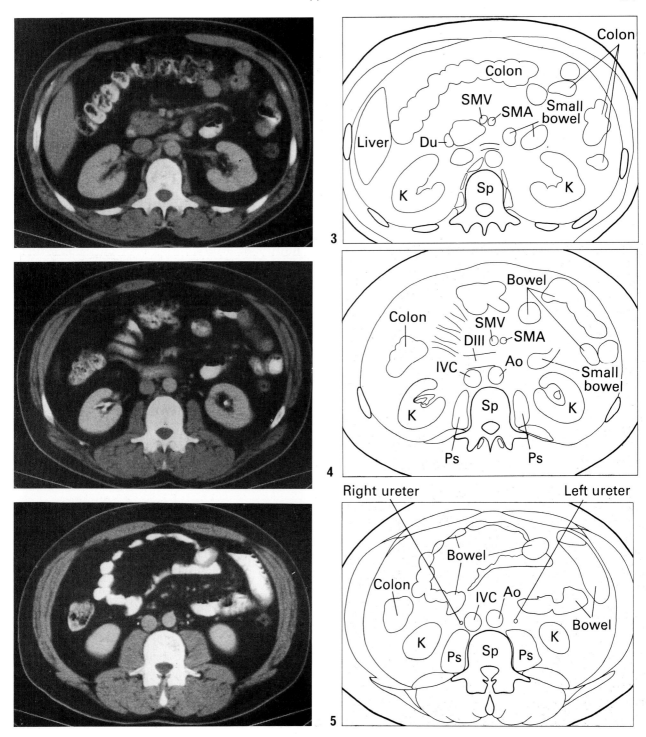

B   Bladder
C   Colon
K   Kidney
Isch. tub Ischial tuberosity
IVC   Inferior vena cava
L. ani   Levator ani
Obt. int. Obturator internus
Ps   Psoas muscle
Sp   Spine
R   Rectum

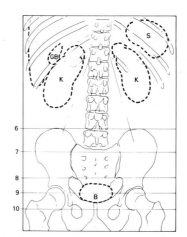

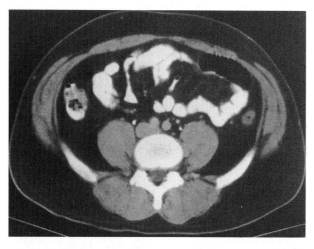

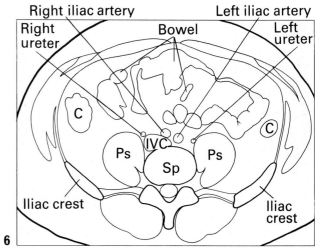

6

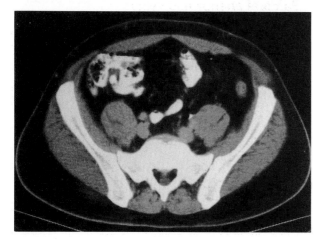

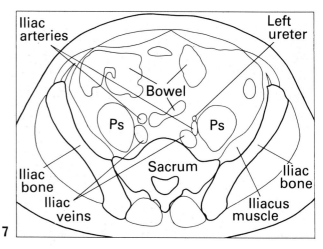

7

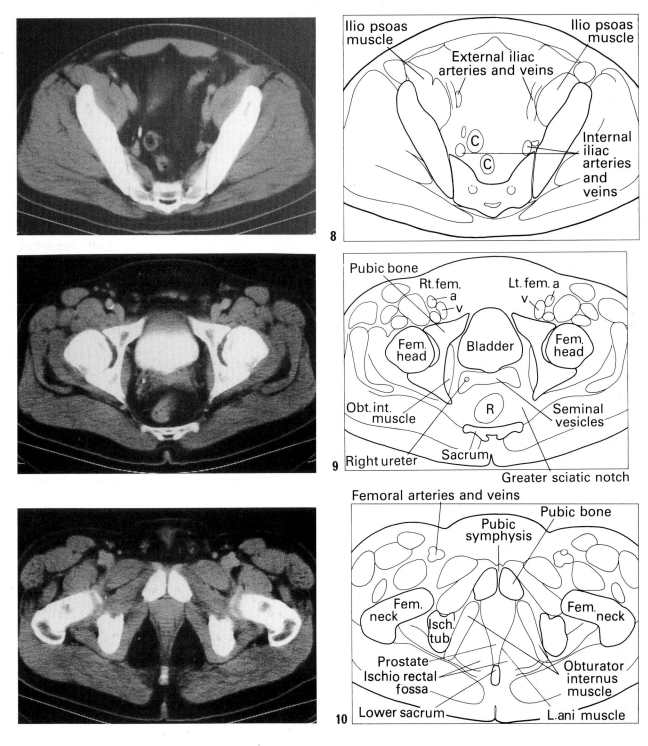

8

Ilio psoas muscle

Ilio psoas muscle

External iliac arteries and veins

Internal iliac arteries and veins

C

C

9

Pubic bone

Rt. fem. a v

Lt. fem. a v

Fem. head

Bladder

Fem. head

Obt. int. muscle

R

Seminal vesicles

Right ureter

Sacrum

Greater sciatic notch

10

Femoral arteries and veins

Pubic symphysis

Pubic bone

Fem. neck

Isch. tub.

Fem. neck

Prostate

Ischio rectal fossa

Obturator internus muscle

Lower sacrum

L. ani muscle

Index

Page references in *italic type* indicate figures.